Natural Health Sciences

Natural Health Sciences: A Comprehensive Guide serves as a valuable resource for both healthcare practitioners and business professionals, supporting ongoing professional development by bridging the gap between proponents of traditional or natural health systems and those who follow scientific or medical perspectives. The book synthesizes existing literature and fosters a more nuanced understanding of the benefits and limitations of natural health practices.

By presenting academic and scientific evidence in an accessible format, it offers evidence-based insights into a broad spectrum of natural health approaches. These include herbal remedies, nutritional strategies, lifestyle interventions, and alternative therapies, covering key areas such as Ayurveda, bioenergetic therapy, music therapy, Traditional Chinese Medicine (TCM), and aromatherapy. It also addresses criticisms, ethical and regulatory concerns, and the future of natural health sciences.

With the increasing awareness of the limitations and side effects of conventional medicine, people are seeking natural, preventive, and personalized approaches to maintain and improve their health. *Natural Health Sciences: A Comprehensive Guide* provides a comprehensive overview of natural health sciences and its various sub-disciplines, allowing readers to gain a deeper understanding of these practices and make informed decisions about their health.

Natural Health Sciences

A Comprehensive Guide

Rasit Dinc

CRC Press
Taylor & Francis Group
Boca Raton London New York

CRC Press is an imprint of the
Taylor & Francis Group, an **informa** business

Designed cover image: Shutterstock

First edition published 2025
by CRC Press
2385 NW Executive Center Drive, Suite 320, Boca Raton FL 33431

and by CRC Press
4 Park Square, Milton Park, Abingdon, Oxon, OX14 4RN

CRC Press is an imprint of Taylor & Francis Group, LLC

ISBN: 978-1-032-85873-9 (hbk)
ISBN: 978-1-032-84530-2 (pbk)
ISBN: 978-1-003-52025-2 (ebk)

DOI: 10.1201/9781003520252

Typeset in Times
by KnowledgeWorks Global Ltd.

Contents

PART I   Health Inspired by Nature: Natural Health Sciences

PART II   Reflection of Natural Health Sciences in the Modern World

Preface

Nature is the oldest source of reference for human health services. Since prehistoric times, plants, animals, and natural minerals have formed the basis of primitive medicines used for treatment and prevention. However, many of these ancient practices have not been tested by the criteria and rigor of modern science. This book aims to be a bridge between these ancient wisdoms offered by the natural health sciences and modern science.

This book is not intended to be a treatment guide or to replace a doctor's recommendations. Rather, it aims to provide information and research that can inform you, the reader's health-related decisions, in an informed way. Considering information based on scientific evidence, you can then better understand the potential benefits and limitations of natural health sciences.

It is important to remember that a healthy lifestyle is an important part of preventive health care. Regular exercise, a balanced and nutritious diet, adequate sleep, and stress management greatly affect the overall health and quality of life of each of us. Natural health sciences can be part of this overall lifestyle approach and help us support our wellness goals.

Every topic covered in this book has been examined in the light of scientific research. With science and nature coming together, there are powerful tools that can be used to achieve a healthy and balanced life. However, it should not be forgotten that the effects of natural health practices and products may vary from person to person. So, before embarking on any natural treatment or incorporating any condition into your health routine, it is extremely important to always consult a healthcare professional.

I wish you a pleasant reading.

Important Notice

This book aims to provide general knowledge in the field of natural health sciences and is not a substitute for professional medical advice. Please consult a healthcare professional before making decisions about your health condition or treatment options. This book is for informational purposes only and should not be used as a referral to a medical diagnosis or treatment.

The information contained in this book has been prepared based on scientific sources and reliable references available at the time of publication. However, medical science is a field that is constantly advancing and changing. Therefore, please note that the information contained in the book may be updated over time.

Although the authors and publishers have made every effort to ensure the accuracy and reliability of the information contained in this book, there may be cases where all or part of the information contained in this book is inaccurate, incomplete, or out of date. Therefore, the authors and publishers cannot be held responsible for any damage or loss resulting from the use of the book or the application of this information.

This book is not a substitute for a medical prescription or treatment plan. If you have concerns about your health problems or symptoms, or if you are considering any treatment options, please consult a healthcare professional. Every individual's health status is different, and a personalized health plan is important for an accurate diagnosis and proper treatment.

By reading this book or using the information it contains, you agree to the warnings and advice set forth above.

About the Author

Prof. Dr. Rasit Dinc holds doctorate degrees in health sciences and business administration and is a distinguished professor of health sciences. He has conducted advanced academic research at some of the world's most prestigious institutions, including Harvard, MIT and Yale, where he gained extensive expertise in his fields. Prof. Dr. Dinc serves as the Chairman of the Board at INVAMED, a globally recognized leader in the development and production of innovative medical devices and healthcare solutions. With over 100 patented medical devices and treatment methods to his name, he has established himself as a prominent scientist in the global healthcare industry, contributing groundbreaking research and advancements to the field of health sciences.

Part I

Health Inspired by Nature
Natural Health Sciences

The first part of the book examines the foundational principles and evolution of natural health practices. The book commences with a historical overview and an examination of the evolution of natural health sciences over time. Readers will investigate the fundamental principles that underpin these practices, the diverse sub-disciplines within the field, and practical strategies for integrating them into a healthy lifestyle. Additionally, the section addresses criticisms, ethical concerns, and regulatory issues related to natural health sciences, and offers insights into future trends. The chapters in this part of the book are listed below.

CHAPTER 1: HISTORICAL PERSPECTIVE AND OVERVIEW OF NATURAL HEALTH SCIENCES

Chapter 1 provides a comprehensive overview of natural health sciences, exploring their historical roots, modern applications, and scientific validation. The evolution of natural health practices from ancient civilizations to the present day, highlighting influential traditions such as Ayurveda and Traditional Chinese Medicine. Readers will gain insight into how these historical practices have shaped current approaches to health and disease management. Chapter 1 also discusses the integration of complementary and alternative medicine (CAM) practices, such as acupuncture and nutrition, into modern healthcare. By emphasizing a holistic approach that respects the body's natural ability to heal, this chapter offers readers an understanding of how natural health sciences can provide effective solutions to complex health problems, support disease prevention, and enhance overall well-being. This basic overview sets the stage for a more in-depth exploration of the scientific evidence and practical applications of natural health disciplines.

CHAPTER 2: BASIC PRINCIPLES OF NATURAL HEALTH PRACTICES

Chapter 2 explores the principles and practices of natural health sciences, emphasizing their relevance and effectiveness in modern healthcare. Readers will explore five core principles: the holistic integration of mind, body, and spirit; proactive disease prevention; the use of natural

DOI: 10.1201/9781003520252-1

remedies; the body's innate ability to heal; and the importance of individualized care. The chapter highlights the holistic approach, which looks at a person's whole context rather than isolated symptoms, and emphasizes the body's ability to heal itself when given the right support. By examining the balance between prevention and treatment, this chapter provides practical insights into how natural health practices – such as herbal remedies, mind–body techniques, and lifestyle changes – can improve overall well-being and complement traditional medical treatments. This comprehensive overview equips readers with the knowledge to make informed decisions about incorporating natural health strategies into their lives.

CHAPTER 3: SUB-DISCIPLINES OF NATURAL HEALTH SCIENCES

Chapter 3 introduces the reader to the diverse and evolving field of natural health sciences, offering a comprehensive exploration of its core sub-disciplines. It presents an in-depth examination of phytotherapy, highlighting the historical and contemporary uses of medicinal plants, as well as their benefits and safety considerations. Readers will gain insight into the principles and practices of homeopathy and naturopathy, discovering how these holistic approaches aim to enhance the body's self-healing abilities. The chapter also explores acupuncture, detailing its scientific basis and effectiveness in treating pain and chronic conditions. It also covers Ayurveda and Traditional Chinese Medicine (TCM), providing historical context and modern applications. By engaging with this chapter, readers will gain a well-rounded understanding of these natural health practices, their therapeutic potential, and their integration into contemporary healthcare.

CHAPTER 4: APPLIED HEALTHY LIVING STRATEGIES

Chapter 4 provides a guide to the essential components of holistic health and wellness. It discusses the importance of a balanced diet and provides practical strategies for optimizing dietary habits to support overall well-being. The chapter emphasizes the role of regular physical activity in maintaining health and improving quality of life. Readers will discover effective methods for managing stress, incorporating appropriate sleep habits, and fostering positive social relationships, all of which are essential to a balanced lifestyle. In addition, the chapter explores detoxification and cleansing practices, highlighting their benefits and considerations. By reading this chapter, individuals will gain valuable insights and actionable steps to improve their health through a well-rounded approach that integrates nutrition, exercise, mental wellness, social support, and detoxification for a more vibrant and harmonious life.

CHAPTER 5: CRITICISMS AND RESPONSES TO NATURAL HEALTH SCIENCES

Chapter 5 addresses the significant criticisms directed at natural health sciences, offering a balanced view of the challenges and responses within this field. It addresses concerns regarding the scientific basis, safety, and efficacy of natural health practices, providing evidence-based responses to common critiques. Readers will have the opportunity to engage with discussions on the scientific validation of herbal remedies, probiotics, acupuncture, and mind–body therapies and to gain insight into how these practices stand up to scrutiny. Furthermore, the chapter addresses issues such as potential adverse effects, the integration of natural and traditional Western medicine, and the necessity for quality control and appropriate training. By engaging with this chapter, readers will gain a nuanced understanding of the ongoing debates surrounding natural health sciences and appreciate the field's evolving nature and its contributions to holistic healthcare.

CHAPTER 6: ETHICAL AND REGULATORY CONCERNS IN NATURAL HEALTH SCIENCES

Chapter 6 examines the pivotal ethical and regulatory issues intrinsic to natural health sciences, establishing parallels with conventional medicine while underscoring distinctive challenges. This chapter addresses a number of ethical issues, including matters pertaining to informed consent, practitioner integrity, and the appropriate balance between traditional practices and modern scientific standards. Furthermore, it analyzes the regulatory aspects of natural health sciences, examining the governance of these practices and the legal frameworks that ensure safety and efficacy. Furthermore, the chapter addresses the professional standards and training requirements for practitioners, emphasizing the necessity for rigorous qualifications and adherence to ethical guidelines. By reading this chapter, individuals will gain a comprehensive understanding of the regulatory landscape and ethical considerations shaping the natural health sciences. This will equip them with the knowledge to navigate these complex issues effectively.

CHAPTER 7: THE FUTURE OF NATURAL HEALTH SCIENCES

Chapter 7 presents an analysis of the future of natural health sciences, with a particular focus on the impact of scientific and technological advancements on the field. Furthermore, it addresses the emergence of personalized medicine, encompassing bespoke approaches to herbal treatments, aromatherapy, acupuncture, and other modalities, which reflect a paradigm shift toward individualized care. The chapter examines integrative health approaches that combine traditional and modern practices and considers how digital health and telemedicine are transforming access to and delivery of natural health therapies. Furthermore, it discusses pioneering research, product development, and the drive toward sustainable and ethical practices. By engaging with this chapter, readers will gain insights into how cutting-edge technologies and research are expanding the possibilities of natural health, improving global healthcare, and offering new, personalized treatment options for diverse needs.

1 Historical Perspective and Overview of Natural Health Sciences

1.1 OVERVIEW OF NATURAL HEALTH SCIENCES

Natural health sciences are a branch of science and art that have deep roots in many cultures and civilizations. Supported by scientific advances, this discipline aims to prevent diseases and support health through a holistic health perspective and natural therapeutic processes [1].

In a large-scale survey of the American public, 38% of Americans used some form of complementary and alternative medicine (CAM) practice [1]. These practices often include various disciplines of the natural health sciences, such as acupuncture, homeopathy, massage therapy, diet, and nutritional counseling.

In many aspects, this branch of science aims to offer alternative solutions to complex health problems that modern medicine cannot materialize today. For example, the addiction crisis caused by opioids used in chronic pain management has brought alternative treatment methods such as acupuncture, which is within the scope of natural health sciences, to the forefront [2].

The basic philosophy of natural health sciences is to respect and support the body's natural healing ability. This includes an approach that focuses on disease prevention and offers strategies to improve the overall health of individuals. Topics such as preventive care, nutrition, detoxification, physical activity, and stress management are important aspects of the natural health sciences.

With a holistic approach, the natural health sciences advocate that the body, mind, and spirit should be considered as a whole. This perspective aims to improve the overall quality of life of individuals. For example, the positive effects of practices such as meditation and yoga on stress management have been demonstrated by scientific research [3].

In this book, we will examine various aspects of the natural health sciences and review the latest scientific research in this field. Scientific evidence can confirm the effectiveness and safety of the natural health sciences as well as guide future applications and research in this field.

1.2 HISTORICAL PERSPECTIVE IN NATURAL HEALTH SCIENCES

The origins of the natural health sciences are as old as the origins of medicine. These sources are often based on the knowledge and experiences that people have gained from nature at various periods of history. Various civilizations have developed their own unique natural health practices that have shaped their understanding of health and disease and methods of treatment [4].

Ancient Egypt is home to the earliest documented examples of natural health practices. For example, the Ebers Papyrus is a text that dates back to 1550 BC and contains more than 700 prescriptions for herbal medicine. These prescriptions describe herbal mixtures used to alleviate the symptoms of diseases and heal the body [5]. The ancient Egyptians used plants, animal products, and minerals to treat diseases [5]. This has formed the basis of modern phytotherapy.

The Ayurvedic tradition of India and the tradition of Traditional Chinese Medicine (TCM) of China are both wide-ranging natural health systems that date back to 2000 BC. India's Ayurvedic tradition treats human health as the totality of body, mind, and spirit. Ayurveda expresses the knowledge (veda) of life (ayur) and emphasizes the integrity of the body, mind, and spirit. One of the

DOI: 10.1201/9781003520252-2

oldest texts of Ayurveda, the "Charaka Samhita," dates back to the 6th century BC and describes natural methods of treatment such as nutrition, lifestyle changes, and herbal remedies [6].

The Chinese tradition of Traditional Chinese Medicine (TCM) balances the flow of energy (qi) in the body and uses natural methods of treatment such as acupuncture, tai chi, qigong, and herbal remedies [7]. An ancient text called "Huangdi Neijing" explains the basic principles and practices of TCM [4].

During the ancient Greek and Roman periods, important medical thinkers such as Hippocrates and Galen adopted natural approaches to health preservation and treatment of diseases and integrated them into their theories of health and disease. Hippocrates' principle of "do no harm first" and Galen's belief that the balance of the four bodily fluids (blood, bile, black bile, and phlegm) determine health and disease shaped the basic principles of the natural health sciences [8, 9].

In medieval Europe, monasteries became centers of knowledge on natural cures and herbal remedies. The monasteries also hosted gardens where many plants were grown and collected. During this period, many manuscript texts were written about the making and use of herbal remedies [10].

In the 19th and 20th centuries, as Western medicine became more technical and specialized, natural health practices such as naturopathy and homeopathy developed and popularized. During this period, individuals such as Benedict Lust, the naturopath, and Samuel Hahnemann, the homeopathic medicine pioneer, developed modern theories and practices of the natural health sciences [11].

At the beginning of the 21st century, a growing interest in scientific research and complementary and alternative medicine (CAM) research has shaped the contemporary practices and philosophy of the natural health sciences. This has helped expand the role of natural health sciences within modern healthcare [1]. For example, mind–body therapies such as yoga and meditation have been recognized and widely accepted as effective tools for stress and anxiety management [3].

REFERENCES

1. P. M. Barnes, B. Bloom and R. L. Nahin, Complementary and Alternative Medicine Use among Adults and Children: United States, 2007, National Health Statistics Reports, Hyattsville, MD, 2008.
2. A. J. Vickers, E. A. Vertosick, G. Lewith, H. MacPherson, N. Foster, K. J. Sherman, D. Irnich, C. M. Witt and K. Linde, "Acupuncture for Chronic Pain: Update of an Individual Patient Data Meta-Analysis," *The Journal of Pain*, vol. 19, no. 5, pp. 455–474, 2018.
3. M. C. Pascoe, D. R. Thompson and C. F. Ski, "Yoga, Mindfulness-Based Stress Reduction and Stress-Related Physiological Measures: A Meta-Analysis," *Psychoneuroendocrinology*, vol. 86, pp. 152–168, 2017.
4. P. U. Unschuld, Huang Di Nei Jing Su Wen: Nature, Knowledge, Imagery in an Ancient Chinese Medical Text: With an Appendix: The Doctrine of the Five Periods and Six Qi in the Huang Di Nei Jing Su Wen, University of California Press, Berkeley, CA, 2003.
5. J. F. Nunn, Ancient Egyptian Medicine, University of Oklahoma Press, Norman, OA 2002.
6. P. Prioreschi, A History of Medicine: Byzantine and Islamic Medicine, Horatius Press, Omaha, 2001.
7. T. Kaptchuk, The Web That Has No Weaver: Understanding Chinese Medicine, McGraw-Hill, New York, NY, 2000.
8. W. H. S. Jones, Hippocrates Vol. 1, G.P. Putnam's Sons, New York, NY, 1923.
9. V. Nutton, Ancient Medicine, Routledge, London, 2004.
10. B. Griggs, Green Pharmacy: The History and Evolution of Western Herbal Medicine, Healing Arts Press, Rochester, VT, 1997.
11. H. A. Baer, Biomedicine and Alternative Healing Systems in America: Issues of Class, Race, Ethnicity, and Gender, University of Wisconsin Press, Madison, WI, 2001.

2 Basic Principles of Natural Health Practices

Natural health practices have gained significant popularity in recent years, as people are increasingly seeking alternative methods to improve their overall well-being. These practices focus on utilizing natural remedies and techniques to promote physical, mental, and emotional health. By understanding the basic principles of natural health practices, individuals can make informed decisions about their own health and well-being [1].

Five principles of natural health practices are the recognition of the interconnectedness of the mind, body, and spirit, the importance of proactive measures to prevent illness and maintain optimal health, prioritizing the use of natural remedies and therapies, the belief in the body's innate ability to heal itself, and lastly, the individualized approach to health [1]. These are further explained below.

Holistic Perspective: Natural health approaches seek to understand the person not only as the sum-total of a disease or symptom, but also within their broader social and environmental context. The holistic view acknowledges the impact of diet, lifestyle, stress levels, and social factors on health [2].

Preventive Approach: Natural health sciences promote measures to prevent the occurrence of diseases and protect one's overall health. This approach includes a balanced diet, regular exercise, stress management, and healthy lifestyle choices [3].

Natural Treatment Methods: Natural health practices emphasize treatment methods that are often found in nature. Natural treatment methods may include herbal remedies, physical therapies, mind-body techniques, and energy-based therapies [2].

Healing Power: Natural health attaches great importance to the body's ability to heal and balance itself. This principle involves the belief that the body can heal on its own when the right support and conditions are provided [4].

Education and Self-Empowerment: Natural health practices encourage individuals to play an informed and active role in their own health status. This principle is achieved through increasing health awareness and adopting healthy lifestyle choices [5].

2.1 HOLISTIC APPROACH

The holistic approach emphasizes a focus on the person and the integration of their body, mind, and spirit in health care. This approach involves evaluating the person not only as a biological system, but also as a whole that interacts with psychological, social, and environmental factors [2].

Central to holistic medicine is the belief that there is constant interaction and adaptation between the biological, psychological, social, and environmental dimensions of the human being. Illness occurs when there is an imbalance in any or more of these four dimensions. Therefore, treatment should be directed at the root of these imbalances rather than focusing solely on symptom relief [1].

For example, if a person is experiencing constant headaches, a holistic approach can assess that person's diet, sleep habits, stress levels, and even potential problems in their personal and professional life, rather than just giving them painkillers. This type of evaluation allows the treatment to be more effective and individually personalized [6].

The holistic approach also encourages the person to take an active role in their own state of health. Patients need to be informed about their own health and empowered to improve their health by making informed decisions in lifestyle choices. This self-management and self-empowerment helps individuals gain more control over their own health outcomes [5].

DOI: 10.1201/9781003520252-3

2.2   THE BODY'S ABILITY TO HEAL ITSELF

The body's ability to heal itself is one of the basic principles of natural health practices. This principle is based on the belief that the body can repair and heal itself when given the right conditions and support [4].

The ability to heal oneself is a mechanism that the body naturally possesses that aims to return to a state of equilibrium, often called homeostasis. As a simple example, consider our body's ability to heal a cut or wound. In this case, the body immediately initiates a series of biological responses to repair the damage and restore wholeness [7].

The same principle applies to the body's ability to cope with more complex situations. For example, in a stressful situation, the body increases the levels of adrenaline and cortisol, which are stress hormones. This increases our ability to react to a dangerous situation (fight or flight response). However, when the stress factor is removed, the body lowers the levels of these hormones and returns to homeostasis [8].

These examples illustrate the power of the body's ability to self-regulate and heal that it naturally possesses. However, in some cases, these mechanisms may be insufficient or may not be enabled. At this point, natural health practices come into play and aim to create conditions that support the body's ability to heal itself. This may include factors such as a balanced diet, adequate sleep, stress management, regular exercise, and natural therapies [9].

2.3   PREVENTION AND TREATMENT OF DISEASE

Prevention and treatment of diseases is one of the main goals of modern medicine. However, the importance of traditional medicine practices and natural health sciences is increasing in the studies carried out in this field. Because both approaches have a significant impact on the prevention and treatment of diseases [10].

Disease prevention is a process that often promotes healthy lifestyle practices. These include factors such as a balanced diet, regular physical activity, sleep patterns, stress management, and the avoidance of exposure to toxins. These practices strengthen the body's natural defense mechanisms and can prevent the development of chronic diseases [11].

In the treatment process, in addition to traditional medicine practices, natural therapies also play an important role. For example, natural health practices such as herbal remedies, acupuncture, massage therapy, meditation, and yoga can alleviate patients' symptoms and improve their quality of life [12].

Natural health sciences take an approach that supports the body's capacity to heal itself in the prevention and treatment of disease. In addition, it advocates addressing not only the symptoms of diseases, but also the underlying causes. This helps to treat and prevent the disease more effectively [1].

REFERENCES

1. R. Snyderman and A. Weil, "Integrative Medicine: Bringing Medicine Back to Its Roots," *Archives of Internal Medicine*, vol. 162, no. 4, pp. 395–397, 2002.
2. V. Maizes, D. Rakel and C. Niemiec, "Integrative Medicine and Patient-Centered Care," *Explore (NY)*, vol. 5, no. 5, pp. 277–289, 2009.
3. W. C. Willett, J. P. Koplan, R. Nugent, C. Dusenbury, P. Puska and T. A. Gaziano, "Prevention of Chronic Disease by Means of Diet and Lifestyle Changes," in Disease Control Priorities in Developing Countries. 2nd edition, edited by D. T. Jamison, J. G. Breman, A. R. Measham, G. Alleyne, M. Claeson, D. B. Evans, P. Jha, A. Mills, and P. Musgrove, Oxford University Press, New York, NY, pp. 833–850, 2006.
4. W. B. Jonas, "Building an Evidence House: Challenges and Solutions to Research in Complementary and Alternative Medicine," *Research in Complementary and Classical Natural Medicine*, vol. 12, no. 3, pp. 159–167, 2005.
5. M. S. Micozzi, Fundamentals of Complementary, Alternative, and Integrative Medicine 5th edition, Saunders, Philadelphia, PA, 2015.

6. I. Bell, O. Caspi, G. E. R. Schwartz, K. L. Grant, T. W. Gaudet, D. L. Rychener, V. Maizes and A. Weil, "Integrative Medicine and Systemic Outcomes Research: Issues in the Emergence of a New Model for Primary Health Care," *Archives of Internal Medicine*, vol. 162, no. 2, pp. 133–140, 2002.

7. D. Servan-Schreiber, Healing Without Freud or Prozac: Natural Approaches to Curing Stress, Anxiety and Depression, Pan MacMillan, London, 2012.

8. R. M. Sapolsky, Why Zebras Don't Get Ulcers, 3rd Edition, Holt Paperbacks, New York, NY, 2004.

9. A. Weil, Spontaneous Healing: How to Discover and Embrace Your Body's Natural Ability to Maintain and Heal Itself, Ballantine Books, New York, NY, 2000.

10. L. H. Kushi, C. Doyle, M. McCullough, C. L. Rock, W. Demark-Wahnefried, E. V. Bandera, S. Gapstur, A. V. Patel, K. Andrews and T. Gansler, "American Cancer Society Guidelines on Nutrition and Physical Activity for Cancer Prevention: Reducing the Risk of Cancer With Healthy Food Choices and Physical Activity," *American Cancer Society Journals*, vol. 62, no. 1, pp. 30–67, 2012.

11. D. Ornish, "Avoiding Revascularization With Lifestyle Changes: The Multicenter Lifestyle Demonstration Project," *The American Journal of Cardiology*, vol. 82, no. 10, pp. 72–76, 1998.

12. P. M. Barnes, B. Bloom and R. L. Nahin, Complementary and Alternative Medicine Use Among Adults and Children: United States, 2007, National Health Statistics Reports, 2008.

3 Sub-Disciplines of Natural Health Sciences

Natural health sciences is a broad field that encompasses many sub-disciplines. These disciplines have emerged from the combination of traditional and modern sciences and have contributed to the development of various natural health practices and treatments. The main sub-disciplines of natural health sciences are as follows:

1. Phytotherapy: This is a branch of science that examines the effects of plants and plant components on health. Modern phytotherapy promotes the safe and effective use of medicinal plants and plant-based products [1].
2. Nutritional Sciences: This is a field that studies the impact of nutrition on health. This discipline explores how foods and diets can be used in the prevention and treatment of diseases [2].
3. Naturopathy: This is a natural and holistic form of medicine that aims to support the body's ability to heal itself. Naturopathy aims to achieve balance between body, mind, and spirit and to treat the causes of the disease, not just its symptoms [3].
4. Acupuncture: This is a practice that was part of ancient Chinese medicine and involves treating health problems by inserting thin needles into specific points on the body. Acupuncture can be effective in pain management and treatment of many chronic conditions [4].
5. Mind–Body Therapies: This includes a range of therapies that recognize that the mind has a significant impact on the health of the body. Techniques such as meditation, yoga, tai chi, and biofeedback fall into this category [5].

3.1 HERBAL TREATMENT (PHYTOTHERAPY)

Phytotherapy is also commonly known as "herbal therapy" or "treatment with plants." This field studies the use of plants for health protection and the treatment of diseases. Mankind may be as old as the history of the use of plants for this purpose, but modern phytotherapy uses and expands this ancient knowledge with scientific methods [6].

In this section, we will discuss the basic principles and historical origins of phytotherapy, an overview of medicinal plants, practical applications, important scientific research on phytotherapy, and safety issues and side effects related to phytotherapy. You will find that phytotherapy is an important natural health science discipline and a field that is expected to play an ongoing greater role in modern medicine.

3.1.1 History and Basic Principles of Phytotherapy

For most of its existence, humanity has used nature as both a source of inspiration and a source of health. Our relationship with plants has been shaped over millions of years of evolution and has played an important role in our survival. In this regard, phytotherapy is one of the oldest and most common forms of enjoying the health benefits of plants [6].

Phytotherapy is derived from the Latin words "*phyto*" (plant) and the Greek words "*therapia*" (treatment). In a broad sense, it refers to the use of plants and herbal ingredients to prevent and treat

DOI: 10.1201/9781003520252-4

health problems. But phytotherapy involves much more than the random or traditional use of plants. Modern phytotherapy applies scientific methods to determine the efficacy, safety, and uses of herbal ingredients [7].

The historical origins of phytotherapy date back to the Stone Age. At that time, people depended on both the nutritional and medicinal values of plants for survival. In later periods, many civilizations, such as the civilizations of Ancient Egypt, Greece, Rome, Islam, and China, further developed and documented the use of medicinal plants. This historical body of knowledge formed the basis of today's modern medicine [8].

Modern phytotherapy combines this ancient knowledge and traditional plant use with scientific research. Clinical studies and laboratory tests are used to test the efficacy and safety of plants. This approach is an important part of scientific evidence-based medicine and has helped phytotherapy gain wider acceptance in the medical field [9].

3.1.1.1 *Historical Development of Phytotherapy*

The development of phytotherapy dates back thousands of years, along with the history of mankind. Since prehistoric times, plants have been used for both nutritional and therapeutic purposes. Archaeological evidence suggests that herbal remedies were used as far back as the Neolithic period and even earlier [6].

In ancient times, various civilizations documented the use of different herbal remedies. In Egypt, the Ebers papyrus is one of the oldest medical texts documenting the use of herbal remedies, dating back to 1550 BC. In ancient Greece and Rome, medical authorities such as Hippocrates and Dioscorides wrote detailed works on the medicinal use of plants [10].

During the Middle Ages, herbal medicine formed the basis of medical practices in Europe, the Middle East, China, and India, that is, both in the west and in the east. Avicenna's *"Canon of Medicine"* and *"Shen-nong's Herbal Classics"* are important medical texts of this period [11, 12].

In the modern era and by the 19th century, thanks to the development of chemistry and pharmacology, herbal medicines became the center of scientific pharmaceutical research. During this period, the active ingredients that formed the basis of many modern medicines were isolated from plants [13, 14].

In the 20th century, the rise of chemical and synthetic drugs caused phytotherapy to be overshadowed for a while. However, in recent years, the importance of phytotherapy has increased again due to the growing demand for a more natural and holistic approach to health [15].

Today, phytotherapy is accepted as a part of modern medicine, and scientific research confirms that phytotherapy is a safe and effective treatment method [1].

3.1.1.2 *Basic Principles of Phytotherapy*

Here are some key elements related to the basic principles of phytotherapy, which are generally based on a natural and holistic approach to health:

1. Benefiting from Nature: Phytotherapy uses the solutions offered by nature in the protection of health and the treatment of diseases. Plants, minerals, and vitamins make up the basic components of natural remedies. These ingredients are often used in their natural form and contain active ingredients that are considered effective [7].
2. Holistic Approach: Phytotherapy does not see the disease or symptom as an isolated condition. Instead, it recognizes that diseases and health conditions are closely related to overall lifestyle, nutrition, and environmental factors. Therefore, overall health status and lifestyle changes play an important role in treatment [7].
3. Preventive Medicine: Phytotherapy focuses on the prevention of disease rather than just treating the symptoms. This often involves diet, lifestyle changes, and the use of herbs that protect and improve overall health [16].

4. Scientific Evidence-Based Practices: Modern phytotherapy uses scientific research to determine the efficacy and safety of plants. This may include clinical trials, epidemiological studies, and laboratory tests. Scientific evidence helps support the effectiveness and safety of herbal remedies and treatments [1].

3.1.2 Medicinal Plants and Their Uses

Medicinal plants are natural resources used to support health and for the prevention and treatment of various diseases. Plants have been the basis of health care in human history, and many of the modern medicines are still based on ingredients derived from plant sources. But the effects and safe use of plants require extensive knowledge and understanding.

In different cultures across the globe, the use of various forms of herbal remedies has been going on for thousands of years. This practice has been intertwined with many areas of modern medicine and, in some cases, has led to the development of modern medicines. For example, aspirin is a drug originally based on salicillin extracted from willow trees [17].

The use of medicinal plants can be a beneficial and cost-effective treatment in many cases. However, the levels of efficacy and safety are often related to the quality, proper use, and dosage of the herbal product. Therefore, it is very important to consult with a healthcare professional before starting any herbal treatment.

3.1.2.1 Examples of Medicinal Plants and Their Uses

To understand the health benefits of herbal remedies, it may be helpful to look at various medicinal plants and their potential uses. Medicinal plants have been used for the prevention and treatment of various diseases for many years. Some examples of various medicinal plants and their uses are given below:

1. Aloe Vera (*Aloe barbadensis*): Used for burns, cuts, and other skin problems. It is also used to relieve stomach upsets [18].
2. Ginger (*Zingiber officinal*): Used to prevent nausea and vomiting. It is also thought to have anti-inflammatory properties and is therefore also used to treat arthritis [19].
3. Lavender (*Lavandula*): Used for relaxation and stress relief. It may also help treat insomnia [20].
4. St. John's Wort (*Hypericum triquetrifolium*): An herb thought to be effective in treating mild to moderate depression. However, it should be used with caution as it may interact with other drugs [21].
5. Thyme (*Thymus vulgaris*): Used especially for respiratory problems and digestive issues. It is believed to have antibacterial and antifungal properties [22].

Please note that although these herbs are used for a variety of health issues, it is important to consult with a healthcare professional before starting any herbal treatment.

3.1.2.2 Plants and Their Contribution to Modern Medicines

Some examples of how plants have contributed to the development of modern medicines are listed below. These examples illustrate the importance of the use of plants in modern medicine and how herbal medicines contribute to the process of drug development. However, a rigorous review based on scientific research is always required for the effectiveness and safety of herbal remedies in specific patient cases.

1. Black Cumin (*Nigella sativa*): Black cumin, derived from Nigella sativa seeds, is used in research on modern cancer drugs due to its anti-inflammatory and anticancer properties [23].
2. Elderberry (*Sambucus nigra*): The antioxidant and antiviral properties of elderberry have been instrumental in the development of modern flu and cold remedies [24].

3. Ergot Fungus (*Claviceps purpurea*): Ergot alkaloids are products of the fungus *Claviceps purpurea* and have formed the basis of modern medicines used to treat migraines and other vascular headaches [25].

4. Fennel (*Foeniculum vulgare*): The antispasmodic effect of fennel has contributed to the development of modern abdominal pain remedies [26].

5. Ginkgo (*Ginkgo biloba*): Ginkgo has been instrumental in the development of modern medicines used to treat neurological disorders [27].

6. Henbane (*Hyoscyamus niger*): Henbane is the main ingredient of drugs used in modern parkinsonian treatments due to its anticholinergic effect [28]. It is also used to treat stomach complaints, toothaches, ulcers, and tumors [27].

7. Lady's Glove (*Digitalis purpurea*): The lady's glove plant, also referred to as foxglove, is the main source of digitalis, which is used in the treatment of congestive heart failure. It has contributed to the development of cardiovascular medicines [27].

8. Opium Poppy (*Papaver somniferum*): The opium poppy plant is the main component of opiate analgesics such as morphine and codeine. It has played an important role in the development of pain medications [14].

9. Willow Tree (*Salix alba*): The main component of aspirin, salicillin, is derived from willow wood and has formed the basis of modern painkillers [14].

3.1.3 Phytotherapy Applications and Research

This section covers phytotherapy applications including herbal teas and infusions, herbal extracts, herbal ointments and creams, herbal steam inhalations, and aromatherapy. This section also covers phytotherapy research including clinical studies, investigation of bioactive components, plant–drug interactions, and the standardization of plant products.

3.1.3.1 *Phytotherapy Applications*

Phytotherapy is a multifaceted field that deals with the use of herbal remedies in the prevention and treatment of health problems. Traditionally, herbal treatment has meant the use of various herbs and plant extracts with a natural and complementary approach.

Phytotherapy applications can take place in a wide range of different forms and for different purposes. Furthermore, scientific research on phytotherapy has an important role to play in understanding the efficacy, safety, and possible side effects of plants.

3.1.3.1.1 *Herbal Teas and Infusions*

Herbal teas and infusions prepared by brewing dried plant materials with boiling water are a common phytotherapy practice. This method allows plants to be effective by passing their active ingredients into the water [29].

Below are 20 examples from scientific research on herbal teas. These examples are based on scientific research on the different health benefits of herbal teas. For more information, please refer to the relevant research in the cited references.

1. Chamomile Tea and Sleep Quality: Chamomile tea has been observed to improve sleep quality and reduce anxiety levels [30].

2. Echinacea Tea and the Common Cold: Echinacea tea has been observed to reduce cold symptoms [31].

3. Elderberry Tea and Viral Infections: Elderberry tea has been found to have a therapeutic effect on viral infections [29].

4. Fennel Tea and Digestion: Fennel tea has been found to have positive effects on the digestive system [32].

5. Ginger Tea and Nausea: Ginger tea has been found to reduce nausea during pregnancy and after chemotherapy [33, 34].
6. Ginkgo Tea and Memory: Ginkgo tea has been found to improve memory and cognitive function [35].
7. Ginseng Tea and Energy: Ginseng tea has been found to increase energy levels and reduce fatigue [36].
8. Green Tea and Metabolism: Green tea has been found to be effective in weight loss by accelerating metabolism [37].
9. Hibiscus Tea and Blood Pressure: Hibiscus tea has been found to be effective in lowering high blood pressure [38].
10. Lavender Tea and Insomnia: Lavender tea has been found to improve sleep quality and alleviate insomnia [39].
11. Lemon Blossom Tea and Stress Reduction: Lemon blossom tea has been found to be effective in reducing stress levels [40].
12. Linden Tea and Sore Throat: Linden tea has been found to have a relieving effect on sore throats [39].
13. Marigold Tea and Anti-inflammation: Marigold tea has been observed to possess anti-inflammatory and antioxidant properties [41].
14. Mint Tea and Digestion: Mint tea has been observed to have a relaxing effect on the digestive system [39].
15. Rosehip Tea and the Immune System: Rosehip tea has been found to have an immune system-strengthening effect [42].
16. Rosemary Tea and Memory: Rosemary tea has been observed to increase memory and learning ability [39].
17. Sage and Concentration: Sage has been observed to increase cognitive function and concentration [39].
18. Sage and Diabetes: Sage has been found to be effective in lowering blood sugar levels [43].
19. Thyme Tea and Antimicrobial Effect: Thyme tea has been observed to have an inhibitory effect on microorganisms [44].
20. White Tea and Antioxidant Effect: White tea has been found to have a high antioxidant capacity [45].

3.1.3.1.2 Herbal Extracts

Herbal extracts are condensed compounds obtained by extracting plant materials with specific solvents. These extracts can be used as supplements in capsule, tablet, or liquid form [46].

Below are 15 examples of herbal extracts. These examples are based on scientific research into the various health benefits of herbal extracts. For more information, please refer to the relevant research in the cited references.

1. Blueberry Extract: Blueberry extract is commonly used to support eye health [47].
2. Dandelion Extract: Dandelion extract is used to maintain liver health [48].
3. Echinacea Extract: Echinacea extract is widely used in the treatment of colds and upper respiratory tract infections [49].
4. Garlic Extract: Garlic extract is used to protect cardiovascular health [50].
5. Ginger Extract: Ginger extract is used in the treatment of rheumatic ailments [27].
6. Ginkgo Biloba Extract: Ginkgo biloba extract is commonly used to support brain function and memory [46].
7. Ginseng Extract: Ginseng root extract is used to increase energy and stamina [46].
8. Horsetail Extract: Horsetail extract is used to reduce joint pain and treat osteoarthritis [51].
9. Kudzu Extract: The effects of kudzu root extract in the treatment of alcohol dependence have been investigated [7].

10. Milk Thistle Extract: Milk thistle extract is used to support liver health [52].
11. Rosemary Extract: The effects of rosemary extract in reducing hair loss have been investigated [7].
12. St. John's Wort Extract: St. John's wort extract is used to treat mild to moderate depression [21].
13. Spearmint Extract: Spearmint extract is used to treat flatulence, food poisoning, fever, cold, flu, rheumatism, sinusitis, earaches, stings, and hiccups [53].
14. Tangle Extract: Tangle extract is used to relieve menopausal symptoms [7].
15. Turmeric Extract: Joint ailments can be treated using turmeric extract due to its anti-inflammatory properties [46].

3.1.3.1.3   Herbal Ointments and Creams

Vegetable oils and extracts are used in the treatment of skin problems by combining them with ointments and creams suitable for direct use on the skin [54]. Examples of herbal ointments and creams include:

1. Aloe Vera Gel: The gel of the aloe vera plant is used for healing skin wounds and reducing skin irritations [55].
2. Arnica Cream: Arnica cream is used to accelerate the healing of injuries and bruises [56].
3. Calendula Cream: Calendula cream is used to relieve skin irritations and reduce inflammation in the skin [57].
4. Chamomile Ointment: Chamomile ointment is used to soothe skin irritations and reduce redness on the skin [58].
5. Cocoa Butter Cream: Cocoa butter cream is used to maintain the skin's moisture balance and relieve skin dryness [59].
6. Coconut Oil Cream: Coconut oil cream helps prevent fungal infections on the skin. It also helps prevent moisture loss in the skin and strengthens the skin barrier [60].
7. Eucalyptus Cream: Eucalyptus cream is used to reduce the symptoms of respiratory conditions.
8. Lavender Ointment: Lavender ointment is effective in relieving skin irritations such as mild burns and insect bites [61].
9. Propolis Cream: Propolis cream is used to accelerate wound healing and prevent skin infections.
10. Rosehip Cream: Rosehip cream is used to relieve redness and irritation on the skin.
11. Rosemary Cream: Rosemary cream is used to treat muscle aches and joint disorders.
12. St. John's Wort Oil Cream: St. John's wort oil cream is used to accelerate the healing of burns and skin wounds.
13. Tea Tree Cream: Tea tree cream is used with antiseptic effect in the treatment of acne and pimples.
14. Turmeric Cream: Turmeric cream is used in the relief of joint inflammations and in the treatment of rheumatoid arthritis.

3.1.3.1.4   Herbal Vapor Inhalations

The method of using herbal vapor inhalations may be effective in treating respiratory ailments by combining vegetable oils with hot water vapor [62].

Below are 20 examples of herbal steam inhalations and their potential health benefits:

1. Cardamom Vapor: Cardamom essential oils may help relieve airway obstruction and shortness of breath.
2. Chamomile Vapor: Chamomile may be effective in relieving respiratory tract inflammations.

3. Clove Vapor: Clove essential oils are thought to have protective effects against respiratory inflammations.
4. Eucalyptus Vapor: Eucalyptus essential oils are an effective option in relieving respiratory ailments.
5. Fennel Vapor: Fennel essential oils can help relieve respiratory tract inflammations and provide an expectorant effect.
6. Fenugreek Vapor: Fenugreek can be used to treat respiratory tract inflammations and coughs.
7. Garlic Vapor: Garlic may be effective against respiratory infections thanks to its antimicrobial properties.
8. Karabash Steam: Karabash herb can be used to reduce respiratory irritation and relieve coughs.
9. Lavender Steam: Lavender steam inhalations may help reduce anxiety and stress.
10. Lemon Balm Vapor: Lemon balm (*Melissa officinalis*) may help relieve respiratory ailments.
11. Licorice Root Vapor: Licorice root may help relieve respiratory irritation [27].
12. Mint Vapor: Essential oils from peppermint leaves may help relieve sinus congestion.
13. Rosehip Vapor: Rosehip may be effective in relieving respiratory irritation.
14. Rosemary Vapor: Rosemary essential oils may help relieve sinus congestion and headaches.
15. Sage Vapor: Sage steam inhalations may help relieve throat inflammations and reduce coughing.
16. Sandalwood Vapor: Sandalwood essential oils can reduce respiratory irritation and coughing.
17. Tea Tree Vapor: Tea tree essential oils can be used to treat respiratory infections.
18. Thyme Vapor: Essential oils of oregano may help treat respiratory infections.
19. White Basil Vapor: White basil has been evaluated to have protective effects against respiratory infections.
20. White Juniper Vapor: White juniper essential oils may help relieve respiratory ailments.

These examples are taken from scientific research in which herbal steam inhalations are used to relieve respiratory ailments and relieve symptoms. However, before making herbal steam inhalations, it is extremely important to take into account the personal state of health and choose the right herbs and methods.

For chronic or persistent respiratory issues, consulting a healthcare professional is strongly advised.

3.1.3.1.5 Aromatherapy
Aromatherapy is a form of phytotherapy that involves the treatment of sensory and emotional health problems through the use of essential oils derived from plants [63].

The 20 examples of plant essential oils derived from plants and used for aromatherapy are:

1. Bergamot Essence: May help relieve anxiety and balance the mood.
2. Chamomile Essence: May improve sleep quality and provide a calming effect.
3. Cinnamon Essence: Used to increase mental alertness and support focus.
4. Eucalyptus Essence: It can be used to facilitate breathing in respiratory tract disorders.
5. Fennel Essence: Used to reduce tension with its calming and relaxing effect.
6. Ginger Essence: May help relieve nausea and promote digestion.
7. Holy Basil (Tulsi) Essence: May contribute to supporting digestion, relieving nausea, healing wounds, lowering blood sugar, easing inflammation, and preventing.
8. Jasmine Essence: May help improve sleep quality and relieve. It may also help to alleviate symptoms of depression.

9. Lavender Essence: Used to reduce stress and anxiety with its relaxing and calming effect.
10. Lemon Essence: May help reduce stress with its energizing and invigorating properties.
11. Licorice Root Essence: It can be used to relieve respiratory tract disorders and reduce cough [27].
12. Mint Essence: May help relieve sinus congestion and relieve headaches.
13. Orange Essence: Can be used to reduce stress with its energizing and invigorating effect.
14. Rose Essence: Can be used to provide spiritual balance with its soothing effect.
15. Rosemary Essence: Used to increase mental alertness and support focus.
16. Sandalwood Essence: Used to relieve stress and tension.
17. Tea Tree Essence: May provide a protective effect against infections due to its antimicrobial properties.
18. Thyme Essence: May help fight infections with its antimicrobial properties.
19. Vanilla Essence: May have soothing and relaxing properties.
20. Ylang Ylang Essence: Can be used to reduce nervous tension and stress.

These examples are taken from scientific research on the various health benefits of plant essences used in aromatherapy. It is therefore important and recommended to consult an aromatherapist or healthcare professional before using it because the effect of aromatherapy can differ depending on personal preferences and health status.

3.1.3.2 *Phytotherapy Research*

3.1.3.2.1 Clinical Trials

Controlled clinical trials are conducted for the efficacy and safety of herbal remedies. Clinical trials are scientific research conducted in the field of medicine and health to evaluate the effectiveness and safety of new treatments, drugs, procedures, or other interventions [64].

These studies may include experiments or observations on human participants and are often designed in the form of randomized controlled trials (RCTs). The aim of clinical studies is to contribute to the solution of health problems by using scientific methods as well as contributing to the development of scientifically safe and effective treatments.

Some basic types of clinical trials include:

1. Randomized Controlled Trial (RCT): Participants are randomly divided into two groups: the trial group and the control group. The trial group receives treatment or intervention, while the control group receives placebo or standard treatment. The effectiveness of the treatment is then evaluated by comparing the results.
2. Observational Studies: Participants are observed in their natural environment without applying the intervention. Observational studies help examine the real-life effects of treatments.
3. Cohort Studies: Groups of people (cohorts) with a particular characteristic or condition are monitored over a long period of time, and their results are evaluated. Such studies can help examine the relationship of certain factors to diseases.
4. Pre-Clinical Trial Studies: Studies on animal or cell culture with the aim of pre-testing the effects of a new treatment or drug on humans.
5. Post-Clinical Trial Studies: Studies conducted to monitor the effects of a treatment after its release and to evaluate side effects.

Protecting the rights of participants and following ethical standards is an important part of clinical trials. In addition, the correct interpretation of the results and their use in the determination of health policies are among the important contributions of clinical studies.

3.1.3.2.2   Investigation of Bioactive Components

Laboratory research on the active ingredients and pharmacological effects of plants is important for understanding the effectiveness of herbal remedies [65]. Bioactive components are chemical compounds found in plants, animals, or microorganisms that have biological effects. These components are usually substances that have nutritional value and have positive effects on health.

The study of bioactive components involves the process of identifying the sources of these components, analyzing their chemical structure, assessing their biological effects, and investigating their potential health benefits. This study may include the following steps:

1. Identification of Plant Sources: Bioactive components are commonly found in plants. Therefore, the study of bioactive components involves identifying plant sources. Determining which plants contain which components is the first step in research.
2. Extraction and Separation Processes: Extraction and separation processes are used to obtain bioactive components from plant materials or other sources. These processes aim to obtain the compounds in a purer form and make them suitable for subsequent analysis.
3. Chemical Analysis: Chemical analyses of bioactive components involve the determination of the chemical structures of compounds. These analyses are performed by spectroscopic techniques, chromatographic methods, and other analytical methods.
4. Biological Activity Tests: Various biological activity tests are performed to evaluate the biological effects of the obtained bioactive components. These tests help determine the anti-inflammatory, antioxidant, anticancer, or other health effects of the compounds.
5. Investigation of Health Potential: Clinical studies are conducted to evaluate the potential health benefits of bioactive ingredients. These studies allow for the more detailed study of the effects of compounds on humans.

The study of bioactive compounds is an important area of research to make new discoveries in the field of health and nutrition. These studies are aimed at contributing to the development of health support products that can be obtained from natural sources and to the prevention or treatment of diseases. However, it is important that such studies are carried out correctly and the results are accurately interpreted. Furthermore, more research needs to be done on the safety and efficacy of bioactive ingredients.

3.1.3.2.3   Plant–Drug Interactions

The interactions of herbal medicines with other drugs are investigated for drug safety [66]. Plant–drug interactions happen when, without notifying their doctor, patients use herbal supplements or herbal products that potentially have negative interactions with the prescription or over-the-counter medications they are taking. Such interactions can occur as a result of the interaction of the effects of drugs with the active ingredients contained in plants and herbal products.

Plant–drug interactions can take several forms:

1. Pharmacokinetic Interactions: Plant compounds can alter the concentration of drugs in the blood by affecting the absorption, distribution, metabolism, or excretion of drugs in the body. This can increase or decrease the effect of the drug.
2. Pharmacodynamic Interactions: Plant compounds and drugs, if they act on the same target organ or mechanism, can interact with each other and cause unwanted side effects when used together.
3. Increased Toxicity: Some plant compounds and drugs can accumulate in the body and cause an increase in toxicity levels when used together.

For example, the consumption of licorice root (*Glycyrrhiza glabra*) can reduce the effect of diuretic drugs, causing blood pressure to rise. St. John's wort (*Hypericum perforatum*) herbal supplements may reduce or enhance the effect of certain antidepressant medications used to treat depression. Likewise, consumption of *Ginkgo biloba* along with blood-thinning medications (e.g., warfarin) may increase the risk of bleeding [27].

The following steps can be taken to avoid plant–drug interactions:

- Patients are advised to always consult their doctor or pharmacist before they start using herbal supplements or herbal products.
- Patients are advised to read the labels of herbal supplements or herbal products and research the active ingredients they contain and possible interactions.
- Patients are advised to take their prescribed medications regularly and talk to a doctor before making dose changes.
- If patients are taking a combination of medications prescribed by more than one doctor or healthcare professional, this is advised to be reported to all relevant doctors and healthcare professionals.
- If any adverse effects or side effects are noticed, the healthcare provider should be contacted without wasting any time.

Plant–drug interactions are important, and it should be noted that such interactions can happen. Providing your healthcare provider with the right information will help ensure that your treatment process is carried out effectively and safely.

3.1.3.2.4 Standardization of Plant Products

Standardization studies are carried out to ensure the quality and reliability of herbal products. Standardization of plant products is the process that involves the regulation and standardization of the bioactive components contained in plants and plant products by scientific methods for quality control and determination of their effectiveness. This process is carried out with the aim of ensuring the safety and quality of herbal products, improving the effectiveness of use, and setting standards for the medical and pharmaceutical use of herbal products [67].

Standardization of vegetable products includes the following steps:

1. Determination of Plant Material: The plant material used for the standardization of plant products should be determined in advance. It is important to use the right plant species and the right plant part (e.g., root, leaf, flower).
2. Identification of Active Ingredients: It is important to identify the active ingredients that contribute to the effectiveness of herbal products. These components are chemicals of plant origin and help determine the quality and effectiveness of plant products.
3. Application of Analytical Methods: Appropriate analytical methods are used to analyze the active ingredients in herbal products. These methods may include spectroscopic techniques, chromatographic methods, and other analytical methods.
4. Determination of Quality Control and Standardization: Standards and quality control procedures are determined to ensure the quality of herbal products. This is done to keep the bioactive ingredient content of plant products and other quality parameters under control.
5. Bioactivity Tests: Bioactivity tests are performed to determine the effectiveness of herbal products. These tests help assess the impact of herbal products against particularly targeted health problems.

The standardization of herbal products includes several types of products, such as herbal remedies, herbal supplements, and cosmetic products. The use of standardized herbal products increases the reliability of the products and helps them achieve more consistent results for users.

In addition, by setting standards for the medical use of herbal products in the health sector, it contributes to the safe and effective execution of treatment processes. Therefore, the standardization of plant products helps to gain wider acceptance and increased use of plant-based products.

3.1.4 Safety and Side Effects of Phytotherapy

Although phytotherapy is a field that includes herbal treatment methods commonly used in natural health sciences, the safety of the plants and herbal products used is an important issue. Herbal treatments are generally natural and carry a low risk of side effects. However, certain plant components and herbal products can have side effects and interactions. Therefore, herbal treatment should be carefully evaluated before being applied, and a healthcare professional should be consulted.

In this section, examples based on scientific studies on phytotherapy applications and research are given. These studies provide a scientific basis for the efficacy and safety of herbal remedies and show how phytotherapy is gaining value in the field of modern medicine. For more information, please refer to the relevant research in the cited references.

3.1.4.1 Safety of Phytotherapy

3.1.4.1.1 Choosing the Right Herb and Dosage

It is important to choose the right herb and dosage in phytotherapy applications. Different plants can have different mechanisms of action. The use of the wrong herb or dosage can therefore lead to undesirable consequences.

3.1.4.1.1.1 Pharmacology and Efficacy Evaluation of Herbal Products

Drug interactions: Herbal products are known to interact with prescription or over-the-counter medications. For example, St. John's Wort (*Hypericum perforatum*) may reduce the effectiveness of certain medications [68].

Effectiveness of herbal products: Clinical studies have evaluated the therapeutic effects of herbal products and their effectiveness compared to other treatment methods. For example, silymarin has been found effective in treating liver diseases [69].

3.1.4.1.1.2 Supporting the Correct Herb and Dosage with Clinical Experience

Harmony of traditional knowledge and scientific research: The traditional uses of some plants have been supported by scientific research. For example, the effects of the Echinacea plant on colds and upper respiratory tract infections have been studied, and its effects on the immune system have been confirmed [70].

3.1.4.1.1.3 Toxicological Assessment and Safety

Toxicological evaluation of plant products: Research is carried out to determine the toxic effects of plant extracts. For example, the use of *Aloe vera* extracts in high doses can cause skin irritation [71].

3.1.4.1.1.4 Individual Tolerance and Conformity

Variation of effects on individuals: Research has shown that the effects of some herbal products on individuals may differ. For example, the effects of Ginkgo biloba on memory may vary depending on personal differences [72].

3.1.4.1.1.5 Quality Control of Herbal Products

Purity and efficacy of herbal products: There may be uncertainties about the safety and efficacy of herbal products that have not been quality controlled. Therefore, quality control of herbal products is important. For example, chemical analysis is carried out to determine the amounts of active ingredients in vegetable products [73].

The information above constitutes a summary of the scientific research on the correct choice of herbs and dosage in phytotherapy. In order to achieve safe and effective results in phytotherapy applications, it is important to choose the right herb and dosage based on scientific research. Therefore, it is crucial for healthcare professionals and phytotherapists to follow the current scientific literature and recommend treatments based on scientific foundations.

3.1.4.1.2   Quality Control

Quality control of plant products is important for determining the quantities and purity of active ingredients in plant extracts. There may be uncertainties about the safety of herbal products without quality control. Quality control is an important step that involves a series of analytical and chemical tests carried out to determine the quantity and purity of the active ingredients contained in herbal products used in phytotherapy.

Quality control of plant extracts and herbal products used in phytotherapy is significant in terms of the safety, efficacy, and clinical applicability of the product. Additionally, quality control ensures the quality and consistency of the product by verifying that the plant components are in the appropriate concentrations to achieve the desired treatment effect.

The following steps and methods can be used for quality control:

1. Chemical Analysis: Chemical analysis of plant products is used to determine the active ingredients in herbal extracts. Analytical methods such as high-performance liquid chromatography (HPLC), gas chromatography (GC), and mass spectrometry (MS) allow the detection of active ingredients in plant products and their quantification to be measured.
2. Microbiological Analysis: Microbiological analysis of plant products is performed to determine the presence of potentially dangerous microorganisms in the product. Such analyses are used to verify that plant products are safe from microbiological contamination such as bacteria, yeast, and mold.
3. Heavy Metal and Pesticide Residue Tests: The presence of heavy metal and pesticide residues in plant products can affect the safety of the product. Therefore, analyses are carried out to verify that vegetable products are free from such contaminants.
4. Herbal Product Purity and Standardization: The purity of herbal products is evaluated by determining the presence of unwanted substances in herbal extracts. Also, the standardization of vegetable products guarantees that the amounts of active ingredients in vegetable products are at the desired level.
5. Quality Certificates: The data obtained as a result of the quality control of herbal products are reported in official documents called quality certificates. These documents ensure reliability and safety between manufacturers and users of herbal products.
6. Good Manufacturing Practices (GMP): The production and quality control of plant products should be carried out in accordance with good manufacturing practices. GMP standards regulate industrial processes to ensure the quality, safety, and effectiveness of herbal products.

Quality control is of paramount importance when it comes to the safety and efficacy of herbal products used in phytotherapy, helping consumers and healthcare professionals achieve the best results from herbal treatments. Quality control contributes to the scientific and reliable application of natural health sciences. Therefore, quality control of herbal products used in phytotherapy is a scientific and ethical responsibility.

3.1.4.1.3   Proper Use

Appropriate use of herbal products shall be carried out in accordance with the label instructions. Recommended dosages should not be exceeded, and doctor control should be ensured with long-term use.

Proper use is an important concept for the effective and safe use of plants and herbal products in phytotherapy applications. Appropriate use in phytotherapy applications based on natural health sciences involves the use of herbal products and correct dosages determined in accordance with the health status of patients. To ensure proper use, the following points should be noted:

1. Assessment of Health Status: Before starting the application of phytotherapy, the patient's health status and existing health problems should be evaluated. Phytotherapy may not be suitable for every health problem, and some herbal products should not be used under certain health conditions.
2. Plant and Herbal Product Selection: After evaluating the health status, the selection of plants or herbal products suitable for the needs of the patient should be made. Different herbs can be effective for different health problems, and not every patient may be suitable for the same herbal product.
3. Proper Dosage and Instructions for Use: Proper dosage and instructions for the use of herbal products should be followed. Dosages should not be exceeded and should be used at the recommended time and frequency. Improper dosage use of herbal products can cause unwanted side effects.
4. Pregnancy and Lactation Period: Care should be taken before the use of herbal products during pregnancy and lactation. Some herbal products can be harmful during pregnancy and lactation and can affect the health of the mother and child.
5. Interactions with Medications: It should be noted that herbal products used in the practice of phytotherapy may interact with prescription or over-the-counter medications. It is important to consult a doctor or pharmacist before the use of herbal products together with medicines.
6. Follow-up of Those with Chronic Diseases: People with chronic diseases should consult their doctors before applying herbal treatment. Some herbal products may affect the course of chronic diseases or interact with other treatments.
7. Individual Tolerances and Reactions: Each person's body structure and metabolism are different. A plant or herbal product may not have the same effect for everyone. Individuals' tolerance and reactions to herbal treatments may vary.
8. Expert Counseling: It is important to get information and advice from a health consultant who is an expert in phytotherapy applications. Healthcare professionals have the appropriate knowledge and experience to ensure proper use of patients and help them achieve the best outcomes.

Proper use is a fundamental element in phytotherapy applications to achieve the desired results and minimize health risks. It is therefore important for people interested in natural health sciences to be aware and educated about proper use.

3.1.4.2   Side Effects of Phytotherapy

Phytotherapy is the use of herbal products and plant extracts used in the field of natural health sciences for therapeutic purposes. Their side effects can often be less compared to traditional medicines because they are usually of natural origin. However, some herbal products can have side effects, and therefore proper use and careful follow-up of phytotherapy are also necessary. This section presents information based on scientific studies on the common side effects of phytotherapy.

The safety and side effects of phytotherapy are important issues for the smooth realization of herbal treatment practices. It is therefore important to consult a healthcare professional before the use of herbal products and to use them with caution. People with any health problem should get information and advice from their doctors or health experts before the use of phytotherapy.

In addition, quality control and proper use of herbal products are essential in terms of preventing possible side effects and protecting the health of the user. Nevertheless, the side effects of phytotherapy should also be considered. Side effects of phytotherapy may vary depending on the content of the herbal product used, the dosage consumed, and the duration of use. Some common side effects include:

3.1.4.2.1   Allergic Reactions

According to research, some herbal products can cause allergic reactions, especially in individuals with allergies. For example, ginger and chamomile can cause allergic reactions in some people. Allergy symptoms can be itching, redness, rash, swelling, and shortness of breath. People at risk of allergies should consult their doctor before using potentially allergic herbal products.

3.1.4.2.2   Gastrointestinal (Intestinal) and Stomach Disorders

Some herbal products used in phytotherapy can lead to stomach upsets and gastrointestinal problems, especially in people with sensitive stomachs. Such side effects include nausea, vomiting, stomach pain, and diarrhea. For example, excessive use of the aloe vera plant can lead to stomach upsets.

3.1.4.2.3   Skin Reactions

Contact with herbal ointments and creams with the skin can lead to skin irritation and allergic reactions in some people. Especially in people with sensitive skin, symptoms including skin redness, itching, and rashes may occur after the use of herbal products. For example, some vegetable oils, such as rosemary oil, can cause skin irritation. For this reason, caution should be exercised, especially to avoid allergic skin reactions.

3.1.4.2.4   Risk of Bleeding

Some herbal products can increase the risk of bleeding by affecting the blood clotting process. Caution should be exercised before the use of herbal products, especially before surgical intervention or in people using blood thinners. For example, overuse of St. John's Wort can affect blood clotting, increasing the risk of bleeding.

3.1.4.2.5   Pregnancy and Lactation Period

During pregnancy and lactation, some herbal products can be harmful and affect the health of mother and child. Therefore, a doctor should be consulted before the use of herbal products during pregnancy and lactation. For example, some herbal products, such as juniper oil, should not be used during pregnancy.

3.1.4.2.6   Drug Interactions

Herbal products may interact with prescription or over-the-counter medications. Some herbal products may reduce or increase the effectiveness of the medications taken. Therefore, it is important to consult a doctor or pharmacist before combining herbal products together with medicines. For example, licorice (glycyrrhizin) may reduce the effectiveness of some medications.

Especially people with chronic diseases or those who regularly use medication should consult their doctors before applying herbal treatment. Also, the right choice of herbs and dosage and proper use can help minimize side effects. Following proper instructions for use and seeking information and advice from healthcare professionals plays an important role in reducing the side effects of phytotherapy.

In summary, side effects of herbal products used in phytotherapy can be found, and therefore correct and careful use is important. People with any health problems should definitely get information and advice from their doctors or health experts before the use of phytotherapy.

3.2   HOMEOPATHY

Homeopathy is a system of alternative medicine that uses natural ingredients for the treatment of diseases. It was developed by Samuel Hahnemann in the 18th century. Homeopathy is based on the idea of treating diseases with substances that cause symptoms similar to those of their symptoms.

3.2.1   What Is Homeopathy?

This chapter covers the history of homeopathy, the ideas of Samuel Hahnemann, and theories of how homeopathy works. It also details the unique principles of homeopathy, the law of the like, the minimum dose, the only solution, and the whole person.

Homeopathy was developed as a system of alternative medicine by German physician Samuel Hahnemann in the 18th century. Hahnemann defined the idea of treating a disease with a substance that has symptoms similar to its symptoms as the law of "similar to similar cures." This idea forms the basis of homeopathy.

Homeopathic remedies are prepared by frequently shaking and diluting a substance in water or alcohol. This process is called "potentization," and homeopaths claim that this process increases the "energy" of medications and reduces their potential harmful side effects [74]. Because of this extreme dilution, most homeopathic products may not have any molecules of the initial active ingredient.

Homeopathy, however, has generally been critically evaluated by the scientific community. Modern science takes a skeptical stance on the biological effectiveness of homeopathic remedies. The biggest reason for the aforementioned criticism is that most homeopathic remedies are diluted to levels that do not contain any molecules of the active substance, which is contrary to Avogadro's law.

Avogadro's law states that the number of molecules in a given volume is constant [75]. This means that after a certain point (potency of 12C, where Avogadro's number is about 6.02×10^{23} molecules/mol), a solution will not contain any molecules of the original substance. Moreover, meta-analyses of many large, controlled, and randomized trials, such as the Cochrane Library, have not shown that homeopathic treatments are more effective than placebo treatment [76].

As a result, homeopathy adopts the method of treatment with substances that have symptoms similar to their symptoms and excessively dilutes these substances. However, the current scientific evidence has not reached a definitive conclusion about the effectiveness and mechanism of homeopathic treatments. Individuals evaluating any treatment option are advised to make a decision in light of the scientific evidence and consultation with a healthcare professional.

3.2.2   How Does Homeopathy Work?

Homeopathic remedies are usually in a very diluted form, and this process is called *"potinization."* This section discusses in detail the preparation and dilution process of homeopathic remedies and theories of how this process increases the "energy" of medicine.

The traditional understanding of how homeopathy works differs significantly from the basic principles accepted by modern science. Therefore, understanding homeopathy is mostly based on traditional principles by which homeopaths describe how this form of treatment works.

Homeopathy is founded on two basic principles:

1. Similia Similibus Curentur (Like Cures Like): This is the most basic principle of homeopathy. This principle implies that when conducting an experiment on a healthy person with a substance, the resulting set of symptoms will resemble the symptoms of the disease. Homeopathy uses substances that can improve these "similar" symptoms.
2. Minimum Dose: During the preparation of homeopathic remedies, the process of constant dilution and shaking of the main substance is called "potency." This process produces a drug that is highly diluted — not even containing molecules of the original substance. Homeopaths believe that this process conserves the "energy" or "essence" of the drug but eliminates its potential toxicity.

However, these principles are incompatible with the basic principles accepted by modern science. The almost complete dilution of homeopathic remedies means that the molecules that determine the effect of a remedy are gone. This, in turn, raises the question of how homeopathic remedies can exert a therapeutic effect.

Some homeopaths suggest that water can conserve the "energy" or "knowledge" of medicine, but this theory has not been scientifically proven. Also, most homeopathic remedies are diluted so much that no molecules of the original substance remain, and this is contrary to Avogadro's law.

Scientific explanations and understandings of how homeopathy works remain inadequate, and examples of how homeopathy is used in practice can help illuminate the basic principles of this form of treatment. However, none of these examples definitively prove the working mechanism of homeopathy. The following are examples of how homeopathy is used:

1. *Allium cepa* (onion) and hay fever: The symptoms experienced when chopping the onion (burning and watering in the eyes, discharge from the nose) are similar to the symptoms of hay fever. Therefore, according to homeopathy, Allium cepa (onion) extract is used to treat the symptoms of hay fever. However, the scientific evidence for homeopathy does not support these claims [77].
2. *Coffea cruda* (raw coffee) and insomnia: Drinking coffee is often associated with a state of wakefulness. However, according to the homeopathy "similar to similar cures" principle, overly diluted raw coffee extract (*Coffea cruda*) is used to treat insomnia. However, there is a lack of conclusive scientific evidence on the effectiveness of this treatment strategy [78].

As always, these and similar examples only illustrate the principles of the practice of homeopathy, not prove the effectiveness or safety of homeopathy treatments. The scientific evidence on homeopathy is often mixed, and it's highly recommended to check with a healthcare professional before trying any homeopathic treatment.

As a result, an understanding of how homeopathy works depends largely on the perspective of those who support this form of treatment and the interpretation of the scientific evidence for homeopathy. In any case, when making a decision to treat a health issue, it is important for individuals to make an informed decision and consult with a healthcare professional.

3.2.3 Use of Homeopathic Remedies

The use of homeopathic remedies depends on the patient's symptoms, general health, age, and a number of other factors. Medicines are usually available in the form of tablets, liquid drops, gels, creams, or lotions [79].

Homeopathic treatment usually requires a personalized approach. This means determining a specific treatment plan based on the patient's symptoms, emotional state, and overall health. This approach is based on the idea that each patient is unique and requires different treatment.

The use of a homeopathic remedy usually involves the following steps:

1. Consultation: Before starting treatment, the homeopath will usually assess the patient's general state of health, symptoms, lifestyle, and emotional state.
2. Drug Selection: Based on the patient's condition and symptoms, the homeopath will choose the most suitable homeopathic remedy.
3. Dosage: Homeopathic remedies are usually extremely diluted and are usually given to the patient once, but in some cases, the medicine may need to be taken more often.
4. Follow-up: The patient's condition should be monitored regularly after the administration of the drug. If symptoms improve, treatment is usually stopped. If symptoms persist or worsen, the homeopath will usually review the treatment plan and adjust it if necessary.

3.3   NATUROPATHY

Naturopathy is a healthcare system that emphasizes natural and holistic approaches. Naturopathic doctors use a variety of therapies and techniques to treat their patients, often aimed at improving natural health and preventing disease.

3.3.1   Principles

Naturopathy is founded on several basic principles including "the healing power of nature," "do-no-harm-first," "treat the cause of the disease," "treat the whole person," and "prevention is better than cure." These are explained as follows.

3.3.1.1   *The Healing Power of Nature* (Vis Medicatrix Naturae)

Naturopathic doctors work to promote and support the body's natural healing ability. This is usually accomplished through the promotion of a healthy lifestyle and diet. "*Vis Medicatrix Naturae*," a Latin term, means "Healing Power of Nature" and is one of the basic principles of naturopathy. This principle focuses on the body's ability to self-heal and return to a natural balance.

Thanks to this principle, naturopathic doctors use a variety of methods to support their patients' bodies' ability to heal themselves and to naturally stimulate healing processes. This often involves making personalized recommendations to improve the patient's lifestyle, nutrition, and overall health practices.

For example, a naturopath may recommend changes in nutrition and sleep patterns to boost a patient's immune system or recommend meditation or other relaxation techniques to overcome chronic stress and improve overall health.

However, the effectiveness of this approach is still controversial, and scientific evidence of naturopathic practices is lacking. Therefore, it is important to consult a healthcare professional before trying any treatment.

3.3.1.2   *Do No Harm First* (Primum Non Nocere)

Naturopaths prefer non-invasive and non-toxic therapies to minimize harm to their patients. "*Primum Non Nocere*," which means "*Do No Harm First*," is one of the basic principles of both naturopathy and general medicine. This principle emphasizes that the safety and well-being of the patient should always be a priority when applying a treatment or intervention.

Naturopathic practitioners apply this principle by preferring non-invasive and non-toxic therapies. This usually involves the use of milder treatments, such as diet and lifestyle changes, herbal remedies, and other natural remedies, rather than surgical intervention or pharmaceutical medications.

However, although the idea of "*Do No Harm First*" is a fundamental part of medical ethics, the important thing is always to carefully evaluate the risks and benefits and determine the most appropriate treatment approach for each individual patient. Also, just because a treatment method is "*natural*" does not automatically mean that it is "*safe*" or "*harmless.*" Therefore, it is extremely important to consult a healthcare professional before trying any treatment.

3.3.1.3   *Treat the Cause of the Disease* (Tolle Causam)

The naturopathic approach aims to find and treat the root cause of the disease rather than relieving symptoms. The principle of "*Tolle Causam*" or "*Treat the Cause*" is a central concept in naturopathy, as in many different medical approaches. This principle emphasizes finding and treating the underlying cause of the disease rather than managing the symptoms.

The "Treat the Cause" approach, within the framework of a broader biopsychosocial model, recognizes that the general lifestyle of the individual and environmental factors play an important role in the development of the disease. Its use can be observed in various areas. For example, in the treatment of depression, treatments such as therapy and lifestyle changes are applied, in addition to the use of antidepressant medications. This approach aims to address the root cause of illnesses, for example, stress or trauma [80].

In the treatment of diabetes, lifestyle changes such as diet and exercise appear to play an important role in medication as well as treatment to address the underlying causes of the disease, including obesity and inactivity [81]. Additionally, in the treatment of osteoarthritis, alongside painkillers, both physical therapy and lifestyle changes like weight loss and exercise target treatment to address the underlying causes of the disease [82].

However, the general acceptance of this principle does not make any inferences about the efficacy or safety of naturopathic treatments. The efficacy and safety of naturopathic treatments should be evaluated separately, and it is important to speak with a healthcare professional before attempting any treatment.

3.3.1.4 *Treat the Whole Person* (Tolle Totum)

Naturopathy considers patients as individual wholes and therefore not only treats physical symptoms, but also considers emotional, mental, and environmental factors. From Latin, *"Tolle Totum"* means *"Treat the Whole"* and this is one of the principles of naturopathy. This principle emphasizes seeing a person not as isolated symptoms or diseases, but as a combination of all body systems, psychological and social state.

Naturopathic doctors apply this principle using a holistic approach that comprehensively assesses their patients' lifestyles, diets, environmental factors, and emotional states. The goal of this approach is to understand how all these factors combine and affect an individual's overall health. For example, when evaluating a patient with chronic pain, a naturopath may consider the physical causes of that pain, as well as factors such as the patient's stress levels, sleep patterns, diet, and physical activity levels.

Scientifically, this "holistic" approach has found support in a number of different areas. For example, the biopsychosocial model emphasizes that the disease is caused by a combination of biological, psychological, and social factors, and therefore all of these factors must be taken into account in the treatment process [83].

However, the effectiveness of this approach often depends on specific applications and treatments, and therefore each treatment must be evaluated individually. It's important to consult a healthcare professional before trying any treatment.

3.3.1.5 *Prevention Is Better than Cure* (Preventare)

Naturopathy attaches great importance to the prevention of diseases and guides its patients to adopt healthy lifestyles and strategies to prevent diseases. *"Preventare,"* or Prevention is Better Than Cure, is a principle unique to naturopathy. It means that focusing on preventing diseases is more effective and less damaging than trying to treat them. This emphasizes preventive health practices such as healthy lifestyles, proper nutrition, and regular exercise.

Scientifically, this principle has found support in a number of areas. It has been widely recognized that healthy lifestyles, proper nutrition, and regular exercise are important in preventing various chronic diseases. For example, ceasing smoking, proper nutrition, and regular exercise are important factors in preventing heart disease, diabetes, and some types of cancer [84]. Furthermore, regular exercise and a healthy diet can help prevent conditions such as obesity, hypertension, and type 2 diabetes [85].

The effectiveness of these preventive health strategies often depends on the individual and their specific situation. Each strategy should be evaluated individually. It's important to speak with a healthcare professional before adopting any preventive health strategy.

Naturopathic treatments can include herbal remedies, acupuncture, hydrotherapy, physical manipulations, diet and lifestyle advice, and more. However, the scientific evidence for naturopathy is varied. Although there are studies on the ability of certain naturopathic therapies (e.g., some herbal remedies) to treat certain conditions or relieve symptoms, more research is needed on the overall efficacy and safety of naturopathy practices [86].

In any case, it's important to speak with a healthcare professional before trying naturopathic treatment.

3.3.2 Examples of Naturopathy Practices

Because of the variety of naturopathy practices, direct examples often include specific treatment strategies or approaches. Below are 30 examples that reflect the wide range of naturopathy practices:

1. Acupuncture: Many naturopaths use acupuncture to balance the flow of energy and relieve pain.
2. Physical manipulations: The use of osteopathy or chiropractic techniques to treat musculoskeletal problems.
3. Herbal remedies: Such as the relaxing effects of chamomile tea.
4. Homeopathy: The use of ultra-diluted substances.
5. Aromatherapy: The use of essential oils.
6. Nutritional counseling: Promoting a healthy diet and helping patients change their eating habits.
7. Stress management techniques: Such as meditation, yoga, and breathing exercises.
8. Hydrotherapy: Such as treatment with water, heated pools, and hot and cold compresses.
9. Detoxification: Diets or cleanses that promote the elimination of toxins from the body.
10. Probiotics: To support gut health.
11. Reiki: Energy healing therapy.
12. Exercise prescription: Personalized exercise programs.
13. Massage therapy: The use of various massage techniques.
14. Biocompatibility test: Some naturopaths may use this test to identify food intolerances or allergies.
15. Neurofeedback: Regulation of brain waves.
16. Ayurveda: Indian healthcare system.
17. Food supplements: Vitamins, minerals, and other food supplements.
18. Stone treatment: The use of minerals and crystals for energy healing purposes.
19. Psychological counseling: Focus on emotional health.
20. Iridology: Trying to identify health problems by looking at the iris of the eye.
21. Reflexology: Applying pressure to the reflex points of the feet, hands, and ears.
22. Shiatsu: Japanese massage technique.
23. Kinesiology: Improving the movement and function of muscles.
24. Immune support treatments: For example, the use of Echinacea for colds.
25. Colon hydrotherapy: Used to cleanse the intestines.
26. Bioresonance: Measurement and regulation of body energy.
27. Balneotherapy: Therapeutic use of mineral waters or sludges.
28. Leech therapy: Used to reduce pain and inflammation.
29. Kupping: Used to improve blood circulation in a specific area.
30. Oxygen therapy: Used to increase oxygen levels in the body.

Many of these techniques and therapies are still being intensively researched today, and the scientific evidence about their effectiveness is varied. Some may be contraindicated because of their potential side effects or risks. Therefore, it is important to consult a healthcare professional before starting any treatment, especially in case of existing health conditions or medication use.

3.4 ACUPUNCTURE

Acupuncture is a Traditional Chinese Medicine practice based on the insertion of fine needles into specific points on the human body. This is a practice to smooth and balance the flow of energy (called Qi) in the body. There are many different types of acupuncture, and they are used to treat a variety of conditions. Acupuncture practices have been used to treat a wide variety of conditions such as pain management, migraines, depression, anxiety, allergies, hypertension, and even infertility in some cases [4, 87].

3.4.1 Scientific Explanation of Acupuncture

According to the principles of Traditional Chinese Medicine (TCM), the effectiveness of acupuncture is achieved by placing needles into energy channels called meridians to regulate the body's energy flow (Qi) and create a balanced state between yin and yang. But these explanations may not be fully compatible with modern science.

Modern scientific explanations base the effects of acupuncture on its effect on the nervous system. Acupuncture has been found to have analgesic (painkiller), sedative, anti-inflammatory, and immunomodulatory (immunomodulating) effects on the central nervous system (brain and spinal cord). Furthermore, acupuncture has also been found to increase the release of neurotransmitters such as endorphins, which are naturally present in the body and help relieve pain [88, 89].

However, it is important to note that the exact mechanism of action of acupuncture is not fully understood, and more research is needed in this area. It has been determined that acupuncture can be effective for some conditions, but this effectiveness usually depends on the situation, the individual, and the acupuncture technique used.

3.4.2 The Use of Acupuncture

The use of acupuncture in many different conditions varies widely. Below are some examples of the effects of acupuncture on certain conditions. These examples are based on general information, while some represent the findings of many studies in this field. As such, the citations of the examples with scientific studies have been listed.

1. Pain management: Acupuncture is often used to manage chronic pain. These include low back pain, neck pain, osteoarthritis, and headaches [4].
2. Migraine: Acupuncture can be effective in reducing migraine pain [90].
3. Anxiety: Some studies have suggested that acupuncture may be effective in reducing symptoms of anxiety [91].
4. Depression: Acupuncture can be used to manage depression as an adjunct approach to antidepressant treatment [87].
5. Insomnia: Some studies have indicated that acupuncture can relieve insomnia symptoms [92].
6. Infertility: Acupuncture can help treat infertility in women and men [93].
7. Obesity: Acupuncture can be used as a tool in weight management [94].
8. Diabetes: In some cases, acupuncture can help relieve the symptoms of diabetes [95].
9. Allergies: Acupuncture can relieve allergic reactions and strengthen the immune system [96].
10. Asthma: Acupuncture can help relieve asthma symptoms [97].
11. Menopause: Acupuncture can help with menopausal symptoms.
12. Fibromyalgia: Acupuncture can help relieve fibromyalgia symptoms.
13. Digestive problems: Acupuncture can help manage digestive problems such as nausea, constipation, and diarrhea.

14. Irritable bowel syndrome (IBS): Acupuncture can help relieve the symptoms of IBS.
15. High blood pressure: Acupuncture can be used in the management of high blood pressure.
16. Low blood pressure: Acupuncture can help relieve the symptoms of low blood pressure.
17. Parkinson's disease: Acupuncture can help relieve the symptoms of Parkinson's disease.
18. Rheumatoid Arthritis: Acupuncture can help relieve the symptoms of rheumatoid arthritis.
19. Joint pain: Acupuncture can be used in the management of joint pain.
20. Chronic fatigue syndrome: Acupuncture can help relieve the symptoms of chronic fatigue syndrome.
21. Sinusitis: Acupuncture can help relieve the symptoms of sinusitis.
22. Tinnitus: Acupuncture can help relieve tinnitus symptoms.
23. TMJ disorders: Acupuncture can help relieve the symptoms of TMJ (temporomandibular joint) disorders.
24. Vertigo: Acupuncture can help relieve the symptoms of vertigo (dizziness).
25. Collar tunnel syndrome: Acupuncture can help relieve the symptoms of collisional tunnel syndrome.
26. Nerve pain: Acupuncture can be used in the management of nerve pain.
27. Edema: Acupuncture can help relieve the symptoms of edema.
28. Menstrual pain: Acupuncture can be used in the management of menstrual pain.
29. Premenstrual syndrome (PMS): Acupuncture can help relieve PMS symptoms.
30. Nausea and vomiting during pregnancy: Acupuncture can relieve nausea and vomiting during pregnancy.
31. Low back and back pain during pregnancy: Acupuncture can relieve low back and back pain during pregnancy.
32. Postpartum depression: Acupuncture can help relieve symptoms of postpartum depression.
33. Sleeping disorders: Acupuncture can help relieve the symptoms of sleeping disorders.
34. Chemotherapy side effects: Acupuncture can alleviate chemotherapy side effects.
35. Ulcerative colitis: Acupuncture can help relieve the symptoms of ulcerative colitis.

The examples with references above represent some scientific studies that acupuncture can be effective for a variety of conditions. However, it should be noted that more research is needed in this regard. The effectiveness of acupuncture usually depends on the situation, the individual, and the acupuncture technique used. Therefore, it is always important to seek professional medical advice when considering any treatment approach.

Acupuncture is a treatment method developed thousands of years ago as part of ancient Chinese medicine. Acupuncture practitioners try to relieve pain and other symptoms by inserting thin needles into specific body points (along energy channels often called "meridians").

Various hypotheses have been put forward to scientifically understand the mechanism of action of acupuncture, and many of these hypotheses are supported by modern science and medicine. They include:

1. Neurohormonal Pathways: When acupuncture is practiced, signals are sent to the body's nervous system, which leads to various interactions in the brain and spinal cord. These interactions stimulate a number of hormones (e.g., endorphins, serotonin, and dopamine) that are secreted by the brain and provide pain relief, peacefulness, and a feeling of general well-being [88].
2. Gate Control Theory: This theory proposes that acupuncture relieves pain by affecting the way the nervous system perceives pain. Acupuncture works by sending impulses to inhibitory nerve endings that "turn off" pain signals at the level of the spinal cord. This prevents pain signals from reaching the brain and therefore reduces the perception of pain [98].
3. Inflammatory Pathways: Acupuncture has also been shown to modulate the body's inflammatory response. There is evidence that acupuncture acts on proteins called inflammatory

cytokines, which increase or decrease inflammation. This means that acupuncture can help relieve pain and inflammation [89].

Each of these theories offers a different perspective on how acupuncture can relieve pain and other symptoms. However, the exact mechanism of action of acupuncture is still not fully understood, and more research is needed in this area.

3.5 AYURVEDA

Ayurveda is a holistic health system that originated in Ancient India and is derived from the Sanskrit roots *"Ayur"* (life) and *"Veda"* (science or wisdom). According to this traditional health system, which is seen more as a lifestyle, health is a result of the harmony between body, mind, spirit, and environment [99].

Ayurveda proposes to understand the individual through the three basic energies or life forces, *"dosha"* (body types). These doshas determine an individual's nature, or *"Prakriti,"* and influence whether they are healthy or diseased [100].

3.5.1 Philosophy of Ayurveda

The basic principle of Ayurveda is that the universe is made up of five main elements (space, air, fire, water, earth), and the human body is a reflection of these elements. In the human body, these elements are represented by the three basic doshas or body types: *Vata* (space and air), *Pitta* (fire and water), and *Kapha* (water and earth). Health depends on these doshas being in balance, and diseases occur when one or more doshas are out of balance [101].

Ayurveda is a term that means *"science of life"* in Sanskrit and offers an in-depth perspective on health and well-being. This system examines the physical, mental, and spiritual health of the individual and the interaction of these three aspects with each other and with the environment. The philosophy of Ayurveda is based on several basic principles:

1. Dosha Theory: Ayurveda describes the body structure and health profile of each individual with three biological energies or doshas (Vata, Pitta, Kapha) derived from the five basic elements (ether, air, fire, water, and earth). Each individual has a unique combination of these three doshas, and this combination determines individual physical and mental characteristics, susceptibility to disease, and even personality traits.
2. Holism: Ayurveda treats the human being as a whole and emphasizes the links between physical, mental, and spiritual health. This approach recognizes that the body, mind, and spirit are in constant interaction with each other and with the environment.
3. The Importance of Balance: Health, according to Ayurveda, is the maintenance of balance between body, mind, and spirit. The disease occurs when this balance is disturbed. Ayurveda recommends maintaining and restoring this balance through methods such as diet, lifestyle changes, herbal remedies, and detoxification procedures.
4. Preventive Health: Ayurveda encourages a proactive approach to health care and emphasizes disease prevention and overall well-being. This involves adjusting the individual's diet and lifestyle habits to fit the dosha balance and the natural rhythm of life.
5. Personalized Care: Ayurveda recognizes that each individual is unique and therefore each of us has our own specific health and well-being needs. Therefore, Ayurvedic treatments and recommendations are often individualized.
6. Connection with Nature: Ayurveda sees people as part of nature and encourages living in harmony with natural rhythms for health and well-being. This includes adapting to seasonal changes and developing habits that are in line with the natural diet and lifestyle.

3.5.2 Ayurveda and Treatment Approaches

Ayurveda includes lifestyle changes, diet, and natural treatments for both the prevention and treatment of disease. These approaches aim to eliminate the cause of disease, support the body's natural healing ability, and improve an individual's overall health and quality of life [99].

The treatment approaches of Ayurveda take into account the unique physical and mental structure of each person, their lifestyle, and their environment. Below are some of Ayurveda's treatment approaches:

1. Diet and Nutrition: Ayurveda is based on the principle of "*we are what we eat*" and emphasizes that diet plays a very important role in maintaining health and treating diseases. Ayurveda recommends foods and dietary styles that are appropriate for certain types of dosha. As a result, the Ayurvedic diet varies depending on each person's dosha balance, lifestyle, and season.
2. Herbal Treatment: Ayurveda uses herbal remedies and formulations in the treatment of various diseases. These formulations usually involve a single herb or a combination of multiple herbs and can be found in a variety of forms (tablets, powders, teas, oils, and so on).
3. Panchakarma: This is one of the most important and comprehensive treatment methods of Ayurveda and includes a series of treatments for detoxification and resuscitation. Panchakarma is used to cleanse the body, remove toxins, and restore dosha balance. This method usually consists of five stages: emesis, enema, cleansing the nose, bloodletting, and purgation.
4. Lifestyle Advice: Ayurveda recognizes that an individual's lifestyle and daily routine have a huge impact on health and well-being. Therefore, Ayurveda emphasizes the importance of factors such as regular exercise, proper sleep patterns, stress management, and emotional balance.
5. Meditation and Yoga: Ayurveda believes that mental and spiritual balance has a significant impact on health. Therefore, practices such as meditation and yoga are encouraged to calm the mind, manage stress, and promote overall well-being. Physical exercise, breathing techniques, and mental concentration aim to manage overall health and stress.
6. Marma Therapy: Marma points are the intersection points of energy channels (*nadis*) in the body, and they play an important role in Ayurveda. Marma therapy uses these points to regulate the flow of energy and promote healing.

Ayurveda recommends various treatment methods and practices for different diseases and conditions. Below are some examples specific to the philosophy and practice of Ayurveda. This information is taken from the vast knowledge base of Ayurveda and should not be considered as medical advice for the treatment of a specific disease or condition. Specific health problems and Ayurvedic treatment options should be discussed with a health professional.

Recommended Ayurveda treatment methods and practices:

1. Dinacharya: Regulates daily routines and lifestyle habits.
2. Ritucharya: Recommends lifestyle and dietary changes according to the seasons.
3. Panchakarma: Detoxification and purification therapy.
4. Abyanga: A type of massage therapy applied to the whole body.
5. Swedana: Therapeutic steam bath to cleanse the body of toxins.
6. Vamana: A type of vomiting therapy for digestive disorders and ailments such as asthma.
7. Virechana: Balances and detoxifies the Pitta dosha.
8. Basti: A type of enema therapy used to balance the Vata dosha.
9. Nasya: A therapy applied to the nose for sinus problems, headaches, and migraines.
10. Raktamokshana: A therapy for the detoxification and purification of blood.

11. Shirodhara: A therapy by pouring hot oil on the forehead to reduce stress and anxiety.
12. Marma Therapy: A therapy that balances energy by applying pressure to energy points in the body.
13. Ayurvedic Diet: Individual nutritional recommendations based on the balance of dosha.
14. Ayurvedic Herbal Treatments: The use of various herbal preparations.
15. Yoga and Meditation: Used to strengthen the mind–body connection and improve overall health.
16. Pranayama: Breathing techniques are used to improve overall energy and health.
17. Ayurvedic Psychology: Guidelines for mental health and balanced living.
18. Jyotish (Vedic Astrology): A system used for personal counseling and referral.
19. Vastu Shastra: A system for thinking about the energy of the home and the environment.
20. Rasayana: A group of Ayurvedic practices that promote youth and longevity.
21. Chyawanprash: An Ayurvedic supplement that promotes overall health and strengthens immunity.
22. Triphala: An Ayurvedic supplement that improves digestion and promotes detoxification.
23. Ashwagandha: An Ayurvedic herb that reduces stress and improves overall health.
24. Turmeric: An anti-inflammatory and antioxidant herb used against many health problems.
25. Ghee: A type of butter used in Ayurveda to boost overall health and the digestive system.
26. Tongue Scraping: A practice for detoxification and overall oral health.
27. Oil Pulling: A practice that improves overall oral health.
28. Ayurvedic Self-Massage: An app to promote overall health and balanced body energy.
29. Aromatherapy: The use of blends made from plant and flower oils to improve mood and overall health.
30. Ayurvedic Sleep Routines: Recommendations for balancing overall health and energy.

Ayurveda is considered one of the oldest health systems in the world, and its history dates back to 5000 BC. Ayurveda has its roots in the Vedic culture of Ancient India. This science has become quite popular in a short period of time and has been recognized as a comprehensive and systematic method of addressing health-related issues [101].

The basic principles and practices of Ayurveda are recorded in detail in the two basic texts, Charaka Samhita and Sushruta Samhita. These texts were written between 1500 BC and 500 AD. Both texts contain comprehensive information about the theories, principles, and practices of Ayurvedic medicine. Charaka Samhita focuses on internal medicine, while Sushruta Samhita is a text that describes surgical procedures and surgical instruments.

After some time, Ayurveda was adopted by scholars in Persia, Arabia, and later in Europe. During this period, the treatment methods and principles of Ayurveda were used in many medical texts and medical education.

However, from the 16th century onward, the influence of Ayurveda in India began to decline. This coincided with British colonization and the introduction of Western medical practices into India. During this period, the practices and training of Ayurveda were largely ignored [100].

By the 20th century, Ayurveda experienced a revival in India and around the world. Today, Ayurveda is considered a traditional and complementary medicine and is used by many people around the world. In addition, efforts are underway to integrate it with modern medicine.

Nowadays, Ayurveda has been accepted and practiced by many people around the world. The limitation of Western medicine in offering a unique and holistic view of the individual has led many people to traditional and holistic health systems such as Ayurveda.

Ayurveda offers a way to maintain a healthy and balanced lifestyle, at a time when life is accelerating, and stress is increasing in the modern world. This usually includes recommendations such as a balanced diet, regular exercise, adequate sleep, stress management, and personal spiritual practices. This holistic approach gives people more control over their overall health and well-being and gives them the tools they need to maintain and improve their health.

However, the current practices of Ayurveda need to be supported by scientific research and evidence. In recent years, a number of scientific studies have been conducted on the effectiveness of some practices of Ayurveda. For example, some studies have shown that some herbal remedies of Ayurveda are effective in treating various diseases [99]. However, much of this research is still a precursor. More comprehensive, well-designed clinical trials are needed.

In particular, the holistic and individualized approach of Ayurveda is thought to complement modern medicine's tendency to take into account genetic and biochemical differences between individuals. It is increasingly recognized that genetic, lifestyle, and environmental factors have a significant impact on the occurrence and development of diseases, which supports the individualized and holistic approach of Ayurveda.

However, in order for Ayurveda to reach its full potential in the modern world, it must be ensured that its safe and effective practices are ensured, supported by scientific research, and appropriate standards of training and certification are established. This will ensure wider acceptance of Ayurveda and help people enjoy the potential benefits that this traditional healthcare system provides.

3.6 TRADITIONAL CHINESE MEDICINE (TCM)

Traditional Chinese Medicine (TCM) represents a view of health that dates back thousands of years and includes the dynamic relationships between nature, the human body, and the universe. TCM deals with the human body as a whole and tries to treat imbalances that occur in the body rather than focusing on the symptoms of a particular disease [102].

The basic principles of TCM are Yin and Yang, Qi (life energy), the five elements theory, and the Zang-Fu organ theory, which are used in the diagnosis and treatment of diseases. TCM includes a variety of treatment methods, such as herbal remedies, acupuncture, Qigong, Tai Chi, and a specific diet [103].

Today, TCM is widely used in China and other Asian countries and is increasingly accepted as an alternative and complementary medicine in Western countries as well. The holistic and individualized approach of TCM complements the more general and standardized approach of modern medicine.

3.6.1 History of Traditional Chinese Medicine

Traditional Chinese Medicine (TCM) dates back nearly 2500 years and is one of the oldest medical systems in the world. This system of medicine has been continuously improved and refined throughout its history and is still widely practiced in modern China.

The roots of the TCM lie in ancient Chinese texts such as Shang Han Lun (Discussion of the Cold Harms) and Huang Di Nei Jing (The Inner Book of the Yellow Emperor). These texts set out the basic principles, theories, and practices of TCM and still play a central role in the education and practice of TCM even today [103, 104].

In the development of TCM, a number of herbal formulas and acupuncture techniques that emerged during various dynastic periods and were used to treat various diseases played an important role. During these periods, medical knowledge and experiences were collected, recorded, and passed on to subsequent generations [105].

In the 19th and 20th centuries, the status of TCM declined as Western medicine spread in China. However, in the middle of the 20th century, TCM began to be taught and practiced along with modern medicine, and various reforms were made to preserve and improve this medical system [106, 107].

Today, TCM is an important part of the healthcare system in China and is offered in many hospitals and clinics. In addition, it is increasingly accepted and practiced in Western countries and throughout the world [108].

It is difficult to determine a specific date of the early practices of Traditional Chinese Medicine (TCM) because this medical system dates back to the history of ancient China. However, the oldest Chinese medical text, the Huangdi Neijing (Inner Book of the Yellow Emperor), was written around 200 BC and contains the basic theories and concepts of the TCM [104].

Among the first treatments mentioned in Huangdi Neijing are acupuncture and herbal remedies used to diagnose and treat diseases. Acupuncture is a technique that stimulates certain points (acupuncture points) on the body. Most of these points are located in pathways called meridians, where energy (Qi) is thought to circulate through the body [103, 109].

Herbal remedies are also an essential component of ancient Chinese medicine. Huangdi Neijing and other ancient Chinese medicinal texts describe in detail the medicinal properties and uses of many plants. These plants are used to treat a variety of diseases and are often combined in a specific formula. These formulas are individually adjusted according to the patient's symptoms and TCM theories [105, 108].

Besides such practices, TCM also includes physical and meditative practices such as Tai Chi and Qigong. These practices aim to keep energy (Qi) in balance and keep the body and mind healthy.

3.6.2 Development of Traditional Chinese Medicine

The development of Traditional Chinese Medicine (TCM) reflects the interaction of different periods, cultures, and philosophical considerations over thousands of years. Throughout this development process, TCM has developed various concepts and theories to understand and explain the relationships between the universe, humans, and nature.

In the early stages, TCM developed a range of treatment modalities that included acupuncture, herbal remedies, massage, and energy exercises. These methods target acupuncture points located in specific areas of the human body and are thought to regulate the flow of energy.

During the Han Dynasty (206 BC–220 AD), the TCM produced a number of important medical texts. These texts have systematically addressed the theoretical foundations and clinical applications of TCM. These texts include classics such as Huangdi Neijing (The Inner Book of the Yellow Emperor) and Shanghan Lun (Discussion of the Cold Harms) [106, 109].

During the Tang (618–907) and Song (960–1279) Dynasties, Traditional Chinese Medicine flourished greatly. Various medical schools and schools of thought emerged at this time with medical knowledge and skills being transferred, expanded, and refined [106, 109].

In the modern era, in the middle of the 20th century, TCM was taught and practiced along with modern medicine. Numerous reforms were made to preserve and improve this medical system [105].

3.6.2.1 Traditional Chinese Medicine (TCM) Practices and Methods

Today, the philosophy and practices of TCM are widely accepted in China and around the world. They are recognized as an effective complementary therapy in the treatment of many diseases [108].

Below is a list of 50 examples of the practices and methods of Traditional Chinese Medicine (TCM) [110–114]:

1. Acupuncture
2. Moxibustion (heat therapy)
3. Tui Na (Chinese massage)
4. Qigong (energy studies)
5. Tai Chi
6. Diet therapy
7. Herbal remedies
8. Cupping (cup therapy)
9. Guasha (skin scraping therapy)
10. Zhen Jiu (combination of acupuncture and moxibustion)

11. Maintaining and restoring balance
12. Yin and Yang balance
13. The theory of the five elements
14. Balance of Qi, blood, and fluids
15. The balance of organ systems (Zang-Fu theory)
16. Tongue and pulse reading for the diagnosis of diseases
17. Meridians and energy pathways
18. Seasonal health practices
19. Sleep regulation
20. Balancing emotions
21. Digestive health
22. Excretory and detoxification
23. Sexual health
24. Women's health (including menstruation and menopause)
25. Children's health
26. Management of aging
27. Respiratory health
28. Dermatological health
29. Mental and emotional health
30. Health of the musculoskeletal system
31. Neurological health
32. Immune health
33. Metabolic health
34. Cardiovascular health
35. Endocrine health
36. Urological health
37. Eye health
38. Otolaryngological (ENT) health
39. Oral and dental health
40. Orthopedic health
41. Oncological health
42. Pain management
43. Rehabilitation
44. Recovery after surgery
45. Stress management
46. Management of chronic diseases
47. Management of acute diseases
48. Management of allergies
49. Management of sleep disorders
50. Management of dependencies

3.6.2.2 *Traditional Chinese Medicine (TCM) Practices and Methods: Brief Descriptions*

The practices and methods of Traditional Chinese Medicine (TCM) are wide and diversified. Each of them is complex in itself and requires detailed examination. However, a general summary of each method is included below. Full scientific descriptions for each item can be found in hundreds of pages of text by scientists researching the TCM.

1. Acupuncture: A practice used to balance and treat the flow of energy by placing thin needles at certain points on the body [112].
2. Moxibustion: The application of heat to acupuncture points, usually done by burning a plant known as *Artemisia Vulgaris* (mugwort) [115].

3. Tui Na: A form of treatment in which manual manipulation and massage techniques are used on the body [116].
4. Qigong: A set of practices that combine breathing, movement, and meditation, aiming to keep energy (Qi) in balance and body and mind healthy [117].
5. Tai Chi: A form of exercise that combines slow, thoughtful movements, breathing, and meditation aims to improve body-mind health [118].
6. Diet therapy: Aims to balance and improve health by using the energetic properties of foods [119].
7. Herbal remedies: Formulas prepared using natural plants and minerals are used to treat various diseases [113].
8. Cupping (cup therapy): Aims to increase blood circulation and relax the muscles with the vacuum effect created by placing a cup in the body and removing the air in it [120].
9. Gua Sha (skin scraping therapy): The practice by which scraping is done on the skin with an instrument to reduce muscle tension and improve blood circulation [121].
10. Zhen Jiu (combination of acupuncture and moxibustion): A form of treatment in which acupuncture and moxibustion methods are used together [122].
11. Management of dependencies: TCM's various tools can help manage dependencies. In particular, acupuncture has been used in the treatment of nicotine and other drug addictions [123].

The relationship between modern medicine and Traditional Chinese Medicine (TCM) has been one of both cooperation and tension. Both practices have their own unique perspectives, practices, and health perspectives, and so they sometimes contradict each other.

Modern medicine is usually aimed at treating a specific symptom or sign of a particular disease. It also focuses on medical tests and evidence-based practices. On the other hand, TCM aims to improve the body's overall health and energy balance. It focuses on improving the overall health of the person, not the symptoms of the disease.

In recent years, there have been many modern medical practitioners who have recognized the importance of alternative medicine, especially in the treatment and prevention of chronic diseases. This has led to some practices of GCT, particularly acupuncture, being accepted as part of modern medicine. Many hospitals and clinics offer integrated medical programs that combine traditional medical practice with modern medical practice.

Nonetheless, contradictions between these two practices still exist. Some modern medical practitioners argue that TCM is not evidence-based and therefore not scientific. Furthermore, research on the efficacy and safety of TCM can be conflicting, and some modern medical practitioners may be skeptical of the use of TCM.

However, many researchers and practitioners are calling for greater collaboration and dialogue between these two medical systems. Combining the two medical systems could provide a more comprehensive and effective treatment for patients, and therefore further research and dialogue in this area is important [124].

REFERENCES

1. M. Ekor, "The Growing Use of Herbal Medicines: Issues Relating to Adverse Reactions and Challenges in Monitoring Safet," *Frontiers in Pharmacology*, vol. 4, p. 177, 2014. doi: 10.3389/fphar.2013.00177.
2. J. O. Hill, "Can a Small-Changes Approach Help Address the Obesity Epidemic? A Report of the Joint Task Force of the American Society for Nutrition, Institute of Food Technologists, and International Food Information Council," *American Journal of Clinical Nutrition*, vol. 89, no. 2, pp. 477–484, 2009.
3. J. Pizzorno and M. Murray, Textbook of Natural Medicine, Churchill Livingstone, 2012.
4. A. J. Vickers, E. A. Vertosick, G. Lewith, H. MacPherson, N. Foster, K. J. Sherman, D. Irnich, C. M. Witt and K. Linde, "Acupuncture for Chronic Pain: Update of an Individual Patient Data Meta-Analysis," *The Journal of Pain*, vol. 19, no. 5, pp. 455–474, 2018.

5. National Center for Complementary and Integrative Health, "Mind and Body Practices," NCCIH Clearinghouse, September 2017. [Online]. Available: https://www.nccih.nih.gov/health/mind-and-body-practices. [Accessed May 2023].

6. F. Capasso, T. S. Gaginella, G. Grandolini and A. A. Izzo, Phytotherapy: A Quick Reference to Herbal Medicine, Springer, 2003.

7. M. Heinrich, J. Barnes, J. Prieto-Garcia, S. Gibbons and E. M. Williamson, Fundamentals of Pharmacognosy and Phytotherapy, Elsevier, 2017.

8. M. Leonti, "The Future Is Written: Impact of Scripts on the Cognition, Selection, Knowledge and Transmission of Medicinal Plant Use and Its Implications for Ethnobotany and Ethnopharmacology. Journal of Ethnopharmacology," *Journal of Ethnopharmacology*, vol. 134, no. 3, pp. 542–555, 2011.

9. M. Heinrich and A. K. Jäger, Ethnopharmacology, Wiley-Blackwell, 2015.

10. L. M. V. Totelin, Hippocratic Recipes: Oral and Written Transmission of Pharmacological Knowledge in Fifth and Fourth Century Greece, ProQuest, 2013.

11. S. Mahdizadeh, M. K. Ghadiri and A. Gorji, "Avicenna's Canon of Medicine: A Review of Analgesics and Anti-Inflammatory Substances," *Avicenna Journal Of Phytomedicine*, vol. 5, no. 3, pp. 182–202, 2015.

12. W. Boericke, Pocket Manual of Homoeopathic Materia Medica, digitallibraryindia, 1901.

13. E. Hsu, "Reflections on the 'Discovery' of the Antimalarial Qinghao," *British Journal of Clinical Pharmacology*, vol. 61, no. 6, pp. 666–70, 2006.

14. R. Arya, "The Role of Medicinal Plants in Development of Modern Medicine," April 2016. [Online]. Available: http://dx.doi.org/10.13140/RG.2.1.4210.4727.

15. E. Ernst, "The Role of Complementary and Alternative Medicine," *BMJ*, vol. 321, no. 7269, pp. 1133–1135, 2000. doi: 10.1136/bmj.321.7269.1133.

16. J. Sarris and J. Wardle, Clinical Naturopathy: An Evidence-Based Guide to Practice, Churchill Livingstone, 2010.

17. J. Vane and R. Botting, "The Mechanism of Action of Aspirin," *Thrombosis Research*, vol. 110, no. 5-6, pp. 255–258, 2003.

18. R. Maenthaisong, N. Chaiyakunapruk, S. Niruntraporn and C. Kongkaew, "The Efficacy of Aloe Vera Used for Burn Wound Healing: A Systematic Review," *Burns*, vol. 33, no. 6, pp. 13–18, 2007.

19. C. D. Black, M. P. Herring, D. J. Hurley and P. J. O'Connor, "Ginger (Zingiber officinale) Reduces Muscle Pain Caused by Eccentric Exercise," *The Journal of Pain*, vol. 11, no. 9, pp. 894–903, 2010.

20. P. H. Koulivand, M. K. Ghadiri and A. Gorji, "Lavender and the nervous system," Evidence-Based Complementary and Alternative Medicine, vol. 2013, p. 681304, 2013. doi: 10.1155/2013/681304.

21. K. Linde, M. Berner and L. Kriston, "St John's Wort for Major Depression," Cochrane Database of Systematic Reviews, vol. 2008, no. 4, p. CD000448, 2008. doi: 10.1002/14651858.CD000448.pub3.

22. M. Sienkiewicz, M. Łysakowska, J. Ciećwierz, P. Denys and E. Kowalczyk, "The Antimicrobial Activity of Thyme Essential Oil Against Multidrug Resistant Clinical Bacterial Strains," *Microbial Drug Resistance*, vol. 18, no. 2, pp. 137–148, 2012.

23. A. Khan, H. Chen, M. Tania and D. Zhang, "Anticancer Activities of Nigella sativa (Black Cumin)," *African Journal of Traditional, Complementary and Alternative Medicines*, vol. 8, no. 5S, pp. 226–232, 2011.

24. M. Mahboubi, "Sambucus nigra (Black Elder) as Alternative Treatment for Cold and Flu," *Advances in Traditional Medicine (ADTM)*, vol. 21, pp. 405–414, 2021.

25. H. Shehata, "Chapter 12: Drugs and Drug Therapy," in Basic Science in Obstetrics and Gynaecology, 4th Edition, edited by Phillip Bennett and Catherine Williamson, Churchill Livingstone, 2010, pp. 259–277. https://doi.org/10.1016/B978-0-443-10281-3.00016-6.

26. S. B. Badgujar, V. V. Patel and A. H. Bandivdekar, "Foeniculum vulgare Mill: A Review of Its Botany, Phytochemistry, Pharmacology, Contemporary Application, and Toxicology," *BioMed Research International*, vol. 2014, p. 842674, 2014. doi: 10.1155/2014/842674.

27. W. M. Hascheck-Hock, C. G. Rousseaux, M. A. Wallig and B. Bolon, Haschek and Rousseaux' s Handbook of Toxicologic Pathology, Volume 3, Academic Press, 2023, pp. 183–303.

28. A. Alizadeh, M. Moshiri, J. Alizadeh and M. Balali-Mood, "Black Henbane and Its Toxicity – A Descriptive Review," *Avicenna Journal of Phytomedicine*, vol. 4, no. 5, pp. 297–311, 2014.

29. K. L. Brown and J. Pollak, Herbal Teas for Lifelong Health, Storey Publishing, 1999.

30. J. K. Srivastava, E. Shankar and S. Gupta, "Chamomile: A Herbal Medicine of the Past With a Bright Future (Review)," *Molecular Medicine Reports*, vol. 3, no. 6, pp. 895–901, 2010.

31. M. Karsch-Völk, B. Barrett, D. Kiefer, R. Bauer and K. L. K. Ardjomand-Woelkart, "Echinacea for Preventing and Treating the Common Cold," *Cochrane Database of Systematic Reviews*, vol. 2014, no. 2, p. CD000530, 2014. doi: 10.1002/14651858.CD000530.pub3.

32. Anonymous, Giant Book Of Herbal Tea Remedies, qasim idrees 2013.

33. J. Choi, J. Lee, K. Kim, H.-K. Choi, S.-A. Lee and H.-J. Lee, "Effects of Ginger Intake on Chemotherapy-Induced Nausea and Vomiting: A Systematic Review of Randomized Clinical Trials," *Nutrients*, vol. 14, no. 23, 2022.

34. J. Stanisiere, P.-Y. Mousset and S. Lafay, "ow Safe Is Ginger Rhizome for Decreasing Nausea and Vomiting in Women During Early Pregnancy?" *Foods (Basel, Switzerland)*, vol. 7, no. 4, p. 50, 2018.

35. B. Field and R. Vadnal, "Ginkgo biloba and Memory: An Overview," *Nutritional Neuroscience*, vol. 1, no. 4, pp. 255–267, 1998.

36. J. Reay, D. Kennedy and A. Scholey, "Single Doses of Panax Ginseng (G115) Reduce Blood Glucose Levels and Improve Cognitive Performance During Sustained Mental Activity," *Journal of Psychopharmacology (Oxford, England)*, vol. 19, no. 4, pp. 357–365, 2005.

37. A. G. Dulloo, C. Duret, D. Rohrer, L. Girardier, N. Mensi, M. Fathi, P. Chantre and J. Vandermander, "Efficacy of a Green Tea Extract Rich in Catechin Polyphenols and Caffeine in Increasing 24-h Energy Expenditure and Fat Oxidation in Humans," *The American Journal of Clinical Nutrition*, vol. 70, no. 6, pp. 1040–1045, 1999.

38. H. Mozaffari-Khosravi, B. Jalali-Khanabadi, M. Afkhami-Ardekani, F. Fatehi and M. Noori-Shadkam, "The Effects of Sour Tea (Hibiscus Sabdariffa) on Hypertension in Patients With Type II Diabetes," *Journal of Human Hypertension*, vol. 23, no. 1, pp. 48–54, 2009.

39. M. M. Marcin, The Complete Book of Herbal Teas, HarperCollins Publishers, 1984.

40. D. O. Kennedy, W. Little and A. B. Scholey, " Attenuation of Laboratory-Induced Stress in Humans after Acute Administration of Melissa officinalis (Lemon Balm)," *Psychosomatic Medicine*, vol. 66, no. 4, pp. 607–613, 2004.

41. P. V. Deeksheetha, S. Gheena, R. Pratibha, S. Rajeshkumar and R. Karthikeyan, "In Vitro Evaluation of Antioxidant and Anti-Inflammatory Potentials of Herbal Formulation Containing Marigold Flower (*Calendula officinalis* L.) Tea," *Cureus*, vol. 15, no. 8, p. e43308, 2023. doi: 10.7759/cureus.43308.

42. H. İlyasoğlu and T. E. Arpa, "Effect of Brewing Conditions on Antioxidant Properties of Rosehip Tea Beverage: Study by Response Surface Methodology," *Journal of Food Science and Technology*, vol. 54, no. 11, pp. 3737–3743, 2017.

43. S. Behradmanesh, F. Derees and M. Rafieian-Kopaei, "Effect of Salvia Officinalis on Diabetic Patients," *Journal of Renal Injury Prevention*, vol. 2, no. 2, pp. 51–54, 2013.

44. B. C. Nzeako, Z. S. Al-Kharousi and Z. Al-Mahrooqui, "Antimicrobial Activities of Clove and Thyme Extracts," *Sultan Qaboos University Medical Journal*, vol. 6, no. 1, pp. 33–39, 2006.

45. T. R. Dias, G. Tomás, N. F. Teixeira, M. G. Alves, P. F. Oliveira and B. M. Silva, "White Tea (*Camellia Sinensis* (L.)): Antioxidant Properties And Beneficial Health Effects," *International Journal of Food Science, Nutrition and Dietetics (IJFS)*, vol. 2, no. 2, pp. 19–26, 2013.

46. D. O. Kennedy and E. L. Wightman, "Herbal Extracts and Phytochemicals: Plant Secondary Metabolites and the Enhancement of Human Brain Function," *Advances in Nutrition*, vol. 2, no. 1, pp. 32–50, 2011.

47. W. Kalt, A. Cassidy, LR. Howard, R. Krikorian, AJ. Stull, F. Tremblay and R. Zamora-Ros, "Recent Research on the Health Benefits of Blueberries and Their Anthocyanins," *Advances in Nutrition*, vol. 11, no. 2, pp. 224–236, 2020.

48. E. Devaraj, "Hepatoprotective Properties of Dandelion: Recent Update," *Journal of Applied Pharmaceutical Science*, vol. 6, no. 4, pp. 202–205, 2016.

49. S. A. Shah, S. Sander, C. M. White, M. Rinaldi and C. I. Coleman, "Evaluation of Echinacea for the Prevention and Treatment of the Common Cold: A Meta-Analysis," *The Lancet. Infectious Diseases*, vol. 7, no. 7, pp. 473–480, 2007.

50. K. Ried, O. R. Frank and N. P. Stocks, "Aged Garlic Extract Lowers Blood Pressure in Patients With Treated but Uncontrolled Hypertension: A Randomised Controlled Trial," *Maturitas*, vol. 67, no. 2, pp. 144–150, 2010.

51. D. Dragos, M. Gilca, L. Gaman, A. Vlad, L. Iosif, I. Stoian and O. Lupescu, "Phytomedicine in Joint Disorders," *Nutrients*, vol. 9, no. 1, 2017.

52. WebMD LLC, "Milk Thistle – Uses, Side Effects, and More," [Online]. Available: https://www.webmd.com/vitamins/ai/ingredientmono-138/milk-thistle. [Accessed 1 August 2023].

53. H. Ullah, A. De Filippis, A. Baldi, M. Dacrema, C. Esposito, E. U. Garzarella, C. Santarcangelo, A. Tantipongpiradet and M. Daglia, "Beneficial Effects of Plant Extracts and Bioactive Food Components in Childhood Supplementation," *Nutrients*, vol. 13, no. 9, 2021.

54. P. Shenefelt, "Herbal Treatment for Dermatologic Disorders," in Herbal Medicine: Biomolecular and Clinical Aspects, 2nd edition, edited by IFF. Benzie and S. Wachtel-Galor, Boca Raton (FL), CRC Press/Taylor & Francis, 2011.

55. M. H. Radha and N. P. Laxmipriya, "Evaluation of Biological Properties and Clinical Effectiveness of *Aloe vera*: A Systematic Review," *Journal of Traditional and Complementary Medicine*, vol. 5, no. 1, pp. 21–26, 2014.

56. P. Kriplani, K. Guarve and U. Baghael, "*Arnica montana* L. – A Plant of Healing: Review," *Journal of Pharmacy and Pharmacology*, vol. 69, no. 8, pp. 925–945, 2017.

57. K. R. Preethi, "Anti-Inflammatory Activity of Flower Extract of *Calendula officinalis* Linn. and Its Possible Mechanism of Action," *Indian Journal of Experimental Biology*, vol. 47, no. 2, pp. 113–120, 2009.

58. A. G. Sah, "A Comprehensive Study of Therapeutic Applications of Chamomile," *Pharmaceuticals (Basel, Switzerland)*, vol. 15, no. 10, p. 1284, 2022.

59. S.-Y. Kang, J.-Y. Um, B.-Y. Chung, S.-Y. Lee, J.-S. Park, J.-C. Kim, C.-W. Park and H.-O. Kim, "Moisturizer in Patients With Inflammatory Skin Diseases," *Medicina*, vol. 58, no. 7, p. 888, 2022.

60. G. Dumancas, L. Viswanath, A. Leon, S. Ramasahayam, R. Maples, R. Hikkaduwa Koralege, U. Don, U. D. N. Perera, J. Langford, A. Shakir and S. Castles, "Chapter 6: Health Benefits of Virgin Coconut Oil," in Vegetable Oil: Properties, Uses and Benefits, edited by Brittany Holt, Nova Science Publishers, pp. 161–194, 2016.

61. K. Vakilian, M. Atarha, R. Bekhradi and R. Chaman, "Healing Advantages of Lavender Essential Oil During Episiotomy Recovery: A Clinical Trial," *Complementary Therapies in Clinical Practice*, vol. 17, no. 1, pp. 50–53, 2011.

62. G. K. Horváth, "Essential Oils in the Treatment of Respiratory Tract Diseases Highlighting Their Role in Bacterial Infections and Their Anti-Inflammatory Action: A Review," *Flavour and Fragrance Journal*, vol. 30, pp. 331–341, 2015.

63. T. R. S. Kurebayashi, "Chinese Phytotherapy to Reduce Stress, Anxiety and Improve Quality of Life: Randomized Controlled Trial," *Revista Da Escola De Enfermagem Da U S P*, vol. 50, no. 5, pp. 853–860, 2016.

64. National Institutes of Health, "NIH's Definition of a Clinical Trial," [Online]. Available: https://grants.nih.gov/policy/clinical-trials/definition.htm.

65. S. Kamiloglu, M. Tomas, T. Ozdal, P. Yolci-Omeroglu and E. Capanoglu, "Bioactive component analysis," in Innovative Food Analysis, edited by Charis M. Galanakis, Academic Press, 2021, pp. 41–65.

66. National Center for Complementary and Integrative Health, "Herb-Drug Interactions," [Online]. Available: https://www.nccih.nih.gov/health/providers/digest/herb-drug-interactions.

67. R. Bauer, "Quality Criteria and Standardization of Phytopharmaceuticals: Can Acceptable Drug Standards Be Achieved?" *Drug Information Journal*, vol. 32, no. 2, pp. 101–110, 1998.

68. A. A. Izzo and E. Ernst, "Interactions Between Herbal Medicines and Prescribed Drugs: An Updated Systematic Review," *Drugs*, vol. 69, no. 13, pp. 1777–1798, 2009.

69. R. Saller, R. Meier, R. Brignoli and J. Melzer, "The Use of Silymarin in the Treatment of Liver Diseases," *Drugs*, vol. 61, no. 4, pp. 2035–2063, 2001.

70. M. Karsch-Völk, B. Barrett and K. Linde, "Echinacea for Preventing and Treating the Common Cold," The Cochrane Database of Systematic Reviews, vol. 2014, no. 2, p. CD000530, 2014. doi: 10.1002/14651858.CD000530.pub3.

71. A. López, M. S. de Tangil and O. Vega-Orellana, "Valorization of *Aloe vera* (*Aloe barbadensis* Miller) Processing by-Products: A Strategy to Improve the Economics of *Aloe vera* Cultivation," *Journal of Cleaner Production*, vol. 55, pp. 1–12, 2013.

72. C. Ramassamy, F. Longpré and Y. Christen, "*Ginkgo biloba* extract (EGb 761) in Alzheimer's disease: is there any evidence?," *Current Alzheimer Research*, vol. 4, no. 3, pp. 253–262, 2007.

73. I. Vermaak, J. H. Hamman and A. M. Viljoen, "Alkaloids in the Genus Amaryllis," *Molecules*, vol. 16, no. 9, pp. 7107–7120, 2011.

74. E. Ernst, "Homeopathy: What Does the "best" Evidence Tell Us?" *Medical Journal of Australia*, vol. 192, no. 8, pp. 458–460, 2010.

75. A. Avogadro, "Testing of a Way of Determining the Relative Masses of the Elementary Molecules of Bodies, and the Proportions According to Which They Enter into These Combinations," *Journal of Physics*, vol. 73, pp. 58–76, 1811.

76. R. Mathie, S. Lloyd, L. Legg, J. Clausen, S. Moss, J. Davidson and I. Ford, "Randomised Placebo-Controlled Trials of Individualised Homeopathic Treatment: Systematic Review and Meta-Analysis," *Systematic Reviews*, vol. 3, p. 142, 2014. doi: 10.1186/2046-4053-3-142.

77. E. Ernst, "A Systematic Review of Systematic Reviews of Homeopathy," *British Journal of Clinical Pharmacology*, vol. 54, no. 6, pp. 577–582, 2002.

78. National Center for Complementary and Integrative Health (NCCIH), "Homeopathy," [Online]. Available: https://www.nccih.nih.gov/health/homeopathy. [Accessed April 2023].

79. National Health and Medical Research Council, "NHMRC Information Paper: Evidence on the effectiveness of homeopathy for treating health conditions," 2015. [Online]. Available: https://www.nhmrc.gov.au/about-us/publications/evidence-effectiveness-homeopathy-treating-health-conditions.
80. P. Cuijpers, A. van Straten, G. Andersson and P. van Oppen, "Psychotherapy for Depression in Adults: A Meta-Analysis of Comparative Outcome Studies," *Journal of Consulting and Clinical Psychology*, vol. 76, no. 6, pp. 909–922, 2008.
81. W. C. Knowler, E. Barrett-Connor, S. E. Fowler, R. F. Hamman, J. M. Lachin, E. A. Walker and D. M. Nathan, "Reduction in the Incidence of Type 2 Diabetes With Lifestyle Intervention or Metformin," *The New England Journal of Medicine*, vol. 346, no. 6, pp. 393–403, 2002.
82. M. C. Hochberg, R. D. Altman, K. T. April, M. Benkhalti, G. Guyatt, J. McGowan, T. Towheed, V. Welch, G. Wells and P. Tugwell, "American College of Rheumatology 2012 Recommendations for the Use of Nonpharmacologic and Pharmacologic Therapies in Osteoarthritis of the Hand, Hip, and Knee," *Arthritis Care & Research*, vol. 64, pp. 465–474, 2012.
83. G. Engel, "The Need for a New Medical Model: A Challenge for Biomedicine," *Science*, vol. 196, no. 4286, pp. 129–136, 1977.
84. E. Kvaavik, G. Batty, G. Ursin, R. Huxley and C. Gale, "Influence of Individual and Combined Health Behaviors on Total and Cause-Specific Mortality in Men and Women: The United Kingdom Health and Lifestyle Survey," *Archives of Internal Medicine*, vol. 170, no. 8, pp. 711–718, 2010.
85. F. B. Hu, J. E. Manson, M. J. Stampfer, G. Colditz, S. Liu, C. G. Solomon and W. C. Willett, "Diet, Lifestyle, and the Risk of Type 2 Diabetes mellitus in Women," *The New England Journal of Medicine*, vol. 345, no. 11, pp. 790–797, 2001.
86. K. Cooley, O. Szczurko, D. Perri, E. J. Mills, B. Bernhardt, Q. Zhou and D. Seely, "Naturopathic Care for Chronic Low Back Pain: A Randomized Trial," *PLoS One*, vol. 4, no. 9, p. e7310, 2019.
87. M. Armour, C. A. Smith, L. Q. Wang, D. Naidoo, G. Y. Yang, H. MacPherson, M. S. Lee and P. Hay, "Acupuncture for Depression: A Systematic Review and Meta-Analysis," *Journal of Clinical Medicine*, vol. 8, no. 8, p. 1140, 2019. doi: 10.3390/jcm8081140.
88. Z. Zhao, "Neural Mechanism Underlying Acupuncture Analgesia," *Progress in Neurobiology*, vol. 85, no. 4, pp. 355–375, 2008.
89. J. L. McDonald, A. W. Cripps and P. K. Smith, "Mediators, Receptors, and Signalling Pathways in the Anti-Inflammatory and Antihyperalgesic Effects of Acupuncture," Evidence-Based Complementary and Alternative Medicine, vol. 2015, p. 975632, 2015. doi: 10.1155/2015/975632.
90. K. Linde, G. Allais, B. Brinkhaus, Y. Fei, M. Mehring, E. A. Vertosick, A. Vickers and A. R. White, "Acupuncture for The Prevention of Episodic Migraine," The Cochrane Database of Systematic Reviews, vol. 2016, no, 6, p. CD001218, 2016. doi:10.1002/14651858.CD001218.pub3.
91. D. Amorim, J. Amado, I. Brito, S. M. Fiuza, N. Amorim, C. Costeira and J. Machado, "Acupuncture and Electroacupuncture for Anxiety Disorders: A Systematic Review of the Clinical Research," *Complementary Therapies in Clinical Practice*, vol. 31, pp. 31–37, 2018.
92. L. J. Cao, "Acupuncture for Treatment of Insomnia: A Systematic Review of Randomized Controlled Trials," *Journal of Alternative and Complementary Medicine*, vol. 15, no. 11, pp. 1171–1186, 2009.
93. M. Y. Qian, "Therapeutic Effect of Acupuncture on the Outcomes of in Vitro Fertilization: A Systematic Review and Meta-Analysis," *Archives of Gynecology and Obstetrics*, vol. 295, no. 3, pp. 543–558, 2017.
94. L. J. Cho, "Acupuncture for Obesity: A Systematic Review and Meta-Analysis," *International Journal of Obesity*, vol. 33, no. 2, pp. 183–196, 2005.
95. W. H. Chen, "Acupuncture for Type 2 Diabetes mellitus: A Systematic Review and Meta-Analysis of Randomized Controlled Trials," *Complementary Therapies in Clinical Practice*, vol. 36, pp. 100–112, 2019.
96. M. B. Taw, W. D. Reddy, F. S. Omole and M. D. Seidman, "Acupuncture and Allergic Rhinitis," *Current Opinion in Otolaryngology & Head and Neck Surgery*, vol. 23, no. 3, pp. 216–220, 2015.
97. H. I. J. Martin, "Efficacy of Acupuncture in Asthma: Systematic Review and Meta-Analysis of Published Data from 11 Randomised Controlled Trials," *The European Respiratory Journal*, vol. 20, no. 4, pp. 846–852, 2002.
98. R. Melzack and P. Wall, "Pain Mechanisms: A New Theory," *Science*, vol. 150, no. 3699, pp. 971–979, 1965.
99. V. Lad, Ayurveda: The Science of Self-Healing: A Practical Guide, Lotus Press, Benllech, 1984.
100. D. Frawley, Ayurvedic Healing, Motilal Banarsidass, Delhi, 2000.
101. M. Tiwari, Ayurveda: A Life of Balance, Healing Arts Press, Rochester, VT 1995.
102. K. Chan and A. C. Lo, "The Role of Chinese Medicine in the Treatment of Chronic Diseases in China," *Planta Medica*, vol. 68, no. 6, pp. 457–462, 2022.

103. P. U. Unschuld, Huang Di Nei Jing Su Wen: Nature, Knowledge, Imagery in an Ancient Chinese Medical Text: With an appendix: The Doctrine of the Five Periods and Six Qi in the Huang Di Nei Jing Su Wen, University of California Press, Berkeley, CA, 2003.
104. M. Ni, The Yellow Emperor's Classic of Medicine: A New Translation of the Neijing Suwen With Commentary, Shambhala Publications, Boston, MA, 1995.
105. E. Hsu, The Transmission of Chinese Medicine, Cambridge University Press, Cambridge, 1999.
106. P. U. Unschuld, Medicine in China: A History of Ideas, University of California Press, Berkeley, CA, 1985.
107. K. Taylor, Chinese Medicine in Early Communist China, 1945-1963: A Medicine of Revolution, Routledge, London, 2005.
108. V. Scheid, Chinese Medicine in Contemporary China: Plurality and Synthesis, Duke University Press, Durham, NC, 2022.
109. G. D. Lu and J. Needham, Celestial Lancets: A History and Rationale of Acupuncture and Moxa, Routledge, London, 2002.
110. T. Kaptchuk, The Web That Has No Weaver: Understanding Chinese Medicine, McGraw-Hill, New York, NY, 2000.
111. G. Maciocia, Foundations of Chinese Medicine: A Comprehensive Text, Elsevier Health Sciences, Edinburgh, 2005.
112. P. Deadman and M. Al-Khafaji, A Manual of Acupuncture, Journal of Chinese Medicine Publications, Vista, CA, 2007.
113. J. K. Chen and T. T. Chen, Chinese Herbal Formulas and Applications, Art of Medicine Press, City of Industry, CA, 2009.
114. B. Flaws, The Treatment of Modern Western Medical Diseases With Chinese Medicine, Blue Poppy Press, Boulder, CO, 2002.
115. M. Coyle, J. L. Shergis, E. T. Huang, X. Guo, Y. M. Di, A. Zhang and C. C. Xue, "Acupuncture Therapies for Chronic Obstructive Pulmonary Disease: A Systematic Review of Randomized, Controlled Trials," *Alternative Therapies in Health and Medicine*, vol. 20, no. 6, pp. 10–23, 2017.
116. I. Z. Chirali, Traditional Chinese Medicine Cupping Therapy, Churchill Livingstone, London, 1999.
117. R. Jahnke, L. Larkey, C. Rogers, J. Etnier and F. Lin, "A Comprehensive Review of Health Benefits of Qigong and Tai Chi," *American Journal of Health Promotion*, vol. 24, no. 6, pp. 1–25, 2010.
118. C. Wang, J. P. Collet and J. Lau, "The Effect of Tai Chi on Health Outcomes in Patients With Chronic Conditions: A Systematic Review," *Archives of Internal Medicine*, vol. 164, no. 5, pp. 493–501, 2004.
119. M. Ni and C. McNease, The Tao of Nutrition, Sevenstar Communications, Ashland, OH, 2009.
120. H. Cao, X. Li and J. Liu, "An Updated Review of the Efficacy of Cupping Therapy," *PLoS One*, vol. 7, no. 2, p. e31793, 2012. doi: 10.1371/journal.pone.0031793.
121. A. Nielsen, N. T. M. Knoblauch, G. J. Dobos, A. Michalsen and T. J. Kaptchuk, "The Effect of Gua Sha Treatment on the Microcirculation of Surface Tissue: A Pilot Study in Healthy Subjects," *Explore*, vol. 3, no. 5, pp. 456–466, 2007.
122. Y. Xiang, X. Wu, J. Lu and X. Hu, "A Comparison of the Ancient Use of Ginseng in Traditional Chinese Medicine With Modern Pharmacological Experiments and Clinical Trials," *Phytotherapy Research*, vol. 32, no. 7, pp. 1235–1245, 2019.
123. J. Tan, A. Molassiotis, T. Wang and L. Suen, "Adverse Events of Auricular Therapy: A Systematic Review," *Evidence-Based Complementary and Alternative Medicine*, vol. 2014, p. 06758, 2014. doi:10.1155/2014/506758
124. T. Hesketh and W. Zhu, "Traditional Chinese Medicine: One Country, Two Systems," *Health in China*, vol. 315, no. 7100, pp. 115–117, 1997.

4 Applied Healthy Living Strategies

This chapter focuses on practical and feasible strategies to support maintaining a healthy lifestyle. Overall health and well-being are often based on basic lifestyle factors such as nutrition, physical activity, stress management, and sleep.

4.1 BALANCING NUTRITION

Nutrition is one of the most important parts of life. Eating a healthy and balanced diet is the key to maintaining optimal energy levels and preventing many diseases. Therefore, the emphasis should be on how to create a balanced diet, which foods are most beneficial for the body, and the best practices in achieving overall nutritional goals.

Nutrition is a lifestyle factor that has a significant impact on our overall health and well-being. Scientific research shows that a balanced and healthy diet plays an important role in the prevention of chronic diseases such as heart disease, diabetes, and some types of cancer [1, 2].

A balanced diet contains all the essential nutrients that function in the body. This includes carbohydrates, proteins, fats, vitamins, minerals, and water [3]. Carbohydrates are the main nutrients used to provide energy. Proteins and fats are involved in the body's growth and repair processes. Vitamins and minerals are important in various metabolic processes, and water ensures the proper functioning of body functions [4].

Having a "balanced" diet means that a person gets all these nutrients in the right proportions. The Academy of Nutrition and Dietetics states that a healthy diet should include a variety of foods. This includes nutrients from different food groups, fruits, vegetables, whole grains, protein sources, and dairy products [5].

A balanced diet requires carefully balancing energy intake and energy consumption to meet energy needs and prevent conditions such as under or overeating [6]. A number of factors, including physical activity level, age, gender, and overall health status, affect energy needs [7].

4.2 REGULAR PHYSICAL ACTIVITY

An active lifestyle is an important part of health and quality of life. Physical activity positively affects many aspects, from heart health to mental health, from energy levels to sleep quality. This section will focus on what types of activities are beneficial, how much exercise should be done, and the effects of exercise on overall health.

Physical activity has a significant impact on overall health and quality of life. Scientific research has shown that regular physical activity can improve both physical and mental health and reduce the risk of chronic diseases such as heart disease, diabetes, and some types of cancer [8].

Physical activity increases energy use, which can have a positive effect on weight management and body composition [9]. In addition, regular exercise strengthens the cardiovascular system, improves bone health, increases muscle strength and flexibility, and improves overall quality of life.

How much and what type of physical activity a person should do depends on his age, gender, general state of health, and personal goals. However, the World Health Organization (WHO) recommends that adults do at least 150 minutes of moderate-intensity aerobic activity per week or 75 minutes of intense aerobic activity. It is also recommended to include muscle-strengthening exercises two or more days a week [10].

DOI: 10.1201/9781003520252-5

Physical activity can be done in a variety of ways that can be integrated into a person's overall lifestyle. This may include activities such as sports, exercise, games, dancing, gardening, housework, or active transportation [9]. The important thing is to do physical activity on a regular basis and choose activities that are usually enjoyed.

4.3 STRESS MANAGEMENT

Stress is an inevitable part of modern life and can have a significant impact on health. Long-term or chronic stress can lead to a number of health problems, including heart disease, hypertension, diabetes, obesity, and psychiatric disorders [11, 12].

Stress management strategies can help reduce stress levels, deal with stress more effectively, and improve overall quality of life. From stress management techniques to meditation and deep breathing techniques, strategies on how to use activities such as yoga and tai chi will be presented [11].

Scientific research has shown that managing and reducing stress can play an important role in preventing these health issues and improving overall health and quality of life. Stress management often involves a number of strategies, including lifestyle changes, physical activity, relaxation techniques, improving mental and emotional skills, and social support [13].

Physical activity plays an important role in managing stress. Exercise promotes the release of chemicals naturally produced in the body to cope with stress and generally produces positive results, such as better mood and better sleep [14]. Good sleep at night is also vital for stress management. Lack of sleep can make stressful situations worse and make us less resilient to the negative effects of stressful situations [15].

Relaxation techniques such as meditation, yoga, and deep breathing can also be effective in reducing stress. These techniques often help reduce the physical symptoms associated with stress and encourage achieving a calmer and relaxed state of mind.

4.4 APPROPRIATE SLEEP HABITS

Sleep is very important for overall health and well-being. Adequate and quality sleep is important for learning, memory, emotional control, immune function, and maintaining overall health [16, 17].

Lack of sleep can have negative effects in many areas, from energy levels to mood and concentration. It is important to prioritize sleep hygiene. It is also important to be familiar with the importance of regular sleep patterns and strategies that can help improve sleep quality.

Lack of sleep, or disorder, is associated with many chronic health problems, including obesity, diabetes, cardiovascular disease, and depression [18, 19]. Lack of sleep can also lead to a decline in concentration, memory, and work performance and even lead to accidents and injuries [20].

Scientific research has shown that regular sleep habits, or sleep hygiene, are effective in promoting adequate and quality sleep [21]. Elements of sleep hygiene include setting a fixed wake-up time, using the bedroom only for sleeping and sexual activity, avoiding excessive consumption of caffeine, nicotine, and alcohol, and establishing a relaxing routine before going to sleep [22].

In conclusion, proper sleep habits are an important strategy for improving overall health and quality of life.

4.5 SOCIAL RELATIONS

Social connections and relationships are important for overall quality of life and health. A good social support network can help manage stress, increase life satisfaction, and improve overall health. In this section, strategies on how to establish and maintain healthy social relationships will be presented.

Social relationships have a significant impact on people's happiness, health, and quality of life. Social connections and support can make it easier to cope with stress, improve psychological well-being, and even extend life expectancy [23–25].

Social isolation and loneliness have been linked to depression, anxiety, and other mental disorders [26]. Also, a lack of social support can have a negative impact on physical health and disease outcomes [27].

Social relationships involve positive and supportive interactions between people. Family, friends, co-workers, and other social groups can form and strengthen bonds between people. Social support can be helpful in coping with stressful situations, sharing problems, and overcoming challenges [28].

A lack of social interaction can have a negative impact on health and happiness. So, developing and maintaining social relationships can help improve overall health and quality of life.

4.6 DETOXIFICATION AND CLEANSING

Detoxification is a process that helps remove toxins from the body. The human body usually carries out this process naturally. Organs such as the kidneys, liver, and sweat glands constantly filter and eliminate waste materials and toxins. However, a combination of environmental factors, unhealthy diets, and lifestyle habits can increase toxin load and interfere with the normal functions of these organs [29].

Detoxification practices often involve lifestyle changes such as nutrition, hydration, exercise, sleep, and stress management. Detox diets often restrict processed foods, additives, refined sugars, and saturated fats. It instead emphasizes whole foods, fresh vegetables and fruits, whole grains, high-quality proteins, and healthy fats [30]. Good hydration also increases toxin excretion from the body, while exercise promotes the elimination of waste materials through sweat [31].

It has also been suggested that detoxification can be achieved by supporting a healthy gut microbiota. A diet enriched with probiotics and prebiotics can improve the gut microbiota, helping the gut increase toxin excretion [32].

However, more scientific evidence is needed on the possible effects of detoxification and cleansing on health. Although anecdotal evidence and some preliminary studies suggest that detoxification diets and lifestyle changes can improve health, more and more comprehensive research is needed to support these results [30].

Examples of detoxification and cleansing include predominantly natural, scientifically supported body functions and certain dietary and lifestyle practices. Here are some of them:

1. Water Consumption: Adequate water consumption helps eliminate toxins in the body [33].
2. Proper Nutrition: Eating a healthy, balanced diet supports the elimination of toxins from the body [34].
3. Exercise: Regular physical activity promotes toxin excretion through sweat [35].
4. Sleep: Adequate sleep supports the body's process of removing toxins [36].
5. Probiotics: Probiotics can increase toxin excretion and support gut health [37].
6. Alcohol Restriction: Limiting or completely abandoning alcohol consumption improves the detoxification functions of the liver [38].
7. Smoking Cessation: Quitting smoking reduces the toxin load on the body and improves overall health [39].
8. Organic Foods: Consuming organic foods reduces the intake of pesticides and other chemicals [40].
9. Antioxidants: Consuming foods that contain antioxidants strengthens the body's defenses against toxins [41].
10. Fiber Foods: Consuming foods high in fiber helps the intestines eliminate toxins [42].
11. Green Tea: Green tea is often recommended because of its antioxidants and other detoxification-promoting ingredients [43].
12. Detox Foot Baths: Although these baths are claimed to be effective in removing toxins, more scientific evidence is needed in this regard [44].
13. Aromatherapy: Some essential oils are thought to promote detoxification, but more research is needed on this topic [45].

14. Stress Management: Chronic stress can increase toxin load, so stress management is important [46].
15. Healing Herbs: Certain herbs may promote detoxification, especially in the liver and kidneys [47].
16. Special Detox Diets: Some diets are designed to *cleanse* the body, but more research is needed on the effectiveness and safety of these diets [30].
17. Sauna: Sauna use is thought to be effective in removing toxins, but more research is needed on this topic [48].
18. Meditation: Meditation can reduce stress, which in turn can indirectly support the detoxification process [49].
19. Homeopathy and Naturopathy: Although homeopathic and naturopathic remedies are claimed to be effective in removing toxins, more scientific evidence is needed in this regard [50].
20. Water fasting: Water fasting is thought to cleanse the body of toxins, but more research is needed on this topic. This practice often requires medical supervision [51].

While each sample represents potential ways to detoxify or cleanse, some are scientifically supported, and some are still controversial. It is always important to speak with healthcare professionals before making any health-related changes.

REFERENCES

1. W. C. Willett and M. J. Stampfer, "Rebuilding the Food Pyramid," *Scientific American*, vol. 288, no. 1, pp. 64–71, 2003.
2. F. B. Hu, "Dietary Pattern Analysis: A New Direction in Nutritional Epidemiology," *Current Opinion in Lipidology*, vol. 13, no. 1, pp. 3–9, 2002.
3. World Health Organization, Diet, Nutrition, and the Prevention of Chronic Diseases: Report of a Joint WHO/FAO Expert Consultation, World Health Organization, 2003.
4. S. S. Gropper, J. L. Smith and J. L. Groff, Advanced Nutrition and Human Metabolism, Cengage Learning, 2008.
5. Academy of Nutrition and Dietetics, Healthy Eating for a Healthy Weight, Academy of Nutrition and Dietetics, 2018. [Online]. Available: https://www.eatright.org/health/wellness/weight-and-body-positivity/back-to-basics-for-healthy-weight-loss.
6. K. D. Hall, S. B. Heymsfield, J. W. Kemnitz, S. Klein, D. A. Schoeller and J. R. Speakman, "Energy Balance and Its Components: Implications for Body Weight Regulation," *The American Journal of Clinical Nutrition*, vol. 95, no. 4, pp. 989–994, 2012.
7. World Health Organization, Healthy Diet, World Health Organization, 2021. [Online]. Available: https://www.who.int/news-room/fact-sheets/detail/healthy-diet.
8. I. M. Lee, E. J. Shiroma, F. Lobelo, P. Puska, S. N. Blair, P. T. Katzmarzyk and Lancet Physical Activity Series Working Group, "Effect of Physical Inactivity on Major non-Communicable Diseases Worldwide: An Analysis of Burden of Disease and Life Expectancy," *The Lancet*, vol. 380, no. 9838, pp. 219–229, 2012.
9. D. E. Warburton, C. W. Nicol and S. S. Bredin. "Health Benefits of Physical Activity: The Evidence," *Canadian Medical Association Journal*, vol. 174, no. 6, pp. 801–809, 2006.
10. World Health Organization, WHO Guidelines on Physical Activity and Sedentary Behaviour, World Health Organization, 2020.
11. S. Cohen, D. Janicki-Deverts and G. E. Miller. "Psychological Stress and Disease," *JAMA*, vol. 298, no. 14, pp. 1685–1687, 2007.
12. B. S. McEwen, "Central Effects of Stress Hormones in Health and Disease: Understanding the Protective and Damaging Effects of Stress and Stress Mediators," *European Journal of Pharmacology*, vol. 583, no. 2-3, pp. 174–185, 2008.
13. S. Cohen, T. Kamarck and R. Mermelstein, "A Global Measure of Perceived Stress," *Journal of Health and Social Behavior*, vol. 24, no. 4, pp. 385–396, 1983.
14. P. Salmon, "Effects of Physical Exercise on Anxiety, Depression, and Sensitivity to Stress: A Unifying Theory," *Clinical Psychology Review*, vol. 21, no. 1, pp. 33–61, 2001.

15. E. J. Kim and J. E. Dimsdale, "The Effect of Psychosocial Stress on Sleep: A Review of Polysomnographic Evidence," *Behavioral Sleep Medicine*, vol. 5, no. 4, pp. 256–278, 2007. doi: 10.1080/15402000701557383

16. M. P. Walker and R. Stickgold, "Sleep, Memory, and Plasticity," *Annual Review of Psychology*, vol. 57, pp. 139–166, 2006.

17. L. Besedovsky, T. Lange and J. Born, "Sleep and Immune Function," *Pflügers Archiv-European Journal of Physiology*, vol. 463, no. 1, pp. 121–137, 2012.

18. F. P. Cappuccio, L. D'Elia, P. Strazzullo and M.A. Miller "Quantity and Quality of Sleep and Incidence of Type 2 Diabetes: A Systematic Review and Meta-Analysis," *Diabetes Care*, vol. 33, no. 2, pp. 414–420, 2010.

19. F. P. Cappuccio, D. Cooper, L. D'Elia, P. Strazzullo and M. A. Miller, "Sleep Duration Predicts Cardiovascular Outcomes: A Systematic Review and Meta-Analysis of Prospective Studies," *European Heart Journal*, vol. 32, no. 12, pp. 1484–1492, 2011. doi: 10.1093/eurheartj/ehr007.

20. J. S. Durmer and D. F. Dinges, "Neurocognitive Consequences of Sleep Deprivation," Seminars in Neurology, vol. 25, no. 1, pp. 117–129, 2005. doi: 10.1055/s-2005-867080.

21. L. A. Irish, C. E. Kline, H. E. Gunn, D. J. Buysse and M. H. Hall, "The Role of Sleep Hygiene in Promoting Public Health: A Review of Empirical Evidence," *Sleep Medicine Reviews*, vol. 22, pp. 23–36, 2015. doi: 10.1016/j.smrv.2014.10.001

22. D. F. Mastin, J. Bryson and R. Corwyn, "Assessment of Sleep Hygiene Using the Sleep Hygiene Index," *Journal of Behavioral Medicine*, vol. 29, no. 3, pp. 223–227, 2006.

23. J. Holt-Lunstad, T. B. Smith and J. B. Layton., "Social Relationships and Mortality Risk: A Meta-Analytic Review," *PLoS Medicine*, Vol. 7, no. 7, p. e1000316, 2010. doi: 10.1371/journal.pmed.1000316

24. L. C. Hawkley and J. T. Cacioppo, "Loneliness Matters: A Theoretical and Empirical Review of Consequences and Mechanisms," *Annals of Behavioral Medicine*, vol. 40, no. 2, pp. 218–227, 2010.

25. J. S. House, K. R. Landis and D. Umberson, "Social Relationships and Health," *Science*, vol. 241, no. 4865, pp. 540–545, 1988.

26. J. T. Cacioppo and S. Cacioppo, "Social Relationships and Health: The Toxic Effects of Perceived Social Isolation," *Social and Personality Psychology Compass*, vol. 8, no. 2, pp. 58–72, 2014.

27. B. N. Uchino, "Understanding the Links between Social Support and Physical Health: A Life-Span Perspective With Emphasis on the Separability of Perceived and Received Support," *Perspectives on Psychological Science*, vol. 4, no. 3, pp. 236–255, 2009.

28. S. Cohen and T.A. Wills, "Stress, Social Support, and the Buffering Hypothesis," *Psychological Bulletin*, vol. 98, no. 2, pp. 310–357, 1985.

29. D. J. Liska, "The Detoxification Enzyme Systems," *Alternative Medicine Review*, vol. 3, no. 3, pp. 187–198, 1998.

30. A. V. Klein and K. Kiat, "Detox Diets for Toxin Elimination and Weight Management: A Critical Review of the Evidence," *Journal of Human Nutrition and Dietetics*, vol. 28, no. 6, pp. 675–686, 2015.

31. R. J. Maughan and S.M. Shirreffs, " Development of Individual Hydration Strategies for Athletes," *International Journal of Sport Nutrition and Exercise Metabolism*, vol. 18, no. 5, pp. 457–472, 2008.

32. S. F. Clarke, E. F. Murphy, O. O'Sullivan, A. J. Lucey, M. Humphreys, A. Hogan, P. Hayes, M. O'Reilly, I. B. Jeffery, R. Wood-Martin, D. M. Kerins, E. Quigley, R. P. Ross, P. W. O'Toole, M. G. Molloy, E. Falvey, F. Shanahan and P. D. Cotter "Exercise and Associated Dietary Extremes Impact on Gut Microbial Diversity," *Gut*, vol. 63, no. 12, pp. 1913–1920, 2014.

33. B. M. Popkin, K. E. D'Anci and I. H. Rosenberg, "Water, Hydration, and Health," *Nutrition Reviews*, vol. 68, no. 8, pp. 439–458, 2010.

34. M. M. Manore, "Exercise and the Institute of Medicine Recommendations for Nutrition," *Current Sports Medicine Reports*, vol. 14, no. 4, pp. 313–319, 2015.

35. J. P. Little, "Effects of High-Intensity Interval Exercise Versus Continuous Moderate-Intensity Exercise on Postprandial Glycemic Control Assessed by Continuous Glucose Monitoring in Obese Adults," *Sports Medicine-Open*, vol. 2, no. 1, pp, pp. 1–11, 2016.

36. L. Xie, H. Kang, Q. Xu, M. J. Chen, Y. Liao, M. Thiyagarajan, J. O'Donnell, D. J. Christensen, C. Nicholson, J. J. Iliff, T. Takano, R. Deane and M. Nedergaard, "Sleep Drives Metabolite Clearance from the Adult Brain," *Science*, vol. 324, no. 6156, pp. 373–377, 2013.

37. M. Kechagia, D. Basoulis, S. Konstantopoulou, D. Dimitriadi, K. Gyftopoulou, N. Skarmoutsou and E. M. Fakiri, "Health Benefits of Probiotics: A Review," *ISRN Nutrition*, vol. 2013, p. 481651, 2013. doi: 10.5402/2013/481651.

38. H. K. Seitz, and P. Becker, "Alcohol Metabolism and Cancer Risk," *Alcohol Research & Health*, vol. 30, no. 1, pp. 38–41, 44–7, 2007.

39. U.S. Department of Health and Human Services (USDHHS), "The Health Consequences of Smoking—50 Years of Progress: A Report of the Surgeon General," 2014.

40. J. Forman, J. Silverstein; Committee on Nutrition; Council on Environmental Health; American Academy of Pediatrics "Organic Foods: Health and Environmental Advantages and Disadvantages," *Pediatrics*, vol. 130, no. 5, pp. 1406–1415, 2012.

41. G. Pizzino, N. Irrera, M. Cucinotta, G. Pallio, F. Mannino, V. Arcoraci, F. Squadrito, D. Altavilla and A. Bitto, "Oxidative Stress: Harms and Benefits for Human Health," Oxidative *Medicine and Cellular Longevity*, vol. 2017,p. 8416763, 2017. doi: 10.1155/2017/8416763.

42. J. Slavin, "Fiber and Prebiotics: Mechanisms and Health Benefits," *Nutrients*, vol. 5, no. 4, pp. 1417–1435, 2013.

43. S. M. Chacko, P. T. Thambi, R. Kuttan and I. Nishigaki "Beneficial Effects of Green Tea: A Literature Review," *Chinese Medicine*, vol. 5, p. 13, 2010.

44. L. M. S. Kim, "Foot Bath of Vinegar and Salt for Fatigue, Stress and Muscle Pain," *The Journal of Korean Oriental Medicine*, vol. 32, no. 3, pp. 153–159, 2011.

45. A. E. Edris, "Pharmaceutical and Therapeutic Potentials of Essential Oils and Their Individual Volatile Constituents: A Review," *Phytotherapy Research: An International Journal Devoted to Pharmacological and Toxicological Evaluation of Natural Product Derivatives*, vol. 21, no. 4, pp. 308–323, 2007.

46. M. Moreno-Smith, S. K. Lutgendorf and A. K. Sood, "Impact of Stress on Cancer Metastasis," *Future Oncology*, vol. 6, no. 12, pp. 1863–1881, 2010.

47. A. H. Gilani, K. H. Janbaz and B. H. Shah, "Quercetin Exhibits Hepatoprotective Activity in Rats," *Biochemical Society Transactions*, vol. 33, no. 6, pp. 1324–1326, 2005.

48. E. S. Hannuksela, "Benefits and Risks of Sauna Bathing," *The American Journal of Medicine*, vol. 110, no. 2, pp. 118–126, 2001.

49. M. C. Pascoe, D. R. Thompson, Z. M. Jenkins and C. F. Ski, "Mindfulness Mediates the Physiological Markers of Stress: Systematic Review and Meta-Analysis," *Journal of Psychiatric Research*, vol. 95, pp. 156–178, 2017.

50. K. Linde, N. Clausius, G. Ramirez, D. Melchart, F. Eitel, L. V. Hedges and W. B. Jonas, "Are the Clinical Effects of Homeopathy Placebo Effects? A Meta-Analysis of Placebo-Controlled Trials," *The Lancet*, vol. 350, no. 9081, pp. 834–843, 1997.

51. G. Fond, A. Macgregor, M. Leboyer and A. Michalsen, "Fasting in Mood Disorders: Neurobiology and Effectiveness. A Review of the Literature," *Psychiatry Research*, vol. 209, no. 3, pp. 253–258, 2013.

5 Criticisms and Responses to Natural Health Sciences

Criticisms of the natural health sciences come from the scientific community, medical profession-als, and the general public. Much of this criticism is that natural health approaches have insufficient scientific basis, can sometimes lead to dangerous side effects, and/or can replace traditional Western medical treatments (allopathic medicine). However, there are responses to every critique, and this section examines some common criticisms and responses to them.

Criticism 1: Lack of Scientific Basis

Some critics point out that natural health sciences are mostly based on anecdotes, experience, and tradi-tions. However, he argues that the efficacy and safety of these approaches must be scientifically proven.

Answer: True, some of the natural health practices are not fully understood by modern science. However, the efficacy and safety of many natural treatments and approaches have been investigated based on rigorous scientific methodologies, such as randomized controlled trials and epidemiological studies [1]. In addition, traditional medicine systems have a large knowledge base based on thousands of years of practical experience and observations.

Criticism 2: Side Effects and Safety Issues

There has been criticism that some treatments used in the natural health sciences can cause side effects, especially when used in conjunction with traditional Western medical therapies.

Answer: While this does not cover all natural remedies, it may be a valid criticism for some. However, many natural treatments are quite safe and mostly well-tolerated [2]. In addition, the side effects of natural treatments are usually milder compared to traditional Western medical treatments [3]. It is important to always be guided by a healthcare professional and to evaluate any type of treatment on an individual basis.

Criticism 3: Use in Place of Traditional Western Medical Treatments

Another criticism of the natural health sciences is that some people may prefer natural treatments over traditional Western medical treatments for serious or life-threatening conditions.

Answer: This can lead to very serious problems without proper information and guidance. However, natu-ral health practices are mostly used in an integrated manner with traditional Western medical treatments, within the framework of complementary and integrative health practices [4]. Such an approach aims to take advantage of both traditional Western and natural treatments as well as individualized patient care.

Criticism 4: Not Knowing the Correct Dosage

It has been criticized that the dosage of natural treatments is not scientifically determined, which can lead to potentially harmful consequences.

Answer: The doses of some natural treatments have not yet been fully determined, which requires further investigation. However, there is a vast body of knowledge regarding the doses of many natural forms of treatment, such as herbal supplements and homeopathy [5].

DOI: 10.1201/9781003520252-6

Criticism 5: Unsubstantiated Claims

Some claims about natural health products and treatments have been criticized as being misleading and not evidence-based.

Answer: There may be misleading claims about some natural products and treatments. However, this problem is not unique to the natural health sciences and can be observed throughout the health sector, including traditional Western medicine. The important point is to assess whether the claims are evidence-based [6].

Criticism 6: Lack of Quality Control

It is stated that there is no uniform standard for the quality and content of natural health products, which can create problems with safety and effectiveness.

Answer: Some natural health products may have limited quality control checks. However, improvements are being made in this regard, and stricter controls and standards have been implemented on natural products in many countries [7].

Criticism 7: Non-Scientific Ways of Thinking

Natural health sciences are criticized as being contrary to scientific ways of thinking, and this situation is unacceptable in a science-based society.

Answer: The natural health sciences generally take a more holistic approach and encompass not only the physical dimension of human health, but also the mental, emotional, and spiritual dimensions. This is complementary, not contrary to scientific thinking [6].

Criticism 8: Incidental Benefits

Some critics claim that the positive results from natural treatments are mostly due to the placebo effect or random circumstances.

Answer: The placebo effect is a valid issue for any type of treatment – allopathic or natural – and this can make it difficult to assess the actual effectiveness of the treatment. However, many forms of natural treatment have proven their effectiveness in placebo-controlled trials [8].

Criticism 9: Lack of Training and Certification

Professionals working in the field of natural health have been criticized for not having enough training and certification.

Answer: The training and certification of professionals working in the natural health sciences may vary depending on the treatment they practice and the country in which they are located. However, in many countries, natural health practitioners are required to reach a certain level of training and certification [7].

Criticism 10: Financial Burden

Natural health products and services are often expensive and not covered by most insurance companies.

Answer: The cost of natural health care can be a concern. However, allopathic medical services and medications can also be quite expensive. Moreover, natural health approaches often focus on preventive care, which can reduce health costs in the long run [9].

Criticism 11: The Slow Effect of Natural Treatments

Some critics argue that natural health practices generally don't offer quick results and are therefore not suitable for acute conditions.

Answer: True, some natural health practices can take time, and this may make them less than ideal for emergencies. However, these treatments can be very effective in managing chronic conditions or improving overall health [10].

Criticism 12: Limited Access to Information

Access to information in the natural health sciences is often limited, making it difficult for consumers to make informed decisions.

Answer: This may be a valid criticism, especially in online sources, due to uncertainties about the quality and accuracy of the information in the references. However, there are many reliable sources of information in the field of natural health, and access to information in this field is constantly evolving [4].

Criticism 13: Multiple Drug Use Problems

It has been criticized that natural health products can interact with prescribed medications, leading to negative consequences.

Answer: Possible interactions between natural products and prescription drugs can pose safety concerns. However, these problems can usually be managed with good communication and accurate information [11].

Criticism 14: Insufficient Research Funding

Research funding for natural health sciences has been criticized as insufficient, which restricts scientific knowledge in the field.

Answer: That's right, research into the natural health sciences is often underfunded. However, this should not underestimate the importance and potential of this field. It is clear that more funding will encourage more high-quality research in this area [12].

Criticism 15: False or Misleading Labeling

It has been criticized that the labeling of natural health products can be misleading and lead consumers to misunderstand or use these products.

Answer: This is an important issue so that consumers can accurately assess the safety and effectiveness of these products. This requires regulatory bodies to exercise tighter controls over the labeling and marketing of natural health products [13].

Criticism 16: Treatments That Are Not Suitable for Everyone

It has been criticized that some natural health practices may not be suitable for everyone, especially those with certain diseases or health conditions.

Answer: Not all forms of treatment are suitable for everyone. This also applies to natural health practices. It therefore requires an individual evaluation and guidance by an appropriate health care professional, and this applies to all health services [14].

Criticism 17: Sharing Incomplete or Misleading Information

Natural health practitioners can mislead patients by providing incomplete or misleading information.

Answer: This points to ethical and professional issues.

Natural health sciences represent a complex and broad area of medicine and are therefore open to criticism. However, responses to these criticisms often highlight the value and potential of natural health practices and the importance of an integrated approach with allopathic medicine. It is therefore important that the best interests of the individual patient are always in mind and that continuous communication with healthcare professionals is maintained.

5.1 EFFECTIVENESS AND SECURITY DISCUSSIONS

Controversies about the efficacy and safety of the natural health sciences have caused widespread debate in the scientific community and among the general public. These discussions often focus on concerns that the effectiveness of natural health practices has not been adequately proven or about the potential side effects and interactions of these treatments.

5.1.1 Effectiveness Discussions

Debates about effectiveness often focus on whether the effectiveness of natural health practices is supported by sufficient scientific evidence. Some studies on this subject support the effectiveness of certain natural treatments, while others have noted that these treatments are no less effective or at all effective than allopathic (traditional) treatment options [5]. However, these debates often suggest the need for more high-quality, double-blind, placebo-controlled studies.

5.1.1.1 Effectiveness Discussions: Concrete Examples

1. St. John's Wort and Depression: St. John's Wort (*Hypericum perforatum*) is widely used to treat depression. However, several studies have presented mixed results on the effects of this herb on major depression disorder. Some have supported its effectiveness, while others have questioned its effectiveness [15].
2. Echinacea and the Common Cold: The effect of Echinacea in relieving the symptoms of colds is controversial. Some studies have found that it relieves symptoms and shortens the duration of the disease, but others do not support these findings [16].
3. Ginkgo Biloba and Dementia: The effectiveness of ginkgo biloba in relieving the symptoms of dementia and Alzheimer's disease has been widely debated. Some studies suggest that certain doses can improve cognitive function, while others have not found this effect during research studies [17].
4. Saw Palmetto and Prostate Enlargement: Saw Palmetto (*Serenoa repens*) is often claimed to be effective in treating benign prostatic hyperplasia. However, some studies have found that this herb does not have an effect on this condition [18].
5. Kava and Anxiety: The effect of kava (*Piper methysticum*) in relieving anxiety symptoms is controversial. Some studies have found kava to be effective in relieving symptoms of anxiety, but others do not support these findings [19].
6. Probiotics and Digestive Health: The effects of probiotics on digestive health issues, especially irritable bowel syndrome (IBS) and inflammatory bowel disease, are still being debated. Some research has found that probiotics may be beneficial for certain conditions, but others have found that they are less effective or not effective at all [20].
7. Yoga and Chronic Pain: The effects of yoga on chronic pain are also discussed. Some studies have found that yoga may be effective in reducing certain types of pain, but others do not support these findings [21].
8. Red Rice Yeast and Cholesterol: Red rice yeast is often claimed to lower LDL cholesterol levels. However, data showing that this effect is clinically significant are inconclusive [22].
9. Aloe Vera and Skin Problems: Aloe Vera is claimed to be effective for a variety of skin problems. However, some studies question the effectiveness of this herb, especially for burns and psoriasis [23].

10. Melatonin and Sleep Disorders: Melatonin is often recommended for sleep disorders. However, studies on the effectiveness of melatonin supplements have yielded mixed results, and there is still widespread debate on this topic [24].

5.1.2 Security Discussions

Discussions about safety often focus on the potential side effects and interactions of natural health products and practices. These concerns often center on the fact that some herbal supplements and other natural products may not be safe for people with certain health conditions or may have harmful interactions with prescription medications [11].

However, these concerns often require further investigation and open communication between natural health practitioners and patients. This is important to ensure that natural health practices are used safely and effectively. Furthermore, having appropriate training and certification of natural health practitioners is critical to ensuring that patients receive safe and effective treatment [2].

Overall, these debates indicate that the natural health sciences need more scientific inquiry and research. This will help us better understand both the effectiveness and safety of these treatments. Furthermore, these controversies also show that natural health practices need more regulation and quality control standards.

5.1.2.1 Security Discussions: Concrete Examples

1. St. John's Wort and Drug Interactions: It is known that St. John's Wort may interact with prescription medications. This herb has been shown to reduce the effectiveness of medications such as oral contraceptives, antidepressants, and anticoagulants [25].
2. Kava and Liver Damage: Kava has been reported to potentially damage the liver. Therefore, caution should be exercised when using kava supplements, and these products should not be used by people with liver disease or taking other medications [26].
3. Ginkgo Biloba and Bleeding Risk: It has been reported that ginkgo biloba may increase the risk of bleeding by interacting with blood thinners. For this reason, people taking blood-thinning medications are advised to speak with their healthcare provider before using ginkgo biloba supplements [27].
4. Yohimbine and Heart Problems: Yohimbine is often used to improve sexual performance, but in some cases it can cause dangerous side effects. A number of side effects have been reported, including high blood pressure, rapid heart rate, and insomnia [28].
5. Ephedra and Cardiovascular Risks: Ephedra is an herb used for weight loss and energy boost. However, ephedra can cause serious cardiovascular side effects that can result in heart attacks, strokes, and even death. In 2004, its sale was banned in the United States [29].
6. Chinese Skullcap and Liver Damage: Chinese Skullcap (*Scutellaria baicalensis*) is often used for a number of health conditions. However, it has been reported that this herb can cause liver damage [30].
7. Aloe Vera and Electrolyte Imbalance: Oral use of Aloe Vera can cause a drop in potassium levels and an electrolyte imbalance in the body. This can affect the heart rhythm and be potentially dangerous [31].
8. Lobelia and Toxicity: High doses of lobelia can be toxic and cause serious health problems such as shortness of breath, rapid heartbeat, and even coma or death [32].
9. Kombucha Tea and Acidosis: Excessive consumption of kombucha tea can cause acidosis (excessive acidity of the blood). This can cause shortness of breath, weakness, dizziness, and loss of consciousness [33].
10. Lycopene and Skin Color Changes: Lycopene is often used to support prostate health. However, excessive consumption of lycopene can cause the skin to become yellowish-orange in color, a condition called lycopenemia [34].

5.2 SCIENTIFIC EVIDENCE AND RESEARCH

A lot of research has been done in the field of natural health sciences, and this research has shown that natural treatment approaches can be effective in some cases. However, it would be misleading to say that every natural treatment method can be an equivalent alternative to medical treatments.

5.2.1 Herbal Remedies

Herbal remedies are often part of traditional medicine, and some have been scientifically shown to be effective. For example, St. John's Wort (*Hypericum perforatum*) has been shown to be effective in treating mild to moderate depression [15]. Similarly, it has been found that Echinacea (*Echinacea purpurea*) can help relieve the symptoms of the common cold [35].

1. St. John's Wort (*Hypericum perforatum*): This herb is widely used, especially in the treatment of depression. The Cochrane review noted that St. John's Wort was effective in treating mild to moderate depression [15].
2. Echinacea (*Echinacea purpurea*): Echinacea is often used to protect against colds and flu. Research has shown that Echinacea can help relieve the symptoms of the common cold [35].
3. Ginkgo Biloba: Ginkgo is used to treat cognitive disorders such as dementia and Alzheimer's disease. Research has shown that ginkgo biloba can improve memory and thinking abilities [36].
4. Garlic (*Allium sativum*): Garlic is used in the treatment and control of cardiovascular diseases. Clinical studies have shown that garlic lowers hypertension and regulates cholesterol levels [37].
5. Ginger (*Zingiber officinale*): Ginger is used against stomach ailments and nausea. It has been shown to be safe and effective for relieving nausea and vomiting in pregnant women [38].
6. Turmeric (*Curcuma longa*): Turmeric is used to treat a variety of conditions due to its anti-inflammatory properties. Research has shown that turmeric can help relieve the symptoms of osteoarthritis [39].
7. Milk Thistle (*Silybum marianum*): Milk thistle is used in the treatment of liver diseases. Clinical studies have shown that milk thistle may help treat some liver diseases [40].
8. Peppermint (*Mentha piperita*): Mint is used to treat digestive ailments. Research has shown that peppermint oil can help relieve irritable bowel syndrome (IBS) symptoms [41].
9. Valerian (*Valeriana officinalis*): Valerian is used in the treatment of sleep disorders. Research has shown that valerian may be effective in treating insomnia [42].
10. Black Cohosh (*Cimicifuga racemosa*): Black Cohosh is used for the relief of menopausal symptoms. Clinical trials have shown that Black Cohosh may be effective in reducing menopausal symptoms [43].

Although herbal remedies have generally been used for thousands of years, many are still not scientifically proven or have not been researched enough for definitive results. Here are some such examples:

1. Kudzu (*Pueraria lobata*): Kudzu is used to treat alcohol dependence. However, there is not enough scientific evidence that this is effective [44].
2. Gotu Kola (*Centella asiatica*): Gotu Kola is used to improve cognitive function. However, reliable evidence about the effectiveness of this herb is lacking [45].
3. Chaparral (*Larrea tridentata*): Chaparral is used to treat cancer and other diseases. However, scientific evidence that it is safe and effective does not yet exist [46].

4. Comfrey (*Symphytum officinale*): Comfrey is used to relieve pain and inflammation when applied topically. However, the general use of this herb is not recommended due to its toxicity potential [47].
5. Lobelia (*Lobelia inflata*): Lobelia is used to treat breathing problems. However, there is no strong scientific evidence that lobelia is effective [48].
6. Colloidal Silver: This product is used to treat a variety of health conditions. However, there is no scientific evidence to support its effectiveness, and long-term use can cause serious side effects [49].
7. Blue Cohosh (*Caulophyllum thalictroides*): This herb is used to induce labor and relieve labor pains. However, scientific support for its use is lacking, and it may cause certain side effects [50].
8. Pennyroyal (*Mentha pulegium*): Pennyroyal is used to treat a variety of health issues. However, scientific evidence on its safety and efficacy is still lacking, and it may cause side effects [51].
9. Mugwort (*Artemisia vulgaris*): This herb is used to treat a variety of health issues. However, scientific evidence for its use is still lacking and may cause certain side effects [52].
10. Ma Huang (*Ephedra sinica*): This herb is used for weight loss and energy boost. However, its use can cause serious side effects, and the scientific evidence on its effectiveness is still controversial [29].

5.2.2 Probiotics

Probiotics are used to regulate the gut microbiota and improve overall health. Various studies have shown that probiotics can improve digestive health, boost the immune system, and even positively affect mood and brain function [53].

Probiotics are microorganisms that are usually bacteria and have health-promoting effects. Probiotics are defined by the World Health Organization (WHO) and the Food and Agriculture Organization (FAO) as "live microorganisms, which, when taken in appropriate amounts, benefit the health of the host" [54].

5.2.2.1 Health Effects of Probiotics

Scientific studies have shown that probiotics have positive effects on digestive system health, immune system functions, mental health, and cardiovascular health [53].

1. Digestive Health: Probiotics play an important role in the management of digestive disorders such as irritable bowel syndrome (IBS), inflammatory bowel disease (IBD), and diarrhea [55]. *Lactobacillus* and *Bifidobacterium* species are often used in the management of these conditions.
2. Immune Health: Probiotics can help regulate the immune system. There is evidence that probiotics have positive effects on the prevention and management of viral infections and allergies [56].
3. Mental Health: In recent years, the effect of probiotics on mental health through the brain-gut axis has attracted more and more attention. Research has shown that certain types of probiotics can relieve symptoms of anxiety and depression [57].
4. Cardiovascular Health: Certain types of probiotics have been shown to have the ability to lower cholesterol levels and regulate blood pressure, indicating that they may have positive effects for cardiovascular health [58].

5.2.2.2 Safety and Side Effects of Probiotics

In general, probiotics are considered safe for healthy individuals. However, the use of probiotics in immunocompromised individuals or patients with serious health problems may bring some risks. These include infections, metabolic effects, and risks of gene transfer [59].

Below are shared specific probiotics and their possible side effects:

1. *Lactobacillus acidophilus*: A well-known type of probiotic. It is often found in yogurt and other fermented foods. Benefits include prevention of diarrhea, alleviation of lactose intolerance, and prevention of vaginal infections. It is generally considered safe but can sometimes cause mild side effects such as gas and bloating [59].
2. *Bifidobacterium bifidum*: It is an important part of the intestinal microflora and is used in the prevention and treatment of diarrhea, irritable bowel syndrome, and certain allergies. It has few side effects, but people with weakened immune systems may be at risk of infection [53].
3. *Saccharomyces boulardii*: This probiotic yeast is effective in preventing antibiotic-associated diarrhea and *Clostridium difficile* infection. It is generally safe but can cause fungemia (fungal infection in the blood) in immunocompromised people [60].
4. *Lactobacillus reuteri*: This probiotic helps improve digestive health and prevent tooth decay. It is generally considered safe but may cause gas and bloating in some people [61].
5. *Streptococcus thermophilus*: Used to make yogurt and cheese and can alleviate lactose intolerance. This probiotic is generally safe, but very rarely can cause infections, especially in people with weakened immune systems [54].
6. *Lactobacillus casei*: This probiotic improves gut health and prevents diarrhea. It is generally considered safe but can cause mild side effects such as bloating and gas in some people [59].
7. *Bifidobacterium longum*: Used for the prevention and treatment of diarrhea, IBS, and lactose intolerance. It is safe for most people but can rarely cause infections in people with weakened immune systems [53].
8. *Lactobacillus rhamnosus GG*: This probiotic supports gut health and specifically prevents diarrhea. It is generally considered safe but may cause mild side effects such as gas and bloating in some people [59].
9. *Bifidobacterium lactis*: This probiotic improves intestinal transit time and prevents constipation. It is generally considered safe but can cause infections in people with weakened immune systems [53].
10. *Lactobacillus plantarum*: This probiotic is used for digestive health, eczema, and the treatment of ulcerative colitis. It is generally considered safe, but it can cause gas and bloating in some individuals [59].
11. *Lactobacillus salivarius*: This type of probiotic is usually found in the mouth and intestines and usually helps prevent tooth decay and periodontal disease. It is generally considered safe but, in some people, it can cause gas and bloating [62].
12. *Lactobacillus gasseri*: May improve digestive health and promote weight loss. It is generally safe but can cause gas and bloating [63].
13. *Bifidobacterium animalis*: It is a type of probiotic usually found in yogurt and can improve digestive health. It is safe for most people but can cause infections in people who are immunosuppressed [64].
14. *Enterococcus faecium*: Supports gut health and may help prevent diarrhea. However, some strains of this strain can be resistant and pose a risk of infection, so caution should be exercised in its use [65].
15. *Bacillus coagulans*: This probiotic improves digestive health and may relieve symptoms of irritable bowel syndrome, rheumatoid arthritis, and vulvovaginal candidiasis. It is generally considered safe but can cause gas and bloating in some people [66].
16. *Leuconostoc mesenteroides*: Often found in fermented foods and improve digestive health. It is safe for most people but can rarely cause infections in people with weakened immune systems [67].
17. *Pediococcus acidilactici*: This probiotic helps balance the gut microbiota and prevent diarrhea. It is generally considered safe but may cause mild side effects such as gas and bloating in some individuals [68].

18. *Bifidobacterium breve*: It is effective in balancing the intestinal microflora and preventing diarrhea. It is generally safe but can cause infections in people with weakened immune systems [69].
19. *Lactobacillus brevis*: This probiotic boosts the immune system and supports digestive health. It is generally considered safe, but it can cause gas and bloating in some people [70].
20. *Lactobacillus paracasei*: Improves gut health and may alleviate allergies. It's generally considered safe, but it can cause mild side effects such as gas and bloating in some people [71].

5.2.3 Acupuncture

Acupuncture is a treatment method based on the placement of fine needles at specific points on the body to treat certain health problems. Acupuncture has been shown to be effective in a number of conditions, particularly pain management and migraine treatment [72].

5.2.4 Mediation and Mind–Body Therapies

Meditation, yoga, and other mind–body therapies are used to manage stress, reduce anxiety, and improve overall quality of life. There is extensive scientific evidence that these therapies have positive effects on both physical and mental health [73].

The examples described in this section illustrate the breadth and diversity of research in the natural health sciences. But the strength and quality of scientific evidence vary greatly and may only apply to certain conditions and populations, not every treatment.

REFERENCES

1. Z. M. Horneber, "How Many Cancer Patients Use Complementary and Alternative Medicine: A Systematic Review and Metaanalysis," *Integrative Cancer Therapies*, vol. 11, no. 3, pp. 187–203, 2012.
2. P. M. Barnes, B. Bloom and R. L. Nahin, Complementary and Alternative Medicine Use Among Adults and Children: United States, 2007, National Health Statistics Reports, Hyattsville, MD, 2008.
3. E. E. Posadzki, "Adverse Effects of Herbal Medicines: An Overview of Systematic Reviews," *Clinical Medicine*, vol. 13, no. 1, pp. 7–12, 2013.
4. National Center for Complementary and Integrative Health (NCCIH), "Complementary, Alternative, or Integrative Health: What's In a Name?," 2018. [Online]. Available: https://www.nccih.nih.gov/health/complementary-alternative-or-integrative-health-whats-in-a-name.
5. E. Ernst, "A Systematic Review of Systematic Reviews of Homeopathy," *British Journal of Clinical Pharmacology*, vol. 54, no. 6, pp. 577–582, 2002.
6. L. G. T. Myers, "The Legitimacy of Academic Complementary Medicine," *The Medical Journal of Australia*, vol. 197, no. 2, pp. 69–70, 2012.
7. Y. Zhao, S.-Q. Zhang, F. Wei, Y.-M. Fan, F. Sun and S. Bai, "Quality Control of Natural Product Medicine and Nutrient Supplements 2014," *Journal of Analytical Methods in Chemistry*, vol. 2014, p. 109068, 2014.
8. J. W. B. Linde, "Are the Clinical Effects of Homeopathy Placebo Effects? A Meta-Analysis of Placebo-Controlled Trials," *The Lancet*, vol. 350, no. 9081, pp. 834–843, 1997.
9. P. Herman, B. Poindexter, C. Witt and D. Eisenberg, "Are Complementary Therapies and Integrative Care Cost-Effective? A Systematic Review of Economic Evaluations," *BMJ Open*, vol. 2, no. 5, p. e001046, 2012.
10. M. Frenkel, E. Ben-Arye and L. Cohen, "Communication in Cancer Care: Discussing Complementary and Alternative Medicine," *Integrative Cancer Therapies*, vol. 9, no. 2, pp. 177–185, 2010.
11. A. A. Izzo and E. Ernst, "Interactions between Herbal Medicines and Prescribed Drugs: An Updated Systematic Review," *Drugs*, vol. 69, no. 13, pp. 1777–1798, 2009.
12. Institute of Medicine (US) Committee on Policies for Allocating Health Sciences Research Funds, "Funding for Health Sciences Research," in Funding Health Sciences Research: A Strategy to Restore Balance, Washington (DC), National Academies Press, 1990.

13. C. Morris and J. Avorn, "Internet Marketing of Herbal Products," *JAMA*, vol. 290, no. 11, pp. 1505–1509, 2003.

14. R. Nahin, J. Dahlhamer and B. Stussman, "Health Need and the Use of Alternative Medicine Among Adults Who Do Not Use Conventional Medicine," *BMC Health Services Research*, vol. 10, p. 220, 2010.

15. K. Linde, M. Berner and L. Kriston, "St John's Wort for Major Depression," *Cochrane Database of Systematic Reviews*, vol. 2008, no. 4, p. CD000448, 2008.

16. M. Karsch-Völk, B. Barrett and K. Linde, "Echinacea for Preventing and Treating the Common Cold," *The Cochrane Database of Systematic Reviews*, vol. 2014, no. 2, p. CD000530, 2014.

17. S. Weinmann, S. Roll, C. Schwarzbach, C. Vauth and S. N. Willich, "Effects of Ginkgo biloba in Dementia: Systematic Review and Meta-Analysis," *BMC Geriatrics*, vol. 10, p. 14, 2010.

18. M. Barry, S. Meleth, J. Lee, K. Kreder, A. Avins, J. Nickel, C. Roehrborn, E. Crawford, H. J. Foster, S. Kaplan, A. McCullough, G. Andriole, M. Naslund, O. Williams, J. Kusek, C. Meyers, J. Betz, A. Cantor and K. McVary, "Complementary and Alternative Medicine for Urological Symptoms (CAMUS) Study Group. Effect of Increasing Doses of Saw Palmetto Extract on Lower Urinary Tract Symptoms: A Randomized Trial," *JAMA*, vol. 306, no. 12, pp. 1344–1351, 2011.

19. J. Sarris, C. Stough, C. Bousman, Z. Wahid, G. Murray, R. Teschke, K. Savage, A. Dowell, C. Ng and I. Schweitzer, "Kava in the Treatment of Generalized Anxiety Disorder: A Double-Blind, Randomized, Placebo-Controlled Study," *Journal of Clinical Psychopharmacology*, vol. 33, no. 5, pp. 643–648, 2013.

20. A. Ford, E. Quigley, B. Lacy, A. Lembo, Y. Saito, L. Schiller, E. Soffer, B. Spiegel and P. Moayyedi, "Efficacy of Prebiotics, Probiotics, and Synbiotics in Irritable Bowel Syndrome and Chronic Idiopathic Constipation: Systematic Review and Meta-Analysis," *The American Journal of Gastroenterology*, vol. 109, no. 10, p. 1547, 2014.

21. A. Büssing, T. Ostermann, R. Lüdtke and A. Michalsen, "Effects of Yoga Interventions on Pain and Pain-Associated Disability: A Meta-Analysis," *The Journal of Pain*, vol. 13, no. 1, pp. 1–9, 2012.

22. J. Liu, J. Zhang, Y. Shi, S. Grimsgaard, T. Alraek and V. Fønnebø, "Chinese Red Yeast Rice (*Monascus purpureus*) for Primary Hyperlipidemia: A Meta-Analysis of Randomized Controlled Trials," *Chinese Medicine*, vol. 1, p. 4, 2006.

23. B. K. Vogler and E. Ernst, "Aloe Vera: A Systematic Review of Its Clinical Effectiveness," *British Journal of General Practice*, vol. 49, no. 447, pp. 823–828, 1999.

24. E. Ferracioli-Oda, A. Qawasmi and M. H. Bloch, "Meta-Analysis: Melatonin for the Treatment of Primary Sleep Disorders," *PLoS One*, vol. 8, no. 5, p. e63773, 2013.

25. A. A. Izzo, "Herb–Drug Interactions: An Overview of the Clinical Evidence," *Fundamental & Clinical Pharmacology*, vol. 18, no. 1, pp. 201–206, 2004.

26. R. Teschke, J. Sarris and V. Lebot, "Kava Hepatotoxicity Solution: A Six-Point Plan for New Kava Standardization," *Phytomedicine*, vol. 18, no. 2–3, pp. 96–103, 2011.

27. J. M. Fessenden, W. Wittenborn and L. Clarke, "Ginkgo Biloba: A Case Report of Herbal Medicine and Bleeding Postoperatively from a Laparoscopic Cholecystectomy," *The American Surgeon*, vol. 68, no. 1, pp. 33–35, 2002.

28. P. A. Cohen, Y. H. Wang, G. Maller, R. DeSouza and I. A. Khan, "Pharmaceutical Quantities of Yohimbine Found in Dietary Supplements in the USA," *Drug Testing and Analysis*, vol. 7, no. 1-2, pp. 83–90, 2015.

29. P. G. Shekelle, M. L. Hardy, S. C. Morton, M. Maglione, W. A. Mojica, M. J. Suttorp and L. Jungvig, "Efficacy and Safety of Ephedra and Ephedrine for Weight Loss and Athletic Performance: A Meta-Analysis," *JAMA*, vol. 289, no. 12, pp. 1537–1545, 2003.

30. M. N. Lai, S. M. Wang, P. C. Chen, Y. Y. Chen and J. D. Wang, "Population-Based Case-Control Study of Chinese Herbal Products Containing Aristolochic Acid and Urinary Tract Cancer Risk," *Journal of the National Cancer Institute*, vol. 102, no. 3, pp. 179–186, 2019.

31. M. D. Boudreau, F. A. Beland, J. A. Nichols and M. Pogribna, "Toxicology and Carcinogenesis Studies of a Nondecolorized [corrected] Whole Leaf Extract of *Aloe barbadensis* Miller (*Aloe vera*) in F344/N Rats and B6C3F1 Mice (Drinking Water Study)," *National Toxicology Program Technical Report Series*, vol. 577, pp. 1–266, 2013.

32. H. A. Spiller and D. B. Willias, "Toxicology of oral Antidiabetic Medications," *The American Journal of Health-System Pharmacy*, vol. 64, no. 10, pp. 1067–1075, 2009.

33. R. Srinivasan, S. Smolinske and D. Greenbaum, "Probable Gastrointestinal Toxicity of Kombucha Tea," *The Journal of General Internal Medicine*, vol. 12, no. 10, pp. 643–644, 1997.

34. E. Perera and A. J. Sinclair, "Hypertension Is a Major Risk Factor for Aortic Root Dilatation in Women With Turner's Syndrome," *Clinical Endocrinology*, vol. 76, no. 1, pp. 151–156, 2012.

35. M. Karsch-Völk, B. Barrett, D. Kiefer, R. Bauer and K. L. K. Ardjomand-Woelkart, "Echinacea for Preventing and Treating the Common Cold," *Cochrane Database of Systematic Reviews*, vol. 2014, no. 2, p. CD000530, 2014.

36. M. S. Tan, J. T. Yu, C. C. Tan, H. F. Wang, D. Miao, Q. Q. Mo and L. Tan, "Efficacy and Adverse Effects of Ginkgo biloba for Cognitive Impairment and Dementia: A Systematic Review and Meta-Analysis," *Journal of Alzheimer's Disease*, vol. 43, no. 2, pp. 589–603, 2015.

37. K. Ried, O. R. Frank and N. P. Stocks, "Aged Garlic Extract Lowers Blood Pressure in Patients With Treated but Uncontrolled Hypertension: A Randomised Controlled Trial," *Maturitas*, vol. 67, no. 2, pp. 144–150, 2010.

38. E. Viljoen, J. Visser, N. Koen and A. Musekiwa, "A Systematic Review and Meta-Analysis of the Effect and Safety of Ginger in the Treatment of Pregnancy-Associated Nausea and Vomiting," *Nutrition Journal*, vol. 13, no. 1, pp. 1–14, 2014.

39. J. W. Daily, M. Yang and S. Park, "Efficacy of Turmeric Extracts and Curcumin for Alleviating the Symptoms of Joint Arthritis: A Systematic Review and Meta-Analysis of Randomized Clinical Trials," *Journal of Medicinal Food*, vol. 19, no. 8, pp. 717–729, 2016.

40. L. Abenavoli, R. Capasso, N. Milic and F. Capasso, "Milk Thistle in Liver Diseases: Past, Present, Future," *Phytotherapy Research*, vol. 24, no. 10, pp. 1423–1432, 2010.

41. R. Khanna, J. K. MacDonald and B. G. Levesque, "Peppermint Oil for the Treatment of Irritable Bowel Syndrome: A Systematic Review and Meta-Analysis," *Journal of Clinical Gastroenterology*, vol. 48, no. 6, pp. 505–512, 2014.

42. S. Bent, A. Padula, D. Moore, M. Patterson and W. Mehling, "Valerian for Sleep: A Systematic Review and Meta-Analysis," *The American Journal of Medicine*, vol. 119, no. 12, pp. 1005–1012, 2006.

43. M. Leach and V. Moore, "Black Cohosh (Cimicifuga Spp.) for Menopausal Symptoms," *Cochrane Database of Systematic Reviews*, vol. 9, 2012.

44. S. E. Lukas, D. Penetar, J. Berko, L. Vicens, C. Palmer, G. Mallya and D. Y. W. Lee, "An Extract of the Chinese Herbal Root Kudzu Reduces Alcohol Drinking by Heavy Drinkers in a Naturalistic Setting," *Alcoholism: Clinical and Experimental Research*, vol. 29, no. 5, pp. 756–762, 2005.

45. C. L. Xu, Q. Z. Wang, L. M. Sun, X. M. Li, J. M. Deng, L. F. Li and W. Wang, "The Effect of Centella asiatica on the Cognitive Function and the TH Expression of Brain Tissues in ADmice," *Traditional Chinese Drug Research & Clinical Pharmacology*, vol. 27, no. 1, pp. 60–64, 2016.

46. R. J. Huxtable, "Physiological Actions of Taurine," *Physiological Reviews*, vol. 72, no. 1, pp. 101–163, 1992.

47. C. Staiger, "Comfrey: A Clinical Overview," *Phytotherapy Research*, vol. 26, no. 10, pp. 1441–1448, 2012.

48. E. Ernst, "The Risk-Benefit Profile of Commonly Used Herbal Therapies: Ginkgo, St. John's Wort, Ginseng, Echinacea, Saw Palmetto, and Kava," *Annals of Internal Medicine*, vol. 136, no. 1, pp. 42–53, 2002.

49. M. Rai, A. Yadav and A. Gade, "Silver Nanoparticles as a New Generation of Antimicrobials," *Biotechnology Advances*, vol. 27, no. 1, pp. 76–83, 2009.

50. T. Low Dog, "The Use of Botanicals During Pregnancy and Lactation," *Alternative Therapies In Health And Medicine*, vol. 15, no. 1, pp. 54–58, 2009.

51. I. B. Anderson, W. H. Mullen, J. E. Meeker, S. C. Khojasteh-Bakht, S. Oishi, S. D. Nelson and P. D. Blanc, "Pennyroyal Toxicity: Measurement of Toxic Metabolite Levels in Two Cases and Review of the Literature," *Annals of Internal Medicine*, vol. 124, no. 8, pp. 726–734, 1996.

52. N. G. Bisset, Herbal Drugs and Phytopharmaceuticals, CRC Press, Boca Raton, FL, 1994.

53. P. Markowiak and K. Śliżewska, "Effects of Probiotics, Prebiotics, and Synbiotics on Human Health," *Nutrients*, vol. 9, no. 9, p. 1021, 2017.

54. C. Hill, F. Guarner, G. Reid, G. R. Gibson, D. J. Merenstein, B. Pot and P. C. Calder, "The International Scientific Association for Probiotics and Prebiotics Consensus Statement on the Scope and Appropriate Use of the Term Probiotic," *Nature Reviews Gastroenterology & Hepatology*, vol. 11, no. 8, pp. 506–514, 2014.

55. E. Dimidi, S. Christodoulides, K. C. Fragkos, S. M. Scott and K. Whelan, "The Effect of Probiotics on Functional Constipation in Adults: A Systematic Review and Meta-Analysis of Randomized Controlled Trials," *The American Journal of Clinical Nutrition*, vol. 110, no. 4, pp. 868–877, 2019.

56. A. T. Vieira, M. M. Teixeira and F. S. Martins, "The Role of Probiotics and Prebiotics in Inducing Gut Immunity," *Frontiers in Immunology*, vol. 4, p. 445, 2013.

57. C. J. Wallace and R. Milev, "The Effects of Probiotics on Depressive Symptoms in Humans: A Systematic Review," *Annals of General Psychiatry*, vol. 16, no. 1, pp. 1–10, 2017.

58. S. Khalesi, J. Sun, N. Buys and R. Jayasinghe, "Effect of Probiotics on Blood Pressure: A Systematic Review and Meta-Analysis of Randomized, Controlled Trials," *Hypertension*, vol. 64, no. 4, pp. 897–903, 2014.

59. S. Doron and D. R. Snydman, "Risk and Safety of Probiotics," *Clinical Infectious Diseases*, vol. 60, no. Supplement 2, pp. S129–S134, 2015.

60. T. Kelesidis and C. Pothoulakis, "Efficacy and Safety of the Probiotic Saccharomyces Boulardii for the Prevention and Therapy of Gastrointestinal Disorders," *Therapeutic Advances in Gastroenterology*, vol. 5, no. 2, pp. 111–125, 2012.

61. C. L. Ohland and W. K. Macnaughton, "Probiotic Bacteria and Intestinal Epithelial Barrier Function," *American Journal of Physiology-Gastrointestinal and Liver Physiology*, vol. 298, no. 6, pp. G807–G819, 2010.

62. S. Twetman, B. Derawi, M. Keller, K. Ekstrand, T. Yucel-Lindberg and C. Stecksen-Blicks, "Short-Term Effect of Chewing Gums Containing Probiotic *Lactobacillus reuteri* on the Levels of Inflammatory Mediators in Gingival Crevicular Fluid," *Acta Odontologica Scandinavica*, vol. 67, no. 1, pp. 19–24, 2009.

63. M. Miyoshi, A. Ogawa, S. Higurashi and Y. Kadooka, "Anti-Obesity Effect of *Lactobacillus gasseri* SBT2055 Accompanied by Inhibition of Pro-Inflammatory Gene Expression in the Visceral Adipose Tissue in Diet-Induced Obese Mice," *European Journal of Nutrition*, vol. 53, no. 2, pp. 599–606, 2014.

64. M. Gagnon, E. E. Kheadr, G. Le Blay and I. Fliss, "In Vitro Inhibition of Escherichia Coli O157:H7 by Bifidobacterial Strains of Human Origin," *International Journal of Food Microbiology*, vol. 92, no. 1, pp. 69–78, 2004.

65. C. J. Kristich, L. B. Rice and C. A. Arias, "Enterococcal Infection—Treatment and Antibiotic Resistance," in Enterococci: From Commensals to Leading Causes of Drug Resistant Infection, edited by M. S. Gilmore, D. B. Clewell, Y. Ike, et al., Boston, MA: Massachusetts Eye and Ear Infirmary, 2014. https://pubmed.ncbi.nlm.nih.gov/24649502/

66. L. Hun, "Bacillus Coagulans Significantly Improved Abdominal Pain and Bloating in Patients With IBS," *Postgraduate Medicine*, vol. 121, no. 2, pp. 119–124, 2015.

67. E. B. Kim and M. L. Marco, "Nonclinical and Clinical Enterococcus Faecium Strains, but Not Enterococcus Faecalis Strains, Have Distinct Structural and Functional Genomic Features," *Applied and Environmental Microbiology*, vol. 80, no. 1, pp. 154–165, 2014.

68. M. Papagianni and S. Anastasiadou, "Pediocins: The Bacteriocins of Pediococci. Sources, Production, Properties and Applications," *Microbial Cell Factories*, vol. 8, no. 1, p. 3, 2009.

69. R. Tojo, A. Suárez, G. Clemente, C. G. De los Reyes-Gavilán, A. Margolles, M. Gueimonde and P. Ruas-Madiedo, "Intestinal Microbiota in Health and Disease: Role of Bifidobacteria in Gut Homeostasis," *World Journal of Gastroenterology: WJG*, vol. 20, no. 41, 2014.

70. M. P. Arena, D. Fiocco, D. Drider, G. Spano and V. Capozzi, "Use of Lactobacillus Plantarum Strains as a Bio-Control Strategy Against Food-Borne Pathogenic Microorganisms," *Frontiers in Microbiology*, vol. 7, p. 464, 2018.

71. S. Nagata, T. Asahara, C. Wang, Y. Suyama, O. Chonan, K. Takano and K. Nomoto, "The Effectiveness of Lactobacillus Beverages in Controlling Infections Among the Residents of an Aged Care Facility: A Randomized Placebo-Controlled Double-Blind Trial," *Annals of Nutrition and Metabolism*, vol. 68, no. 1, pp. 51–59, 2016.

72. K. Linde, G. Allais, B. Brinkhaus, Y. Fei, M. Mehring, E. A. Vertosick, A. Vickers and A. R. White, "Acupuncture for the Prevention of Episodic Migraine," *The Cochrane Database of Systematic Reviews*, vol. 6, p. CD001218, 2016.

73. M. Goyal, S. Singh and E. M. Sibinga, "Meditation Programs for Psychological Stress and Well-Being: A Systematic Review and Meta-Analysis," *JAMA Internal Medicine*, vol. 174, no. 3, pp. 357–368, 2014.

SUGGESTED READINGS

Abdel-Tawab, M., O. Werz, and M. Schubert-Zsilavecz, "*Boswellia serrata*: An Overall Assessment of in Vitro, Preclinical, Pharmacokinetic and Clinical Data," *Clinical Pharmacokinetics*, vol. 50, no. 6, pp. 349–369, 2011. doi:10.2165/11586800-000000000-00000

Aggarwal, B. B., and H. Ichikawa, "Molecular Targets and Anticancer Potential of Indole-3-Carbinol and Its Derivatives," *Cell Cycle*, vol. 4, no. 9, pp. 1201–1215, 2005.

Aissaoui, A., S. Zizi, Z. H. Israel, and B. Lyoussi, "Hypoglycemic and Hypolipidemic Effects of *Coriandrum sativum* L. in Meriones Shawi Rats," *Journal of Ethnopharmacology*, vol. 137, no. 1, pp. 652–661, 2011.

Amagase, H., and N. R. Farnsworth, "A Review of Botanical Characteristics, Phytochemistry, Clinical Relevance in Efficacy and Safety of *Lycium barbarum* Fruit (Goji)," *Food Research International*, vol. 44, no. 7, pp. 1702–1717, 2011. doi:10.1016/j.foodres.2011.03.008

Amenta, F., L. Parnetti, V. Gallai, and A. Wallin, "Treatment of Cognitive Dysfunction Associated With Alzheimer's Disease With Cholinergic Precursors. Ineffective Treatments or Inappropriate Approaches?" *Mechanisms of Development and Aging*, vol. 122, no. 16, pp. 2025–2040, 2001.

Anand David, A. V., R. Arulmoli, and S. Parasuraman, "Overviews of Biological Importance of Quercetin: A Bioactive Flavonoid," *Pharmacognosy Reviews*, vol. 10, no. 20, pp. 84–89, 2016.

Asian Ginseng. National Center for Complementary and Integrative Health, U.S. Department of Health and Human Services, 1 Sept. 2020, www.nccih.nih.gov/health/asian-ginseng.

Astragalus. National Center for Complementary and Integrative Health, U.S. Department of Health and Human Services, 1 Sept. 2020, www.nccih.nih.gov/health/astragalus.

Astragalus. WebMD. https://www.webmd.com/vitamins/ai/ingredientmono-963/astragalus.

Auld, F., E. L. Maschauer, I. Morrison, D. J. Skene, and R. L. Riha, "Evidence for the Efficacy of Melatonin in the Treatment of Primary Adult Sleep Disorders," *Sleep Medicine Reviews*, vol. 34, pp. 10–22, 2017. doi:10.1016/j.smrv.2016.06.005.

Barnes, J., L. A. Anderson, and J. David Phillipson, "St John's Wort (*Hypericum perforatum* L.): A Review of Its Chemistry, Pharmacology and Clinical Properties," *Journal of Pharmacy and Pharmacology*, vol. 53, no. 5, pp. 583–600, 2001. doi:10.1211/0022357011775910.

Bent, S., A. Padula, D. Moore, M. Patterson, and W. Mehling, "Valerian for Sleep: A Systematic Review and Meta-Analysis," *The American Journal of Medicine*, vol. 119, no. 12, pp. 1005–1012, 2006. doi:10.1016/j.amjmed.2006.02.026.

Bereczki, D., and I. Fekete, "Vinpocetine for Acute Ischaemic Stroke," *The Cochrane Database of Systematic Reviews*, no. 1, p. CD000480, 2008.

Bhat, J., A. Damle, P. P. Vaishnav, R. Albers, M. Joshi, and G. Banerjee, "In Vivo Enhancement of Natural Killer Cell Activity Through Tea Fortified With Ayurvedic Herbs," *Phytotherapy Research*, vol. 24, no. 1, 2010, p. 129–135. doi:10.1002/ptr.2889.

Bick, R. L., and R. A. Yeager, "Antithrombotic Efficacy of Cilostazol Plus Aspirin, Aspirin Alone, and Aspirin Plus Warfarin in the Rabbit Venous Thrombosis Model," *Thrombosis Research*, vol. 105, no. 2, pp. 125–30, 2002.

Birketvedt, G. S., M. Shimshi, T. Erling, and J. Florholmen, "Experiences With Three Different Fiber Supplements in Weight Reduction," *Medical Science Monitor: International Medical Journal of Experimental and Clinical Research*, vol. 11, no. 1, pp. PI5–PI8, 2005. https://pubmed.ncbi.nlm.nih.gov/15614200/

Blessing, E. M., M. M. Steenkamp, J. Manzanares, and C. R. Marmar, "Cannabidiol as a Potential Treatment for Anxiety Disorders," *Neurotherapeutics*, vol. 12, no. 4, 2015, p. 825–836. doi:10.1007/s13311-015-0387-1.

Boels, D., A. Landreau, C. Bruneau, R. Garnier, C. Pulce, M. Labadie, L. de Haro, and P. Harry, "Shiitake Dermatitis Recorded by French Poison Control Centers – New Case Series with Clinical Observations," *Clinical Toxicology (Philadelphia, Pa.)*, vol. 52, no. 6, pp. 625–628, 2014. doi: 10.3109/15563650.2014.923905.

Borzelleca, J. F., D. Peters, and W. Hall, "A 13-Week Dietary Toxicity and Toxicokinetic Study With l-Theanine in Rats," *Food and Chemical Toxicology*, vol. 44, no. 7, pp. 1158–1166, 2006. doi:10.1016/j.fct.2006.03.014

Bottiglieri, T., "S-Adenosyl-L-Methionine (SAMe): from the Bench to the Bedside–Molecular Basis of a Pleiotrophic Molecule," *The American Journal of Clinical Nutrition*, vol. 76, no. 5, pp. 1151S–1157S, 2002. doi:10.1093/ajcn/76.5.1151S

Bundy, R., A. F. Walker, R. W. Middleton, G. Marakis, and J. C. Booth, "Artichoke Leaf Extract Reduces Symptoms of Irritable Bowel Syndrome and Improves Quality of Life in Otherwise Healthy Volunteers Suffering from Concomitant Dyspepsia: A Subset Analysis," *Journal of Alternative and Complementary Medicine*, vol. 10, no. 4, pp. 667–669, 2004.

Canter, P. H., and E. Ernst, "Anthocyanosides of *Vaccinium myrtillus* (bilberry) for Night Vision—A Systematic Review of Placebo-Controlled Trials," *Survey of Ophthalmology*, vol. 49, no. 1, pp. 38–50, 2004. doi:10.1016/j.survophthal.2003.10.006

Carr, A. C., and S. Maggini, "Vitamin C and Immune Function," *Nutrients*, vol. 9, no. 11, p. 1211, 2017. doi: 10.3390/nu9111211.

Chan, Y. S., L. N. Cheng, J. H. Wu, E. Chan, Y. W. Kwan, S. M. Lee, G. P. Leung, P. H. Yu, and S. W. Chan, "A Review of the Pharmacological Effects of Arctium Lappa (burdock)," *Inflammopharmacology*, vol. 19, no. 5, pp. 245–254, 2011.

Charlebois, D., Elderberry as a Medicinal Plant. In J. Janick and A. Whipkey (eds.), Issues in New Crops and New Uses. ASHS Press, Alexandria, VA, 2007.

Choudhary, D., S. Bhattacharyya, and S. Bose, "Efficacy and Safety of Ashwagandha (*Withania somnifera* (L.) Dunal) Root Extract in Improving Memory and Cognitive Functions," *Journal of Dietary Supplements*, vol. 14, no. 6, p. 599–612, 2017. doi:10.1080/19390211.2017.1284970.

Clare, B. A., R. S. Conroy, and K. Spelman, "The Diuretic Effect in Human Subjects of an Extract of Taraxacum officinale folium Over a Single Day," *Journal of Alternative and Complementary Medicine*, vol. 15, no. 8, pp. 929–934, 2009.

Clifford, T., G. Howatson, D. J. West, and E. J. Stevenson, "The Potential Benefits of Red Beetroot Supplementation in Health and Disease," *Nutrients*, vol. 7, no. 4, pp. 2801–2822, 2015.

Cohen, M. M., "Tulsi – *Ocimum sanctum*: A Herb for All Reasons," *Journal of Ayurveda and Integrative Medicine*, vol. 5, no. 4, pp. 251–259, 2014. doi:10.4103/0975-9476.146554.

Dai, X., J. M. Stanilka, C. A. Rowe, E. A. Esteves, C. Nieves Jr, S. J. Spaiser, M. C. Christman, B. Langkamp-Henken, and S. S. Percival, "Consuming Lentinula Edodes (Shiitake) Mushrooms Daily Improves Human Immunity: A Randomized Dietary Intervention in Healthy Young Adults," *Journal of the American College of Nutrition*, vol. 34, no. 6, pp. 478–487, 2015. doi:10.1080/07315724.2014.950391.

Daily, J. W., M. Yang, and S. Park, "Efficacy of Turmeric Extracts and Curcumin for Alleviating the Symptoms of Joint Arthritis: A Systematic Review and Meta-Analysis of Randomized Clinical Trials," *Journal of Medicinal Food*, vol. 19, no. 8, pp. 717–729, 2016.

Dalli, E., J. Milara, J. Cortijo, E. J. Morcillo, and J. Cosín-Sales, "Crataegus laevigata Decreases Neutrophil Elastase and Has Hypolipidemic Effect: A Randomized, Double-Blind, Placebo-Controlled Trial," *Phytomedicine*, vol. 20, no. 8-9, pp. 692–701, 2013. doi:10.1016/j.phymed.2013.02.014

Daniele, C., G. Mazzanti, M. H. Pittler, and E. Ernst, "Adverse-Event Profile of Crataegus Spp.: A Systematic Review," *Drug Safety*, vol. 29, no. 6, pp. 523–535, 2006. doi:10.2165/00002018-200629060-00006

Darbinyan, V., G. Aslanyan, E. Amroyan, E. Gabrielyan, C. Malmström, and A. G. Panossian, "Clinical Trial of *Rhodiola rosea* L. Extract SHR-5 in the Treatment of Mild to Moderate Depression," *Nordic Journal of Psychiatry*, vol. 61, no. 5, p. 343–348, 2007. doi:10.1080/08039480701643290.

Davis, P. A., and W. Yokoyama, "Cinnamon Intake Lowers Fasting Blood Glucose: Meta-Analysis," *Journal of Medicinal Food*, vol. 14, no. 9, pp. 884–889, 2011.

De Jesus Moreno Moreno, M., "Cognitive Improvement in Mild to Moderate Alzheimer's Dementia after Treatment With the Acetylcholine Precursor Choline Alfoscerate: A Multicenter, Double-Blind, Randomized, Placebo-Controlled Trial," *Clinical Therapeutics*, vol. 25, no. 1, pp. 178–193, 2003.

Devinsky, O., E. Marsh, D. Friedman, E. Thiele, L. Laux, J. Sullivan, I. Miller, R. Flamini, A. Wilfong, F. Filloux, M. Wong, N. Tilton, P. Bruno, J. Bluvstein, J. Hedlund, R. Kamens, J. Maclean, S. Nangia, N. S. Singhal, C. A. Wilson, A. Patel, and M. R. Cilio, "Cannabidiol in Patients With Treatment-Resistant Epilepsy: An Open-Label Interventional Trial," *Lancet Neurology*, vol. 15, no. 3, p. 270–278, 2016. doi:10.1016/S1474-4422(15)00379-8.

Dong Quai, National Center for Complementary and Integrative Health, U.S. Department of Health and Human Services, 1 Sept. 2020, www.nccih.nih.gov/health/dong-quai.

Doron, S., and D. R. Snydman, "Risk and Safety of Probiotics," *Clinical Infectious Diseases*, vol. 60, no. Suppl 2, pp. S129–S134, 2015. doi:10.1093/cid/civ085.

Echinacea, National Center for Complementary and Integrative Health, U.S. Department of Health and Human Services, 1 Sept. 2020, www.nccih.nih.gov/health/echinacea.

Ernst, E., and M. H. Pittler, "Efficacy of Ginger for Nausea and Vomiting: A Systematic Review of Randomized Clinical Trials," *The British Journal of Anaesthesia*, vol. 84, no. 3, pp. 367–371, 2000.

Ernst, E., and M. H. Pittler, "Yohimbine for Erectile Dysfunction: A Systematic Review and Meta-Analysis of Randomized Clinical Trials," *Journal of Urology*, vol. 159, no. 2, pp. 433–436, 1998. doi:10.1016/S0022-5347(01)63953-3.

Ewing, L. E., C. M. Skinner, C. M. Quick, S. Kennon-McGill, M. R. McGill, L. A. Walker, M. A. ElSohly, B. J. Gurley, and I. Koturbash, "Hepatotoxicity of a Cannabidiol-Rich Cannabis Extract in the Mouse Model," *Molecules*, vol. 24, no. 9, p. 1694, 2019. doi:10.3390/molecules24091694.

Feringa, H. H., D. A. Laskey, J. E. Dickson, and C. I. Coleman, "The Effect of Grape Seed Extract on Cardiovascular Risk Markers: A Meta-Analysis of Randomized Controlled Trials," *Journal of the American Dietetic Association*, vol. 111, no. 8, pp. 1173–1181, 2011.

Fiocchi, A., P. Sarratud, L. Terracciano, E. Vacca, R. Bernardini, and C. Ballabio, "Assessment of the Allergenic Potential of Herbal Medicinal Products: A Blinded Study," *Pediatric Allergy and Immunology*, vol. 29, no. 1, pp. 98–101, 2018.

Flemish, Z., S. Pellechia-Clarke, B. Bailey, and M. McGuigan, "Unintentional Exposure of Young Children to Camphor and Eucalyptus Oils," *Paediatrics & Child Health*, vol. 6, no. 2, pp. 80–83, 2001.

Frank, M., T. J. Weckman, T. Wood, W. E. Woods, C. L. Tai, S-L. Chang, A. Ewing, J. W. Blake, and T. Tobin, "Hordenine: Pharmacology, Pharmacokinetics and Behavioural Effects in the Horse," *Equine Veterinary Journal*, vol. 22, no. 6, pp. 437–441, 1990.

Galizia, I., L. Oldani, K. Macritchie, E. Amari, D. Dougall, T. N. Jones, R. W. Lam, G. J. Massei, L. N. Yatham, and A. H. Young, "S-Adenosyl Methionine (SAMe) for Depression in Adults," *The Cochrane Database of Systematic Reviews*, vol. 2016, no. 10, p. CD011286, 2016. doi:10.1002/14651858.CD011286.pub2

Gibson, G. R., R. Hutkins, M. E. Sanders, S. L. Prescott, R. A. Reimer, S. J. Salminen, K. Scott, C. Stanton, K. S. Swanson, P. D. Cani, K. Verbeke, and G. Reid, "Expert Consensus Document: The International Scientific Association for Probiotics and Prebiotics (ISAPP) Consensus Statement on the Definition and Scope of Prebiotics," *Nature Reviews Gastroenterology & Hepatology*, vol. 14, no. 8, pp. 491–502, 2017. doi:10.1038/nrgastro.2017.75.

Gibson, G. R., K. P. Scott, R. A. Rastall, K. M. Tuohy, A. Hotchkiss, A. Dubert-Ferrandon, M. Gareau, E. F. Murphy, D. Saulnier, G. Loh, S. Macfarlane, N. Delzenne, Y. Ringel, G. Kozianowski, R. Dickmann, I. Lenoir-Wijnkoop, C. Walker, and R. Buddington, "Dietary Prebiotics: Current Status and New Definition," *Food Science and Technology Bulletin: Functional Foods*, vol. 7, no. 1, pp. 1–19, 2010. doi:10.1616/1476-2137.15880.

Ginkgo, National Center for Complementary and Integrative Health, U.S. Department of Health and Human Services, 1 Sept. 2020, www.nccih.nih.gov/health/ginkgo.

Glade, M. J., and K. Smith, "Phosphatidylserine and the Human Brain," *Nutrition*, vol. 31, no. 6, pp. 781–786, 2015.

Göbel, H., G. Schmidt, and D. Soyka, "Effect of Peppermint and Eucalyptus Oil Preparations on Neurophysiological and Experimental Algesimetric Headache Parameters," *Cephalalgia*, vol. 14, no. 3, pp. 228–234, 1994.

Gonzales, G. F., "Ethnobiology and Ethnopharmacology of *Lepidium meyenii* (Maca), a Plant from the Peruvian Highlands," *Evidence-Based Complementary and Alternative Medicine*, vol. 2012, p. 193496, 2012.

Gotu Kola, National Center for Complementary and Integrative Health, U.S. Department of Health and Human Services, 1 Sept. 2020, www.nccih.nih.gov/health/gotu-kola.

Green tea, National Center for Complementary and Integrative Health, U.S. Department of Health and Human Services, 1 Sept. 2020, www.nccih.nih.gov/health/green-tea.

Harvard, T. H., Chan School of Public Health, anthocyanins, 2021

Harvard, T. H. Chan School of Public Health, Omega-3 Fatty Acids: An Essential Contribution, 2021.

Harvard, T. H., Chan School of Public Health, Omega-6 Fatty Acids: An Essential Role, 2021.

Harvard, T. H., Chan School of Public Health, The Nutrition Source – Protein, 2021.

Hausenblas, H. A., D. Saha, P. J. Dubyak, and S. D. Anton, "Saffron (*Crocus sativus* L.) and Major Depressive Disorder: A Meta-Analysis of Randomized Clinical Trials," *Journal of Integrative Medicine*, vol. 11, no. 6, pp. 377–383, 2013.

Hawkins, J., C. Baker, L. Cherry, and E. Dunne, "Black Elderberry (*Sambucus nigra*) Supplementation Effectively Treats Upper Respiratory Symptoms: A Meta-Analysis of Randomized, Controlled Clinical Trials," *Complementary Therapies in Medicine*, vol. 42, pp. 361–365, 2019. doi:10.1016/j.ctim.2018.12.004

Hawrelak, J. A., and S. P. Myers, "Effects of Two Natural Medicine Formulations on Irritable Bowel Syndrome Symptoms: A Pilot Study," *Journal of Alternative and Complementary Medicine*, vol. 16, no. 10, pp. 1065–1071, 2010.

Heymann, E. W., and A. Muñoz, "Foraging at a New Feeding Site by Spider Monkeys (*Ateles paniscus* Chamek): A Test of Directed Social Learning," *Folia Primatologica*, vol. 70, no. 6, pp. 351–353, 1999. doi:10.1159/000021711

Heymsfield, S. B., D. B. Allison, J. R. Vasselli, A. Pietrobelli, D. Greenfield, and C. Nunez, "Garcinia Cambogia (Hydroxycitric Acid) as a Potential Antiobesity Agent: S Randomized Controlled Trial," *JAMA*, vol. 280, no. 18, pp. 1596–1600, 1998. doi:10.1001/jama.280.18.1596

Hirsch, K. R., A. E. Smith-Ryan, E. J. Roelofs, E. T. Trexler, and M. G. Mock, "*Cordyceps militaris* Improves Tolerance to High-Intensity Exercise After Acute and Chronic Supplementation," *Journal of Dietary Supplements*, vol. 14, no. 1, pp. 42–53, 2017. doi:10.1080/19390211.2016.1203386.

Holick, M. F., "Vitamin D Deficiency," *The New England Journal of Medicine*, vol. 357, pp. 266–281, 2007

Holubarsch, C. J., W. S. Colucci, T. Meinertz, W. Gaus, and M. Tendera, "The Efficacy and Safety of Crataegus Extract WS® 1442 in Patients With Heart Failure: the SPICE Trial," *European Journal of Heart Failure*, vol. 10, no. 12, pp. 1255–1263, 2008. doi:10.1016/j.ejheart.2008.10.004

Howatson, G., P. G. Bell, J. Tallent, B. Middleton, M. P. McHugh, and J. Ellis, "Effect of Tart Cherry Juice (Prunus cerasus) on Melatonin Levels and Enhanced Sleep Quality," *European Journal of Nutrition*, vol. 51, no. 8, pp. 909–916, 2012.

Huang, J., Y. Zhang, L. Dong, Q. Gao, L. Yin, H. Quan, and M. Dai, "Ethnopharmacology, Phytochemistry, and Pharmacology of Chinese Salvia Species: A Review," *Journal of Ethnopharmacology*, vol. 206, pp. 62–91, 2017. doi:10.1016/j.jep.2017.05.028

Huseini, H. F., S. Kianbakht, R. Hajiaghaee, and F. H. Dabaghian, "Anti-Hyperglycemic and Anti-Hypercholesterolemic Effects of Aloe vera Leaf Gel in Hyperlipidemic Type 2 Diabetic Patients: A Randomized Double-Blind Placebo-Controlled Clinical Trial," *Planta Medica*, vol. 78, no. 4, pp. 311–316, 2012.

Iffland, K., and F. Grotenhermen, "An Update on Safety and Side Effects of Cannabidiol: A Review of Clinical Data and Relevant Animal Studies," *Cannabis and Cannabinoid Research*, vol. 2, no. 1, pp. 139–154, 2017. doi:10.1089/can.2016.0034.

Inoue, N., F. Sugihara, and X. Wang, "Ingestion of Bioactive Collagen Hydrolysates Enhance Facial Skin Moisture and Elasticity and Reduce Facial Aging Signs in a Randomised Double-Blind Placebo-Controlled Clinical Study," *The Journal of the Science of Food and Agriculture*, *vol.* 96, pp. 4077–4081, 2016. doi:10.1002/jsfa.7606

Isbrucker, R. A., and G. A. Burdock, "Risk and Safety Assessment on the Consumption of Licorice Root (Glycyrrhiza Sp.), Its Extract and Powder as a Food Ingredient, With Emphasis on the Pharmacology and Toxicology of Glycyrrhizin," *Regulatory Toxicology and Pharmacology*, vol. 46, no. 3, pp. 167–192, 2006.

Ishaque, S., L. Shamseer, C. Bukutu, and S. Vohra, "*Rhodiola Rosea* for Physical and Mental Fatigue: A Systematic Review," BMC Complementary and Alternative Medicine, vol. 12, p. 70, 2012. doi:10.1186/1472-6882-12-70.

Izzo, A. A., "Drug Interactions With St. John's Wort (Hypericum perforatum): A Review of the Clinical Evidence," *International Journal of Clinical Pharmacology and Therapeutics*, vol. 42, no. 03, pp. 139–148, 2004. doi:10.5414/CPP42139

Jackman, S. R., O. C. Witard, A. Philp, G. A. Wallis, K. Baar, and K. D. Tipton, "Branched-Chain Amino Acid Ingestion Stimulates Muscle Myofibrillar Protein Synthesis Following Resistance Exercise in Humans," *Frontiers in Physiology*, vol. 8, p. 390, 2017. doi:10.3389/fphys.2017.00390.

Jepson, R. G., G. Williams, and J. C. Craig, "Cranberries for Preventing Urinary Tract Infections," *Cochrane Database Systematic Reviews*, vol. 10, no. 10, p. CD001321, 2012.

Jin, X., J. Ruiz Beguerie, D. M. Sze, and G. C. Chan, "*Ganoderma lucidum* (Reishi Mushroom) for Cancer Treatment," *Cochrane Database of Systematic Reviews*, vol. 4 no. 4, p. CD007731, 2016. doi:10.1002/14651858.CD007731.pub3.

Jorissen, B. L., F. Brouns, M. P. Van Boxtel, R. W. Ponds, F. R. Verhey, J. Jolles, and W. J. Riedel, "Safety of Soy-Derived Phosphatidylserine in Elderly People," *Nutritional Neuroscience*, vol. 5, no. 5, pp. 337–343, 2002.

Kapetanovic, I. M., M. Muzzio, Z. Huang, T. N. Thompson, and D. L. McCormick, "Pharmacokinetics, oral Bioavailability, and Metabolic Profile of Resveratrol and Its Dimethylether Analog, Pterostilbene, in Rats," *Cancer Chemotherapy and Pharmacology*, vol. 68, no. 3, pp. 593–601, 2011.

Keithley, J., and B. Swanson, "Glucomannan and Obesity: A Critical Review," *Alternative Therapies in Health and Medicine*, vol. 11, no. 6, pp. 30–34, 2005. https://pubmed.ncbi.nlm.nih.gov/16320857/

Khanna, R., J. K. MacDonald, and B. G. Levesque, "Peppermint Oil for the Treatment of Irritable Bowel Syndrome: A Systematic Review and Meta-Analysis," *Journal of Clinical Gastroenterology*, vol. 48, no. 6, pp. 505–512, 2014.

Khoo, H. E., A. Azlan, S. T. Tang, and S. M. Lim, "Anthocyanidins and Anthocyanins: Colored Pigments as Food, Pharmaceutical Ingredients, and the Potential Health Benefits," *Food & Nutrition Research*, vol. 61, no. 1, p. 1361779, 2017.

Kim, K. J., W. S. Sung, B. K. Suh, S. K. Moon, J. S. Choi, J. G. Kim, and D. G. Lee, "Antifungal Activity and Mode of Action of Silver Nano-Particles on Candida albicans," *Biometals*, vol. 22, no. 2, pp. 235–242, 2009.

Kimmatkar, N., V. Thawani, L. Hingorani, and R. Khiyani, "Efficacy and Tolerability of *Boswellia serrata* Extract in Treatment of Osteoarthritis of Knee – A Randomized Double Blind Placebo Controlled Trial," *Phytomedicine*, vol. 10, no. 1, pp. 3–7, 2003. doi:10.1078/094471103321648593

Kimura, K., M. Ozeki, L. R. Juneja, and H. Ohira, "L-Theanine Reduces Psychological and Physiological Stress Responses," *Biological Psychology*, vol. 74, no. 1, pp. 39–45, 2007. doi:10.1016/j.biopsycho.2006.06.006

Koehler, K., M. K. Parr, H. Geyer, J. Mester, and W. Schänzer, "Serum Testosterone and Urinary Excretion of Steroid Hormone Metabolites after Administration of a High-Dose Zinc Supplement," *European Journal of Clinical Nutrition*, vol. 63, no. 1, pp. 65–70, 2009.

Kolehmainen, M., O. Mykkänen, P. V. Kirjavainen, T. Leppänen, E. Moilanen, M. Adriaens, and L. Pulkkinen, "Bilberries Reduce Low-Grade Inflammation in Individuals With Features of Metabolic Syndrome," *Molecular Nutrition & Food Research*, vol. 56, no. 10, pp. 1501–1510, 2012. doi:10.1002/mnfr.201200195

Kreider, R. B., D. S. Kalman, J. Antonio, T. N. Ziegenfuss, R. Wildman, R. Collins, D. G. Candow, S. M. Kleiner, A. L. Almada, and H. L. Lopez, "International Society of Sports Nutrition Position Stand: Safety and Efficacy of Creatine Supplementation in Exercise, Sport, and Medicine," *Journal of the International Society of Sports Nutrition*, vol. 14, p. 18, 2017. doi:10.1186/s12970-017-0173-z.

Le, H. T., C. M. Schaldach, G. L. Firestone, and L. F. Bjeldanes, "Plant-Derived 3,3'-Diindolylmethane Is a Strong Androgen Antagonist in Human Prostate Cancer Cells," *Journal of Biological Chemistry*, vol. 278, no. 23, pp. 21136–21145, 2003.

Leach, M. J., and V. Moore, "Black Cohosh (Cimicifuga Spp.) for Menopausal Symptoms," *The Cochrane Database of Systematic Reviews*, vol. 2012, no. 9, p. CD007244, 2012. doi:10.1002/14651858.CD007244.pub2

Li, S. P., G. H. Zhang, Q. Zeng, Z. G. Huang, Y. T. Wang, T. T. X. Dong, and K. W. K. Tsim, "Hypoglycemic Activity of Polysaccharide, With Antioxidation, Isolated from Cultured *Cordyceps mycelia*," *Phytomedicine*, vol. 13, no. 6, 2006, pp. 428–433. doi:10.1016/j.phymed.2005.02.002.

Liu, X., G. C. Machado, J. P. Eyles, V. Ravi, and D. J. Hunter, "Dietary Supplements for Treating Osteoarthritis: A Systematic Review and Meta-Analysis," *British Journal of Sports Medicine*, vol. 52, no. 3, pp. 167–175, 2018.

Lukas, S. E., D. Penetar, J. Berko, L. Vicens, C. Palmer, G. Mallya, and D. Y. Lee, "An Extract of the Chinese Herbal Root Kudzu Reduces Alcohol Drinking by Heavy Drinkers in a Naturalistic Setting," *Alcoholism: Clinical and Experimental Research*, vol. 29, no. 5, pp. 756–762, 2005. doi:10.1097/01.ALC.0000163499.64347.92

Mahady, G. B., "Goldenseal (*Hydrastis canadensis*): Is There Enough Scientific Evidence to Support Safety and Efficacy?" *Nutrition in Clinical Care: An Official Publication of Tufts University*, vol. 4, no. 5, pp. 243–249, 2001.

Mahady, G. B., J. Parrot, C. Lee, G. S. Yun, and A. Dan, "Botanical Dietary Supplement Use in Peri- and Postmenopausal Women," *Menopause*, vol. 10, no. 1, pp. 65–72, 2003. doi:10.1097/00042192-200310010-00011

Markowiak, P., and K. Śliżewska, "Effects of Probiotics, Prebiotics, and Synbiotics on Human Health," *Nutrients*, vol. 9, no. 9, p. 1021, 2017. doi:10.3390/nu9091021.

Marles, R. J., M. L. Barrett, J. Barnes, M. L. Chavez, P. Gardiner, R. Ko, G. B. Mahady, T. Low Dog, N. D. Sarma, G. I. Giancaspro, M. Sharaf, and J. Griffiths, "United States Pharmacopeia Safety Evaluation of Spirulina," *Critical Reviews in Food Science and Nutrition*, vol. 51, no. 7, pp. 593–604, 2011. doi:10.1080/10408391003721719.

Martinez-Zapata, M. J., R. W. Vernooij, S. M. Uriona Tuma, A. T. Stein, R. M. Moreno, E. Vargas, D. Capellà, and X. Bonfill Cosp, "Phlebotonics for Venous Insufficiency," *Cochrane Database of Systematic Reviews*, no. 4, p. CD003229, 2016.

Mayo Clinic, Caffeine: How much is too much? Mayo Foundation for Medical Education and Research, 8 March 2020, www.mayoclinic.org/healthy-lifestyle/nutrition-and-healthy-eating/in-depth/caffeine/art-20045678.

Mazzanti, G., F. Menniti-Ippolito, P. A. Moro, F. Cassetti, R. Raschetti, C. Santuccio, and S. Mastrangelo, "Hepatotoxicity from Green Tea: A Review of the Literature and Two Unpublished Cases," *The European Journal of Clinical Pharmacology*, vol. 65, no. 4, pp. 331–341, 2009. doi:10.1007/s00228-008-0610-7.

McCormack, D., and D. McFadden, "Pterostilbene and Cancer: Current Review," *Journal of Surgical Research*, vol. 173, no. 2, pp. e53–e61, 2012.

McLean, A. Jr., D. D. Cardenas, D. Burgess, and E. Gamzu, "Placebo-Controlled Study of Pramiracetam in Young Males With Memory and Cognitive Problems Resulting from Head Injury and Anoxia," *Brain Injury*, vol. 5, no. 4, pp. 375–380, 1991.

McRorie, J. W. Jr., and N. M. McKeown, "Understanding the Physics of Functional Fibers in the Gastrointestinal Tract: An Evidence-Based Approach to Resolving Enduring Misconceptions About Insoluble and Soluble Fiber," *Journal of the Academy of Nutrition and Dietetics*, vol. 117, no. 2, pp. 251–264, 2017. doi:10.1016/j.jand.2016.09.021.

Melatonin: What You Need To Know, National Center for Complementary and Integrative Health, U.S. Department of Health and Human Services, 1 Sept. 2020, www.nccih.nih.gov/health/melatonin-what-you-need-to-know.

Mirzoian, R. S., and T. S. Gan'shina, "[The Use of Pikamilon in the Treatment of Anxiety Disorders]," *Zh Nevrol Psychiatrist Im S S Korsakova*, vol. 106, no. 12, pp. 52–56, 2006. (Russian)

Mori, K., Y. Obara, M. Hirota, Y. Azumi, S. Kinugasa, S. Inatomi, and N. Nakahata, "Nerve Growth Factor-Inducing Activity of *Hericium erinaceus* in 1321N1 Human Astrocytoma Cells," *Biological and Pharmaceutical Bulletin*, vol. 31, no. 9, pp. 1727–1732, 2008. doi:10.1248/bpb.31.1727.

Nakamura, K., "Aniracetam: Its Novel Therapeutic Potential in Cerebral Dysfunctional Disorders Based on Recent Pharmacological Discoveries," *CNS Drug Reviews*, vol. 8, no. 1, pp. 70–89, 2002.

Nakano, S., H. Takekoshi, and M. Nakano, "Chlorella (*Chlorella pyrenoidosa*) Supplementation Decreases Dioxin and Increases Immunoglobulin A Concentrations in Breast Milk," *Journal of Medicinal Food*, vol. 10, pp. 134–42, 2007. doi:10.1089/jmf.2006.023.

National Center for Complementary and Integrative Health (NCCIH), bilberry, 2016. https://nccih.nih.gov/health/bilberry

National Center for Complementary and Integrative Health (NCCIH), black cohosh, 2020. https://nccih.nih.gov/health/blackcohosh/ataglance.htm

National Center for Complementary and Integrative Health (NCCIH), Horse Chestnut, 2016. https://nccih.nih.gov/health/horsechestnut

National Center for Complementary and Integrative Health (NCCIH), Red Clover, 2016. https://nccih.nih.gov/health/redclover/ataglance.htm

Nawrot, P., S. Jordan, J. Eastwood, J. Rotstein, A. Hugenholtz, and M. Feeley, "Effects of Caffeine on Human Health," *Food Additives & Contaminants*, vol. 20, no. 1, pp. 1–30, 2003. doi:10.1080/0265203021000007840.

Neelakantan, N., M. Narayanan, R. J. de Souza, and R. M. van Dam, "Effect of Fenugreek (*Trigonella foenum-graecum* L.) Intake on Glycemia: A Meta-Analysis of Clinical Trials," *Nutrition Journal*, vol. 13, p. 7, 2014. doi:10.1186/1475-2891-13-7

Nirvanashetty, S., S. K. Panda, and S. Jackson-Michel, "Safety Evaluation of Oleoresin-Based Turmeric Formulation: Assessment of Genotoxicity and Acute and Subchronic Oral Toxicity," *BioMed Research International*, eCollection, 2022. doi:10.1155/2022/5281660.

Nohr, L. A., L. B. Rasmussen, and J. Straand, "Resin from the mukul Myrrh Tree, Guggul, can It Be Used for Treating Hypercholesterolemia? A Randomized, Controlled Study," *Complementary Therapies in Medicine*, vol. 17, no. 1, pp. 16–22, 2009.

Nostro, A., and T. Papalia, "Antimicrobial Activity of Carvacrol: Current Progress and Future Prospectives," *Recent Patents on Anti-infective Drug Discovery*, vol. 7, no. 1, pp. 28–35, 2012.

Obolskiy, D., I. Pischel, N. Siriwatanametanon, and M. Heinrich, "Garcinia Mangostana L.: A Phytochemical and Pharmacological Review," *Phytotherapy Research*, vol. 23, no. 8, pp. 1047–1065, 2009. doi:10.1002/ptr.2730

Oliveira de Souza, M., M. Silva, M. E. Silva, O. R. de Paula, and M. L. Pedrosa, "Diet Supplementation With Acai (*Euterpe oleracea* Mart.) Pulp Improves Biomarkers of Oxidative Stress and the serum Lipid Profile in Rats," *Nutrition*, vol. 26, no. 7-8, pp. 804–810, 2010. doi:10.1016/j.nut.2009.09.007

Onakpoya, I., S. K. Hung, R. Perry, B. Wider, and E. Ernst, "The Use of Garcinia Extract (hydroxycitric Acid) as a Weight Loss Supplement: A Systematic Review and Meta-Analysis of Randomized Clinical Trials," *Journal of Obesity*, vol. 2011, p. 509038, 2011. doi:10.1155/2011/509038

Onakpoya, I., R. Terry, and E. Ernst, "The Use of Green Coffee Extract as a Weight Loss Supplement: A Systematic Review and Meta-Analysis of Randomized Clinical Trials," *Gastroenterology Research and Practice*, vol. 2011, p. 382852, 2011.

Ostad, S. N., M. Soodi, M. Shariffzadeh, N. Khorshidi, and H. Marzban, "The Effect of Fennel Essential Oil on Uterine Contraction as a Model for Dysmenorrhea, Pharmacology and Toxicology Study," *Journal of Ethnopharmacology*, vol. 76, no. 3, pp. 299–304, 2001.

Ostrovskaya, R. U., M. A. Gruden, N. A. Bobkova, R. D. Sewell, T. A. Gudasheva, A. N. Samokhin, S. B. Seredinin, W. Noppe, V. V. Sherstnev, and L. A. Morozova-Roche, "The Nootropic and Neuroprotective

Proline-Containing Dipeptide Noopept Restores Spatial Memory and Increases Immunoreactivity to Amyloid in an Alzheimer's Disease Model," *Journal of Psychopharmacology*, vol. 21, no. 6, pp. 611–619, 2007.

Pahlavani, N., M. Jafari, O. Sadeghi, M. Rezaei, H. Rasad, H. A. Rahdar, and M. H. Entezari, "L-Arginine Supplementation and Risk Factors of Cardiovascular Diseases in Healthy Men: A Double-Blind Randomized Clinical Trial," *F1000Research*, vol. 3, p. 306, 2017. doi:10.12688/f1000research.5877.2

Panossian, A., and G. Wikman, "Pharmacology of Schisandra chinensis Bail.: An Overview of Russian Research and Uses in Medicine," *J Ethnopharmacol*, vol. 118, no. Jul 23;2, pp. 183–212, 2008.

Pasiakos, S. M., T. M. McLellan, and H. R. Lieberman, "The Effects of Protein Supplements on Muscle Mass, Strength, and Aerobic and Anaerobic Power in Healthy Adults: A Systematic Review," *Sports Medicine*, vol. 45, no. 1, pp. 111–131, 2015.

Patel, K. R., E. Scott, V. A. Brown, A. J. Gescher, W. P. Steward, and K. Brown, "Clinical Trials of Resveratrol," *Annals of the New York Academy of Sciences*, vol. 1215, no. 1, pp. 161–169, 2011.

Patel, S., and A. Goyal, "Recent Developments in Mushrooms as Anti-Cancer Therapeutics: A Review," *3 Biotech*, vol. 2, no. 1, pp. 1–15, 2012.

Pattanayak, P., P. Behera, D. Das, and S. K. Panda, "Ocimum sanctum Linn. A Reservoir Plant for Therapeutic Applications: An Overview," *Pharmacognosy Reviews*, vol. 4, no. 7, 2010, p. 95–105. doi:10.4103/0973-7847.65323.

Pawlus, A. D., and A. D. Kinghorn, "Review of the Ethnobotany, Chemistry, Biological Activity and Safety of the Botanical Dietary Supplement *Morinda citrifolia* (noni)," *Journal of Pharmacy and Pharmacology*, vol. 59, no. 12, pp. 1587–1609, 2007. doi:10.1211/jpp.59.12.0001

Pedraza-Chaverri, J., N. Cárdenas-Rodríguez, M. Orozco-Ibarra, and J. M. Pérez-Rojas, "Medicinal Properties of Mangosteen (*Garcinia mangostana*)," *Food and Chemical Toxicology*, vol. 46, no. 10, pp. 3227–3239, 2008. doi:10.1016/j.fct.2008.07.024

Penniston, K. L., and S. A. Tanumihardjo, "The Acute and Chronic Toxic Effects of Vitamin A," *The American Journal of Clinical Nutrition*, vol. 83, no. 2, pp. 191–201, 2006. doi: 10.1093/ajcn/83.2.191.

Peterson, C. T., K. Denniston, and D. Chopra, "Therapeutic Uses of Triphala in Ayurvedic Medicine," *The Journal of Alternative and Complementary Medicine*, vol. 23, no. 8, pp. 607–614, 2017.

Petropoulos, S., F. Di Gioia, G. Polizzi, M. Papademetriou, S. Sampaio, A. Alexopoulos, V. Gkoutzioulias, and K. Tzima, "Fenugreek (*Trigonella foenum-graecum* L.): An Overview of the Past and a look into the Future," *Food Reviews International*, vol. 37, no. 1, pp. 77–125, 2021. doi:10.1080/87559129.2020.1743734

Piscoya, J., Z. Rodriguez, S. A. Bustamante, N. N. Okuhama, M. J. Miller, and M. Sandoval, "Efficacy and Safety of Freeze-Dried cat's Claw in Osteoarthritis of the Knee: Mechanisms of Action of the Species Uncaria guianensis," *Inflammation Research*, vol. 50, no. 9, pp. 442–448, 2001.

Pittler, M. H., and E. Ernst, "Horse Chestnut Seed Extract for Chronic Venous Insufficiency," *The Cochrane Database of Systematic Reviews*, vol. 2012, no. 11, p. CD003230, 2012. doi:10.1002/14651858.CD003230.pub4

Pittler, M. H., and E. Ernst, "Feverfew for Preventing Migraine," *The Cochrane Database of Systematic Reviews*, no. 1, p. CD002286, 2004.

Pittler, M. H., and E. Ernst, "Kava Extract for Treating Anxiety," *The Cochrane Database of Systematic Reviews*, no. 1, p. CD003383, 2003. doi:10.1002/14651858.cd003383.

Pittler, M. H., R. Guo, and E. Ernst, "Hawthorn Extract for Treating Chronic Heart Failure," *The Cochrane Database of Systematic Reviews*, no. 1, p. CD005312, 2008. doi:10.1002/14651858.CD005312.pub2

Potterat, O., "Goji (*Lycium barbarum* and *L. chinense*): Phytochemistry, Pharmacology and Safety in the Perspective of Traditional Uses and Recent Popularity," *Planta Medica*, vol. 76, no. 1, pp. 7–19, 2010. doi:10.1055/s-0029-1186218

Pratte, M. A., K. B. Nanavati, V. Young, and C. P. Morley, "An Alternative Treatment for Anxiety: A Systematic Review of Human Trial Results Reported for the Ayurvedic Herb Ashwagandha (*Withania somnifera*)," *The Journal of Alternative and Complementary Medicine*, vol. 20, no. 12, pp. 901–908, 2014. doi:10.1089/acm.2014.0177.

Prebiotics: What You Need to Know, Mayo Clinic, Mayo Foundation for Medical Education and Research, 7 Oct. 2020, www.mayoclinic.org/prebiotics-probiotics-and-your-health/art-20390058.

Probiotics: What You Need to Know, National Center for Complementary and Integrative Health, U.S. Department of Health and Human Services, 1 Aug. 2019, www.nccih.nih.gov/health/probiotics-what-you-need-to-know.

Proksch, E., D. Segger, J. Degwert, M. Schunck, V. Zague, and S. Oesser, "Oral Supplementation of Specific Collagen Peptides Has Beneficial Effects on Human Skin Physiology: A Double-Blind, Placebo-Controlled Study," *Skin Pharmacology and Physiology*, vol. 27, no. 1, pp. 47–55, 2014. doi:10.1159/000351376

Rafii, M. S., S. Walsh, J. T. Little, K. Behan, B. Reynolds, C. Ward, S. Jin, R. Thomas, and P. S. Aisen, "A Phase II Trial of Huperzine A in Mild to Moderate Alzheimer's Disease," *Neurology*, vol. 76, no. Apr 19;16, pp. 1389–1394, 2011.

Rajoria, S., R. Suriano, A. Shanmugam, Y. L. Wilson, S. P. Schantz, J. Geliebter, and R. K. Tiwari, "Metastatic Phenotype Is Regulated by Estrogen in Thyroid Cells," *Thyroid*, vol. 20, no. 1, pp. 33–41, 2010.

Ried, K., C. Toben, and P. Fakler, "Effect of Garlic on serum Lipids: An Updated Meta-Analysis," *Nutrition Reviews*, vol. 71, no. 5, pp. 282–299, 2013.

Rohdewald, P., "A Review of the French Maritime Pine Bark Extract (Pycnogenol), a Herbal Medication With a Diverse Clinical Pharmacology," *International Journal of Clinical Pharmacology and Therapeutics*, vol. 40, no. 4, pp. 158–168, 2002. doi:10.5414/cpp40158

Roodenrys, S., D. Booth, S. Bulzomi, A. Phipps, C. Micallef, and J. Smoker, "Chronic Effects of Brahmi (*Bacopa monnieri*) on Human Memory," *Neuropsychopharmacology*, vol. 27, no. 2, pp. 279–81, 2002.

Sabelli, H., P. Fink, J. Fawcett, and C. Tom, "Sustained Antidepressant Effect of PEA Replacement," *The Journal of Neuropsychiatry and Clinical Neurosciences*, vol. 8, no. 2, pp. 168–171, 1996.

Sadlon, A. E., and D. W. Lamson, "Immune-Modifying and Antimicrobial Effects of Eucalyptus Oil and Simple Inhalation Devices," *Alternative Medicine Review*, vol. 15, no. 1, pp. 33–47, 2010.

Saller, R., J., Reichling, R. Brignoli, and R. Meier, "An Updated Systematic Review of the Pharmacology of Silymarin," *Forschende Komplementärmedizin/Research in Complementary Medicine*, vol. 13, no. 2, 2006, p. 20–29. doi:10.1159/000093765.

Schapowal, A., P. Klein, and S. L. Johnston, "Echinacea Reduces the Risk of Recurrent Respiratory Tract Infections and Complications: A Meta-Analysis of Randomized Controlled Trials," *Advances in Therapy*, vol. 32, no. 3, pp. 187–200. doi:10.1007/s12325-015-0194-4.

Schauss, A. G., X. Wu, R. L. Prior, B. Ou, D. Patel, D. Huang, and J. P. Kababick, "Phytochemical and Nutrient Composition of the Freeze-Dried Amazonian Palm Berry, Euterpe Oleraceae Mart. (Acai)," *Journal of Agricultural and Food Chemistry*, vol. 54, no. 22, pp. 8598–8603, 2006. doi:10.1021/jf060976g

Schoonees, A., J. Visser, A. Musekiwa, and J. Volmink, "Pycnogenol® (Extract of French Maritime Pine Bark) for the Treatment of Chronic Disorders," *Cochrane Database System Rev*, vol. 2012, no. 4, p. CD008294, 2012. doi:10.1002/14651858.CD008294.pub4

Schwab, U., A. Törrönen, L. Toppinen, G. Alfthan, M. Saarinen, A. Aro, and M. Uusitupa, "Betaine Supplementation Decreases Plasma Homocysteine Concentrations but Does Not Affect Body Weight, Body Composition, or Resting Energy Expenditure in Human Subjects," *The American Journal of Clinical Nutrition*, vol. 76, no. 5, pp. 961–967, 2002.

Schwedhelm, E., R. Maas, R. Freese, D. Jung, Z. Lukacs, A. Jambrecina, and R. H. Böger, "Pharmacokinetic and Pharmacodynamic Properties of Oral L-Citrulline and L-Arginine: Impact on Nitric Oxide Metabolism," *British Journal of Clinical Pharmacology*, vol. 65, no. 1, pp. 51–59, 2008. doi:10.1111/j.1365-2125.2007.02990.x

Shams, T., M. S. Setia, R. Hemmings, J. McCusker, M. Sewitch, and A. Ciampi, "Efficacy of Black Cohosh-Containing Preparations on Menopausal Symptoms: A Meta-Analysis," *Alternative Therapies in Health and Medicine*, vol. 16, no. 1, pp. 36–44, 2010.

Shara, M., and S. J. Stohs, "Efficacy and Safety of White Willow Bark (Salix alba) Extracts," *Phytotherapy Research*, vol. 29, no. 8, pp. 1112–1116, 2015. doi:10.1002/ptr.5377

Shergis, J. L., A. L. Zhang, W. Zhou, and C. C. Xue, "Panax Ginseng in Randomized Controlled Trials: A Systematic Review," *Phytotherapy Research*, vol. 27, no. 7, pp. 949–965, 2013. doi:10.1002/ptr.4832.

Shoskes, D. A., S. I. Zeitlin, A. Shahed, and J. Rajfer, "Quercetin in Men With Category III Chronic Prostatitis: A Preliminary Prospective, Double-Blind, Placebo-Controlled Trial," *Urology*, vol. 54, no. 6, pp. 960–963, 1999.

Silveri, M. M., J. Dikan, A. J. Ross, J. E. Jensen, T. Kamiya, Y. Kawada, P. F. Renshaw, and D. A. Yurgelun-Todd, "Citicoline Enhances Frontal Lobe Bioenergetics as Measured by Phosphorus Magnetic Resonance Spectroscopy," *NMR in Biomedicine: An International Journal Devoted to the Development and Application of Magnetic Resonance In vivo*, vol. 21, no. 10, pp. 1066–1075, 2008.

Sinescu, I., P. Geavlete, R. Multescu, C. Gangu, F. Miclea, I. Coman, I. Ioiart, V. Ambert, T. Constantin, B. Petrut, and B. Feriche, "Long-Term Efficacy of Serenoa repens Treatment in Patients With Mild and Moderate Symptomatic Benign Prostatic Hyperplasia," *Urologia Internationalis*, vol. 86, no. 3, 2011, p. 284–289. doi:10.1159/000322645.

Spirulina, National Center for Complementary and Integrative Health, U.S. Department of Health and Human Services, 1 Sept. 2020, www.nccih.nih.gov/health/spirulina.

Srinivasan, K., "Biological Activities of Red Pepper (Capsicum annuum) and Its Pungent Principle Capsaicin: A Review," *Critical Reviews in Food Science and Nutrition*, vol. 56, no. 9, pp. 1488–1500, 2016.

Srinivasan, K., "Black Pepper and Its Pungent Principle-Piperine: A Review of Diverse Physiological Effects," *Critical Reviews in Food Science and Nutrition*, vol. 47, no. 8, pp. 735–748, 2007.

Srivastava, J. K., E. Shankar, and S. Gupta, "Chamomile: A Herbal Medicine of the Past With a Bright Future (Review)," *Molecular Medicine Reports*, vol. 3, no. 6, pp. 895–901, 2010.

St. John's Wort and Depression: In Depth, National Center for Complementary and Integrative Health, U.S. Department of Health and Human Services, 1 Sept. 2020, www.nccih.nih.gov/health/st-johns-wort-and-depression-in-depth.

Stabler, S. P., "Vitamin B12 Deficiency," *The New England Journal of Medicine*, vol. 368, pp. 149–160, 2013.

Stohs, S. J., and M. J. Hartman, "Review of the Safety and Efficacy of Moringa oleifera," *Phytotherapy Research*, vol. 29, no. 6, pp. 796–804, 2015. doi:10.1002/ptr.5325.

Subiza, J., J. L. Subiza, M. Hinojosa, R. Garcia, M. Jerez, R. Valdivieso, and E. Subiza, "Anaphylactic Reaction after the Ingestion of Chamomile Tea; a Study of Cross-Reactivity With Other Composite Pollens," *Journal of Allergy and Clinical Immunology*, vol. 74, no. 2, pp. 269–272, 1994.

Suryawan, A., J. W. Hawes, R. A. Harris, Y. Shimomura, A. E. Jenkins, and S. M. Hutson, "A Molecular Model of Human Branched-Chain Amino Acid Metabolism," *The American Journal of Clinical Nutrition*, vol. 68, no. 1, pp. 72–81, 1998. doi:10.1093/ajcn/68.1.72.

Susalit, E., N. Agus, I. Effendi, R. R. Tjandrawinata, D. Nofiarny, T. Perrinjaquet-Moccetti, and M. Verbruggen, "Olive (Olea europaea) Leaf Extract Effective in Patients With Stage-1 Hypertension: Comparison With Captopril," *Phytomedicine*, vol. 18, no. 4, pp. 251–258, 2011.

Sutovska, M., G. Nosalova, J. Sutovsky, L. Franova, L. Prisenzňaková, and P. Capek, "Possible Mechanisms of Dose-Dependent Cough Suppressive Effect of Althaea officinalis Rhamnogalacturonan in Guinea Pigs Test System," *International Journal of Biological Macromolecules*, vol. 45, no. 1, pp. 27–32, 2009.

Swanson, D., R. Block, and S. A. Mousa, "Omega-3 Fatty Acids EPA and DHA: Health Benefits Throughout Life," *Advances in Nutrition*, vol. 3, no. 1, pp. 1–7, 2012. doi:10.3945/an.111.000893

Taku, K., M. K. Melby, F. Kronenberg, M. S. Kurzer, and M. Messina, "Extracted or Synthesized Soybean Isoflavones Reduce Menopausal Hot Flash Frequency and Severity: Systematic Review and Meta-Analysis of Randomized Controlled Trials," *Menopause*, vol. 19, no. 7, pp. 776–790, 2012.

Talbott, S. M., J. A. Talbott, T. L. Talbott, and E. Dingler, "β-Glucan Supplementation, Allergy Symptoms, and Quality of Life in Self-Described Ragweed Allergy Sufferers," *Food Science & Nutrition*, vol. 1, no. 1, pp. 90–101, 2013.

Tan, M. S., J. T. Yu, C. C. Tan, H. F. Wang, X. F. Meng, C. Wang, T. Jiang, X. C. Zhu, and L. Tan, "Efficacy and Adverse Effects of Ginkgo biloba for Cognitive Impairment and Dementia: A Systematic Review and Meta- Analysis," *Journal of Alzheimer's Disease*, vol. 43, no. 2, pp. 589–603, 2015. doi:10.3233/JAD-140837.

Tankanow, R., H. R. Tamer, D. S. Streetman, S. G. Smith, J. L. Welton, T. Annesley, and B. E. Bleske, "Interaction Study between Digoxin and a Preparation of Hawthorn (Crataegus oxyacantha)," *Journal of Clinical Pharmacology*, vol. 43, no. 6, pp. 637–642, 2003. doi:10.1177/0091270003043006009

Tarozzi, A., C. Angeloni, M. Malaguti, F. Morroni, S. Hrelia, and P. Hrelia, "Sulforaphane as a Potential Protective Phytochemical Against Neurodegenerative Diseases," *Oxidative Medicine and Cellular Longevity*, vol. 2013, p. 415078, 2013.

Tice, J. A., B. Ettinger, K. Ensrud, R. Wallace, T. Blackwell, and S. R. Cummings, "Phytoestrogen Supplements for the Treatment of Hot Flashes: The Isoflavone Clover Extract (ICE) Study: A Randomized Controlled Trial," *JAMA*, vol. 290, no. 2, pp. 207–214, 2003. doi:10.1001/jama.290.2.207

Unfer, V., F. Facchinetti, B. Orrù, B. Giordani, and J. Nestler, "Myo-Inositol Effects in Women With PCOS: A Meta-Analysis of Randomized Controlled Trials," *Endocrine Connections*, vol. 6, no. 8, pp. 647–658, 2017.

Verma, S. K., V. Jain, and S. S. Katewa, "Blood Pressure Lowering, Fibrinolysis Enhancing and Antioxidant Activities of Cardamom (Elettaria Cardamomum)," *The Indian Journal of Biochemistry and Biophysics*, vol. 46, no. 6, pp. 503–6, 2009.

Traber, M. G., "Vitamin E Inadequacy in Humans: Causes and Consequences," *Advances in Nutrition*, vol. 5, no. 5, pp. 503–514, 2014. doi: 10.3945/an.114.006254

Wachtel-Galor, S., Y. T. Szeto, B. Tomlinson, and I. F. Benzie, "*Ganoderma lucidum* ('Lingzhi'); Acute and Short-Term Biomarker Response to Supplementation," *International Journal of Food Sciences and Nutrition*, vol. 55, no. 1, 2004, p. 75–83. doi:10.1080/09637480310001642510.

Wadhera, A., and M. Fung, "Systemic Argyria Associated With Ingestion of Colloidal Silver," *Dermatology Online Journal*, vol. 11, no. 1, p. 12, 2005.

Wang, Y., X. Han, Y. D. Li, Y. Wang, S. Y. Zhao, D. J. Zhang, and Y. Lu, "Lentinan Dose Dependence between Immunoprophylaxis and Promotion of the Murine Liver Cancer," *Oncotarget.*, vol. 8, no. 56, pp. 95152–95162, 2017. doi:10.18632/oncotarget.19808

Watson, H., and S. Mitra, "Safety Profile of Omega-3 Fatty Acid Supplements," *Omega-3 Fatty Acids*, 139–149. doi:10.1007/978-3-030-10519-8_9

West, B. J., S. Deng, A. K. Palu, and C. J. Jensen, "*Morinda citrifolia* (Noni) Improves Athlete Endurance: Its Mechanisms of Action," *Journal of Dietary Supplements*, vol. 6, no. 3, pp. 247–258, 2009. doi:10.1080/19390210903070819

Widrig, R., A. Suter, R. Saller, and J. Melzer, "Choosing between NSAID and Arnica for Topical Treatment of Hand Osteoarthritis in a Randomised, Double-Blind Study," *Rheumatology International*, vol. 27, no. 6, pp. 585–591, 2007.

Wilson, J. M., P. J. Fitschen, B. Campbell, G. J. Wilson, N. Zanchi, L. Taylor, C. Wilborn, D. S. Kalman, J. R. Stout, J. R. Hoffman, T. N. Ziegenfuss, H. L. Lopez, R. B. Kreider, A. E. Smith-Ryan, and J. Antonio, "International Society of Sports Nutrition Position Stand: Beta-Hydroxy-Beta-Methylbutyrate (HMB)," *Journal of the International Society of Sports Nutrition*, vol. 10, no. 1, p. 6, 2013.

Zakay-Rones, Z., E. Thom, T. Wollan, and J. Wadstein, "Randomized Study of the Efficacy and Safety of Oral Elderberry Extract in the Treatment of Influenza A and B Virus Infections," *Journal of International Medical Research*, vol. 32, no. 2, pp. 132–140, 2004. doi:10.1177/147323000403200205

Zare, R., F. Heshmati, H. Fallahzadeh, and A. Nadjarzadeh, "Effect of Cumin Powder on Body Composition and Lipid Profile in Overweight and Obese Women," *Complementary Therapies in Clinical Practice*, vol. 20, no. 4, pp. 297–301, 2014.

Zeisel, S. H., and K. A. da Costa, "Choline: An Essential Nutrient for Public Health," *Nutrition Reviews*, vol. 67, no. 11, pp. 615–623, 2009.

Zhang, Y., and L. Tang, "Discovery and Development of Sulforaphane as a Cancer Chemopreventive Phytochemical," *Acta Pharmacologica Sinica*, vol. 28, no. 9, pp. 1343–1354, 2007.

Ziegler, D., A. Ametov, A. Barinov, P. J. Dyck, I. Gurieva, P. A. Low, U. Munzel, N. Yakhno, I. Raz, M. Novosadova, J. Maus, and R. Samigullin, "Oral Treatment With Alpha-Lipoic Acid Improves Symptomatic Diabetic Polyneuropathy: The SYDNEY 2 Trial," *Diabetes Care*, vol. 29, no. 11, pp. 2365–2370, 2006.

Zvejniece, L., B. Svalbe, G. Veinberg, S. Grinberga, M. Vorona, I. Kalvinsh, and M. Dambrova, "Investigation into Stereoselective Pharmacological Activity of Phenotropil," *Basic & Clinical Pharmacology & Toxicology*, vol. 109, no. 4, pp. 407–412, 2011.

6 Ethical and Regulatory Concerns in Natural Health Sciences

Ethical and regulatory issues in the natural health sciences often parallel the ethical and regulatory issues of traditional medicine and scientific methodology. However, the natural health sciences have some characteristics that sometimes differ from traditional medicine, and this raises its own unique ethical and regulatory issues.

6.1 ETHICAL MATTERS

The ethical issues of the natural health sciences often focus on issues such as consumer awareness, information sharing, lack of scientific evidence, and misleading marketing practices.

6.1.1 Consumer Awareness

Users of natural health products and practices often have incomplete or misleading information about the safety and efficacy of the products. This raises the responsibility of natural health practitioners to provide their patients with complete and accurate information about the potential risks and limitations of these products [1].

Consumer awareness has a critical role to play in the natural health sciences. When it comes to both traditional and alternative health practices, it is important for individuals to be informed in their decision-making process, to choose the right options and to receive effective treatment.

Users of natural health products and therapies often have incomplete or misleading information about the safety and efficacy of products and practices. This raises the responsibility of natural health practitioners to provide their patients with complete and accurate information about the potential risks and limitations of these products [1]. This has become the health practitioner's ethical obligation as part of sharing information.

If product labels and descriptions are misleading or incomplete, it may be possible for consumers to have a misleading perception of a product's effectiveness, safety, and potential side effects. This can lead consumers to use potentially harmful or ineffective products and make the wrong decisions that can worsen their health [2].

Lack of information, misleading information, or incomprehensible information can make it difficult or even impossible for consumers to make the right health decisions. Therefore, it is the responsibility of natural health practitioners, regulators, and policymakers to ensure that consumers have access to accurate and understandable information. This awareness-raising process is necessary for users to be able to make informed decisions about natural health products and therapies [1].

Consumer awareness also enables natural health practitioners to deliver their services in an ethical and professional manner. When patients receive the information, they need to understand treatment options and actively participate in treatment processes, they can achieve better health outcomes [2].

DOI: 10.1201/9781003520252-7

6.1.2   Information Sharing

Natural health practitioners have an obligation to provide their patients and other health care providers with clear and accurate information about the natural health practices and products used. They should also provide the information needed to enable patients to make informed decisions about their own health conditions and treatment options [2].

Sharing information is an important ethical issue in the natural health sciences. An open and honest exchange of information between practitioners and consumers promotes effective and safe treatment processes. Information sharing helps practitioners and consumers make informed decisions about healthcare, treatment options, and potential risks.

Natural health practitioners have an obligation to provide their patients and other health care providers with clear and accurate information about the natural health practices and products used. This information may be about how effective a treatment is, under what conditions it should be used, its potential side effects and risks, and how it interacts with other treatment options [2].

However, for information sharing to be effective, information must be accurate, up-to-date, and based on scientific evidence. Misleading, incomplete, or outdated information can cause consumers to make erroneous decisions or be unnecessarily skeptical of healthcare.

Another aspect of information sharing is its enablement of patients to make informed decisions about their own health conditions and treatment options. When sharing information with their patients, practitioners need to communicate in a language and style that patients can understand. Thus, patients can better understand treatment processes and possible outcomes and have more control over their own health status [1].

There are numerous studies that emphasize the importance of information sharing in natural health sciences. These studies show that sharing information can positively influence patients' treatment processes and outcomes. Therefore, information sharing is recognized as a fundamental part of ethical practices in the natural health sciences [2].

6.1.3   Lack of Scientific Evidence

Natural health products and practices generally do not face the same level of scrutiny and regulation as scientifically proven treatment methods. This can make it difficult for users and practitioners to determine whether a treatment really works or is potentially harmful [1].

6.1.4   Misleading Marketing Practices

Some natural health products and services may be marketed with misleading or exaggerated claims. This can lead consumers to purchase and use harmful or ineffective products [2].

6.2   REGULATORY AFFAIRS

The regulatory issues of the natural health sciences often include issues such as the regulation of products and services, licensing, education and standards, and the circulation of counterfeit products.

In the natural health sciences, regulatory bodies play an important role in determining the safety, effectiveness, and quality of practices and products in this field. However, regulation of natural health practices and products can be handled differently in various countries, which can affect both practitioners and consumers.

The primary regulatory issues relate to how the safety and efficacy of natural health practices and products are proven and evaluated. In many countries, the issue of whether natural health products and practices are subject to the same regulatory standards as other health products, such as medicines and medical devices, is controversial [3].

Many countries have specific regulations on the marketing and sale of natural health products. However, these regulations often vary from country to country and often allow conclusions to be drawn about the safety or effectiveness of a product without sufficient scientific evidence [3].

Regulation of natural health practices also includes training and certification of practitioners. In many countries, natural health practitioners are subject to regulations that require them to have a certain level of education and to provide practices that meet certain standards. The enforcement and supervision of these regulations depend, in most cases, on regulatory authorities [3].

Dissolving regulatory issues in the natural health sciences is important to ensure the safety and effectiveness of practices and products in this field. However, this requires practitioners, regulators, and policymakers to work together to ensure the scientifically proven safety and efficacy of natural health practices and products [3].

6.2.1 Regulation of Products and Services

Regulation of natural health products and services is often important to ensure consumer reassurance. However, the inadequacy or lack of these regulations can lead to the provision of potentially harmful or ineffective products and services to consumers [1, 4].

In the natural health sciences, products and services are often regulated differently than traditional medical practices and products. This is mainly because natural health products and services are often based on long-standing traditions and are generally not supported by scientific research or to a lesser extent supported.

Regulation of natural health products, in most countries, includes certain categories, such as nutritional supplements, herbal remedies, and homeopathic products. There are various regulations on the labeling, safety standards, marketing practices, and production processes of these products [5]. These regulations are generally intended to provide safe and effective products to consumers.

The regulation of natural health care often focuses on practitioners, which requires specific training and certification. Practices such as acupuncture, massage therapy, naturopathy, and chiropractic are generally subject to specific training and licensing requirements [6]. However, these regulations may vary from country to country.

The regulation of both natural health products and services is aimed at protecting the consumer and protecting public health. However, the effectiveness and enforceability of these regulations depend on several factors, such as the scientific evidence of products and services, the training of practitioners, and the supervisory ability of regulatory authorities.

6.2.2 Licensing

The training and licensing requirements for natural health practitioners are often not the same as those for traditional medical practitioners. This means that there can be a wide variation between education and skill levels which can pose a potential risk to consumers [2].

Licensing in natural health sciences is a process that certifies that practitioners have reached a certain level of education and provide services that meet certain standards. Licensing usually results in a document or certificate that demonstrates that a practitioner is skilled in a particular natural health discipline and is working in accordance with a code of ethics [6].

The licensing process typically requires education, experience, and usually the completion of an exam. This process is usually managed by one or more supervisory boards that evaluate a practitioner's knowledge and skills in a particular natural health discipline.

Licensing provides consumers with the ability to document practitioners' competencies and integrity. It also allows regulatory agencies to monitor practitioners' professional behavior and practices and implement disciplinary measures as needed.

However, the licensing process and requirements can vary greatly from natural health discipline to discipline and from country to country. For example, in some countries, there may be a certain level of education and certification requirement for natural health practitioners, while in other countries these requirements may be less stringent or not at all [6].

However, the licensing process provides consumers with a degree of assurance that practitioners are proficient in a particular natural health discipline. This is especially important where there is widespread uncertainty about the quality and effectiveness of natural health practices and products.

6.2.3   Training and Standards

The lack of training and standards in the natural health sciences means that there can be wide variation between practitioners' abilities and ethical obligations. This can make it difficult to provide consumers with accurate and effective treatments (Ernst, 2002).

Education and standards in the natural health sciences play an important role in determining practitioners' competencies and the quality of natural health practices and products. Training helps practitioners develop their knowledge and skills in a particular natural health discipline, while standards determine how those knowledge and skills are to be applied [6].

Training for natural health practitioners often involves developing a thorough knowledge and understanding of a particular natural health discipline. This usually includes basic medical issues such as human anatomy and physiology, diagnosis and treatment of diseases, patient care, and ethics, as well as certain natural health practices such as herbal remedies, nutrition, acupuncture, or massage therapy.

Standards determine how practitioners should practice in a particular natural health discipline. This usually includes issues such as patient assessment and care, application techniques, informing patients and obtaining their consent, and ethical rules. Standards can also cover areas such as the production, labeling, and marketing of natural health products.

Training and standards help practitioners provide consumers with safe and effective natural health practices and products. However, education and standards can vary from natural health discipline to discipline and from country to country. This creates both opportunities and challenges for natural health practitioners, consumers, and regulators [6].

Example 1: Acupuncture Training and Standards

Acupuncture is a licensed practice in many countries and requires intensive training, usually lasting 3-4 years. This training usually includes human anatomy, physiology, and diseases, as well as the theory and practice of acupuncture. Acupuncture standards generally cover issues such as needle application, sterilization techniques, evaluation, and approval of patients [7].

Example 2: Herbal Medicine Education and Standards

Herbal medicine practitioners often receive extensive education about the medicinal uses of herbs and their potential side effects. Herbal medicine standards generally cover issues such as the correct and safe use of herbal products, product quality and labeling, and informing patients and obtaining their consent [8].

Example 3: Massage Therapy Training and Standards

Massage therapists usually receive extensive training in human anatomy, physiology and biomechanics, massage and bodywork techniques, ethics, and business practices. Massage therapy standards usually cover topics such as massage techniques, evaluation and approval of patients, hygiene, and ethical rules [9].

Example 4: Homeopathy Training and Standards

Homeopathic practitioners receive extensive training in homeopathic principles, homeopathic uses of substances, patient evaluation and management, and ethical and professional practices. Homeopathy standards generally cover issues such as the correct and safe use of homeopathic products, product quality and labeling, and informing patients and obtaining their consent [10].

6.2.4   Circulation of Counterfeit Products

Misleading labeling, misleading marketing practices, and counterfeit products are major issues in the regulation of natural health products and services. Such practices can put consumers' health at risk and damage the reputation of natural health sciences [1].

In the natural health sciences, the circulation of counterfeit products is a serious issue that threatens the health and safety of consumers. This is often characterized by fake, counterfeit, or misleading labeling or marketing practices. Counterfeit products often contain low-quality or contaminated natural health products that are neither effective nor safe as stated on their labels [11].

Some counterfeit products may contain misleading or incomplete information about when the ingredients they contain are not in the correct dose or at all. This can lead consumers to use potentially harmful or ineffective products based on misleading information. In addition, counterfeit products can often have low manufacturing standards, which can lead to contamination or other safety issues.

The issue of counterfeit products being circulated is a major concern for regulatory agencies, consumers, and natural health practitioners. This topic illustrates the importance and complexity of ethical and regulatory issues in the field of natural health sciences.

Regulators have developed various strategies to remove counterfeit products from circulation and inform consumers of the possible dangers of these products. However, for these efforts to be effective, consumers and practitioners need to become more aware of this issue, and their ability to recognize counterfeit products needs to be improved [11].

6.3   PROFESSIONAL STANDARDS AND TRAINING

In the professional practice of the natural health sciences, standards and training determine practitioners' levels of competence, ethical behavior, and ultimately patient outcomes. It also assures consumers of the quality and reliability of natural health services.

Professional standards are rules and guidelines that determine the knowledge, skills, and ethical behavior of natural health care providers. These are usually set by professional associations or regulatory bodies and cover topics such as the implementation of natural health care, patient care, education, continuous professional development, and ethical practices. Standards are vital to ensure the quality and reliability of services and practices [6].

The training provides natural health care providers with the necessary knowledge and skills. Education often includes a broad and in-depth knowledge and understanding of a particular natural health discipline. This usually includes basic medical issues such as human anatomy and physiology, diagnosis and treatment of diseases, patient care, and ethics, as well as certain natural health practices such as herbal remedies, nutrition, acupuncture, or massage therapy. Education is also important for continuous professional development and the maintenance of professional competencies [5].

6.3.1   Professional Standards

Professional standards determine how practitioners should practice in a particular natural health discipline. This usually includes issues such as patient assessment and care, application techniques, informing patients and obtaining their consent, and ethical rules. Standards can also cover areas such as the production, labeling, and marketing of natural health products.

Some natural health disciplines require their practitioners to have a certain level of education and/or a specific certification. For example, acupuncture practitioners usually must have completed a specific training program and passed a certification exam [7].

Professional standards are rules and guidelines established to determine the appropriateness and ethics of practitioners in the natural health sciences. These standards regulate practitioners' professional skill levels, knowledge, and approaches to patient care. These standards are often created by professional associations or regulatory bodies [12].

Professional standards for natural health practitioners cover a variety of areas. Some of these areas include:

1. Clinical Practice: Professional standards regulate practitioners' clinical practice. This includes topics such as the assessment, diagnosis and treatment of a patient, patient services, and practice techniques.
2. Training and Certification: Professional standards often determine the training and certification requirements of practitioners. This may include the need for a specific level of education or completion of a certificate program.
3. Code of Ethics: Professional standards determine the ethical behavior of practitioners. This includes issues such as protecting patients' privacy, obtaining consent, and providing accurate information.
4. Continuous Professional Development: Professional standards often set requirements for continuous professional development for practitioners to keep their professional knowledge and skills up-to-date.

Professional standards for natural health practitioners ensure that patients are safe and receive the highest quality care. In addition, these standards help promote broader acceptance of natural health practices in society and reassure consumers of practitioners' competencies and ethics [6].

Examples of Professional Standards

1. Clinical Practice: The American Association of Naturopathic Physicians requires its members to follow certain standards when evaluating patients, making diagnoses, and creating treatment plans. This includes a complete evaluation of the patient's medical history, appropriate laboratory tests, and other diagnostic procedures [13].
2. Training and Certification: The American Massage Therapy Association requires that certified massage therapists have reached a certain level of training and attend continuing education courses. This ensures that the knowledge and skills of massage therapists are constantly updated and improved [14].
3. Code of Ethics: The American Holistic Nurses Association has published a code of ethics that requires its members to protect patients' privacy, provide them with complete and accurate information, and always have their patients' best interests in mind [15].
4. Continuing Professional Development: The American Association of Acupuncture and Oriental Medicine requires acupuncture and oriental medicine practitioners to attend continuing professional development courses and complete a certain number of training hours over a specified period of time. This ensures that practitioners' knowledge and skills are up-to-date and effective [16].

6.3.2 Education

Training enables natural health practitioners to gain competence in a specific discipline. Training programs usually cover a range of topics, ensuring that the practitioner has a comprehensive knowledge and skill set. These topics often include anatomy, physiology, pathology, medical ethics and law, medical terms, pharmacology, and techniques in the specific discipline.

Education is essential for the practitioner to be able to effectively assess patients, make the correct diagnosis, and create an effective treatment plan. The training also helps the practitioner understand their ethical and legal responsibilities and practice in accordance with professional standards [5].

Education is an important part of the professional standards in the field of natural health sciences. The right training and certification ensure that natural health practitioners are skilled and knowledgeable in their profession. Education also helps practitioners provide safe and effective care to their patients [12].

Education in the natural health sciences generally covers the following areas:

1. Basic Medical Knowledge: Natural health practitioners often receive extensive training in basic medical knowledge. This includes topics such as anatomy, physiology, biochemistry, and pathology.
2. Unique Knowledge and Skills: Each natural health discipline is based on the requirement to have its own unique set of knowledge and skills. This may include various massage techniques for a massage therapist, herbal remedies and diet therapies for a naturopath, or understanding traditional Chinese medical theories and acupuncture points for an acupuncturist.
3. Clinical Experience: Natural health education often includes clinical experience or an internship. This allows practitioners to have the opportunity to work with real patients, under the supervision of an experienced mentor.
4. Continuing Education: Natural health practitioners are often required to attend continuing education courses to keep their professional knowledge and skills up-to-date.

The training gives natural health practitioners the ability to provide the best care to their patients and also helps practitioners keep abreast of developments and research in their profession. This helps promote wider acceptance of natural health sciences in society and reassures consumers of practitioners' qualifications and training [6].

Some important organizations that provide education in natural health sciences are:

1. Bastyr University (USA): Founded in 1978, Bastyr offers degrees in naturopathy, acupuncture and oriental medicine, nutrition, herbal sciences, Ayurveda, and psychology in science [17].
2. National University of Natural Medicine (USA): Founded in 1956, this university offers degrees in naturopathic medicine, classical Chinese medicine, nutrition, global health, and integrative health research [18].
3. Australian College of Natural Medicine (Australia): One of Australia's leading schools of natural medicine. It offers training in the fields of acupuncture, naturopathy, nutrition, and Western herbal medicine [19].
4. Canadian College of Naturopathic Medicine (Canada): Founded in 1978, this college is one of the few institutions in Canada that trains naturopathic doctors [20].
5. Beijing University of Chinese Medicine (China): This university is the largest and oldest traditional Chinese medicine university in the world and offers education to both local and international students [21].
6. University of Westminster (UK): The Department of Relevance and Natural Health Sciences at this university offers a range of courses on herbal medicine and naturopathy [22].

6.4   LEGAL AND REGULATORY FRAMEWORKS

Because the natural health sciences are a thriving field, regulations and legal frameworks can vary from country to country and even from region to region. Nevertheless, specific legal and regulatory frameworks are important for the safety of consumers and the protection of product quality.

1. Product and Service Regulations: Natural health products and services are generally subject to a set of regulations, such as medical products and services. For example, in the

United States, the Food and Drug Administration (FDA) regulates dietary supplements and homeopathic remedies, while the Federal Trade Commission (FTC) regulates the marketing of these products [23, 24]. These regulations ensure the safety and effectiveness of products and protect consumers from misleading claims.

2. Licensing and Certification: Most natural health practitioners must obtain licensing or certification to certify that they are complying with professional standards. For example, in many states, naturopathic doctors can become licensed provided they have reached a certain level of education and passed an exam. Such requirements ensure the competence of practitioners and their compliance with professional standards [25].

3. Ethical Standards and Professional Rules: Professional associations in the field of natural health sciences generally establish ethical standards and professional rules that their members adhere to. This is important to protect the rights of patients and elevate the reputation of the profession [5].

4. Research and Clinical Trial Arrangements: Research and clinical trials in the natural health sciences are also often regulated. These regulations ensure that research complies with ethical and scientific standards and help protect patients [5].

Although regulations depend on the country and region, there is a general sense of respect and acceptance in the field of natural health sciences around the world. This is important both to protect consumers and to ensure the quality and effectiveness of natural health services.

REFERENCES

1. E. Ernst, "The Role of Complementary and Alternative Medicine," *BMJ*, vol. 321, no. 7269, pp. 1133–1135, 2000.
2. M. H. Cohen, Complementary & Alternative Medicine: Legal Boundaries and Regulatory Perspectives, Johns Hopkins University Press, Baltimore, MD, 2002.
3. World Health Organization, "National Policy on Traditional Medicine and Regulation of Herbal Medicines: Report of a WHO Global Survey," 2005.
4. E. Ernst, "A Systematic Review of Systematic Reviews of Homeopathy," *British Journal of Clinical Pharmacology*, vol. 54, no. 6, pp. 577–582, 2002.
5. World Health Organization, "WHO Traditional Medicine Strategy: 2014-2023," 2013. [Online]. Available: https://apps.who.int/iris/bitstream/handle/10665/92455/9789241506090_eng.pdf.
6. Federation of State Medical Boards, "Model Guidelines for the Use of Complementary and Alternative Therapies in Medical Practice," 2018.
7. National Certification Commission for Acupuncture and Oriental Medicine, 2017.
8. American Herbalists Guild, *AHG Guide to Getting an Herbal Education*, 2018.
9. American Massage Therapy Association, *Standards of Practice*, 2017.
10. Council for Homeopathic Certification, *CHC Certificants Professional Code of Conduct and Standards of Practice,* 2020.
11. World Health Organization, *Substandard and Falsified Medical Products,* 2017.
12. National Center for Complementary and Integrative Health (NCCIH), "Complementary, Alternative, or Integrative Health: What's In a Name?," 2018. [Online]. Available: https://www.nccih.nih.gov/health/complementary-alternative-or-integrative-health-whats-in-a-name.
13. American Association of Naturopathic Physicians, *Naturopathic Medical Standards of Practice*, 2017.
14. American Massage Therapy Association, *Standards of Practice*, 2022.
15. American Holistic Nurses Association, *Code of Ethics*, 2017.
16. American Association of Acupuncture and Oriental Medicine, *Continuing Education Requirements,* 2021.
17. Bastyr University, "Academics," [Online]. Available: https://www.bastyr.edu/academics.
18. National University of Natural Medicine, "Academics," [Online]. Available: https://nunm.edu/academics/.
19. Australian College of Natural Medicine, "Courses," [Online]. Available: https://www.acnm.edu.au/courses/.
20. Canadian College of Naturopathic Medicine, "Doctor of Naturopathy," [Online]. Available: https://www.ccnm.edu/programs/doctor-naturopathy.

21. Beijing University of Chinese Medicine, "Programs," [Online]. Available: http://www.bucm.edu.cn/col/col2244/index.html.
22. University of Westminster, "Complementary and Natural Healthcare," [Online]. Available: https://www.westminster.ac.uk/courses/subjects/complementary-medicines-and-therapies.
23. U.S. Food and Drug Administration, Dietary Supplements, FDA, 2021. [Online]. Available: https://www.fda.gov/food/dietary-supplements.
24. Federal Trade Commission, Advertising and Marketing, FTC, 2021. [Online]. Available: https://www.ftc.gov/tips-advice/business-center/advertising-and-marketing.
25. National Center for Complementary and Integrative Health, Credentialing, Licensing, and Education, NCCIH, 2021. [Online]. Available: https://www.nccih.nih.gov/health/credentialing-licensing-and-education.

SUGGESTED READINGS

Adolphe, J. L., S. J. Whiting, B. H. Juurlink, L. U. Thorpe, and J. Alcorn, "Health Effects With Consumption of the Flax Lignan Secoisolariciresinol Diglucoside," *British Journal of Nutrition*, vol. 103, no. 7, pp. 929–938, 2010.

Agah, S., A. M. Taleb, R. Moeini, N. Gorji, and H. Nikbakht, "Cumin Extract for Symptom Control in Patients With Irritable Bowel Syndrome: A Case Series," *Middle East Journal of Digestive Diseases*, vol. 5, no. 4, pp. 217–222, 2013.

Aissaoui, A., S. Zizi, Z. H. Israel, and B. Lyoussi, "Hypoglycemic and Hypolipidemic Effects of *Coriandrum sativum* L. in Meriones Shawi Rats," *Journal of Ethnopharmacology*, vol. 137, no. 1, pp. 652–661, 2011.

Akhondzadeh, S., H. R. Naghavi, M. Vazirian, A. Shayeganpour, H. Rashidi, and M. Khani, "Passionflower in the Treatment of Generalized Anxiety: A Pilot Double-Blind Randomized Controlled Trial With Oxazepam," *Journal of Clinical Pharmacy and Therapeutics*, vol. 26, no. 5, pp. 363–367, 2001.

Akhondzadeh, S., M. Noroozian, M. Mohammadi, S. Ohadinia, A. H. Jamshidi, and M. Khani, "Salvia officinalis Extract in the Treatment of Patients With Mild to Moderate Alzheimer's Disease: A Double Blind, Randomized and Placebo-Controlled Trial," *Journal of Clinical Pharmacy and Therapeutics*, vol. 28, no. 1, pp. 53–59, 2003.

Akilen, R., A. Tsiami, D. Devendra, and N. Robinson, "Cinnamon in Glycaemic Control: Systematic Review and Meta Analysis," *Clinical Nutrition*, vol. 31, no. 5, pp. 609–15, 2012.

Alexandrovich, I., O. Rakovitskaya, E. Kolmo, T. Sidorova, and S. Shushunov, "The Effect of Fennel (Foeniculum vulgare) Seed Oil Emulsion in Infantile Colic: A Randomized, Placebo-Controlled Study," *Alternative Therapies in Health and Medicine*, vol. 9, no. 4, pp. 58–61, 2003.

Alzohairy, M. A., "Therapeutics Role of *Azadirachta indica* (Neem) and Their Active Constituents in Diseases Prevention and Treatment," *Evidence-Based Complementary and Alternative Medicine*, vol. 2016, p. 7382506, 2016.

Amagase, H., B. Sun, and C. Borek, "*Lycium barbarum* (Goji) Juice Improves in Vivo Antioxidant Biomarkers in serum of Healthy Adults," *Nutrition Research (New York, N.Y.)*, vol. 29, no. 1, pp. 19–25, 2009.

American Urological Association Education and Research, Inc. Management of Benign Prostatic Hyperplasia (BPH). 2011.

Anderson, J. W., L. D. Allgood, A. Lawrence, L. A. Altringer, G. R. Jerdack, D. A. Hengehold, and J. G. Morel, "Cholesterol-Lowering Effects of psyllium Intake Adjunctive to Diet Therapy in Men and Women With Hypercholesterolemia: Meta-Analysis of 8 Controlled Trials," *The American Journal of Clinical Nutrition*, vol. 71, no. 2, pp. 472–479, 2000.

Asl, M. N., and H. Hosseinzadeh, "Review of Pharmacological Effects of Glycyrrhiza Sp. and Its Bioactive Compounds," *Phytotherapy Research*, vol. 22, no. 6, pp. 709–724, 2008.

Bae, J., J. Kim, R. Choue, and H. Lim, "Dietary Intake and serum Levels of Trans-9,trans-11 Conjugated Linoleic Acid Are Associated With the Risk of Metabolic Syndrome in Men but Not in Women," *British Journal of Nutrition*, vol. 111, no. 7, pp. 1181–1187, 2014.

Bagchi, D., M. Bagchi, S. J. Stohs, D. K. Das, S. D. Ray, C. A. Kuszynski, and H. G. Preuss, "Free Radicals and Grape Seed Proanthocyanidin Extract: Importance in Human Health and Disease Prevention," *Toxicology*, vol. 148, no. 2-3, pp. 187–197, 2000.

Bagchi, D., A. Garg, R. L. Krohn, M. Bagchi, M. X. Tran, and S. J. Stohs, "Oxygen Free Radical Scavenging Abilities of Vitamins C and E, and a Grape Seed Proanthocyanidin Extract in Vitro," *Research Communications in Molecular Pathology and Pharmacology*, vol. 95, no. 2, pp. 179–189, 1997.

Bamosa, A. O., H. Kaatabi, F. M. Lebdaa, A. M. Elq, and A. Al-Sultanb, "Effect of Nigella sativa Seeds on the Glycemic Control of Patients With Type 2 Diabetes mellitus," *Indian Journal of Physiology and Pharmacology*, vol. 54, no. 4, pp. 344–354, 2010.

Barnes, J., L. A. Anderson, S. Gibbons, and J. D. Phillipson, "Echinacea Species (Echinacea angustifolia (DC.) Hell., Echinacea pallida (Nutt.) Nutt., *Echinacea purpurea* (L.) Moench): A Review of Their Chemistry, Pharmacology and Clinical Properties," *Journal of Pharmacy and Pharmacology*, vol. 57, no. 8, pp. 929–954, 2005.

Bartels, E. M., V. N. Folmer, H. Bliddal, R. D. Altman, C. Juhl, S. Tarp, and R. Christensen, "Efficacy and Safety of Ginger in Osteoarthritis Patients: A Meta-Analysis of Randomized Placebo-Controlled Trials," *Osteoarthritis and Cartilage*, vol. 23, no. 1, pp. 13–21, 2015.

Barton, D. L., H. Liu, S. R. Dakhil, et al. Wisconsin Ginseng (*Panax quinquefolius*) to Improve Cancer-Related Fatigue: A Randomized, Double-Blind Trial, N07C2. *Journal of the National Cancer Institute*, vol. 105, no. 16, pp. 1230–1238, 2013.

Baur, J. A., and D. A. Sinclair, "Therapeutic Potential of Resveratrol: The in Vivo Evidence," *Nature Reviews Drug Discovery*, vol. 5, no. 6, pp. 493–506, 2006.

Beer, A. M., and T. Wegener, "Willow Bark Extract (*Salicis cortex*) for Gonarthrosis and Coxarthrosis – Results of a Cohort Study With a Control Group," *Phytomedicine*, vol. 15, no. 11, pp. 907–913, 2008.

Benlhabib, E., J. I. Baker, D. E. Keyler, and A. K. Singh, "Effects of Purified Puerarin on Voluntary Alcohol Intake and Alcohol Withdrawal Symptoms in Prats Receiving Free Access to Water and Alcohol," *Journal of Medicinal Food*, vol. 7, no. 2, pp. 180–186, 2004.

Benson, S., L. A. Downey, C. Stough, M. Wetherell, A. Zangara, and A. Scholey, "An Acute, Double-Blind, Placebo-Controlled Cross-Over Study of 320 Mg and 640 Mg Doses of *Bacopa monnieri* (CDRI 08) on Multitasking Stress Response and Mood," *Phytotherapy Research*, vol. 28, no. 4, pp. 551–559, 2014.

Bent, S., A. Padula, D. Moore, M. Patterson, and W. Mehling, "Valerian for Sleep: A Systematic Review and Meta-Analysis," *The American Journal of Medicine*, vol. 119, no. 12, pp. 1005–1012, 2006.

Bhardwaj, P., and D. Khanna, "Green Tea Catechins: Defensive Role in Cardiovascular Disorders," *Chinese Journal of Natural Medicines*, vol. 11, no. 4, pp. 345–353, 2013.

Bommer, S., P. Klein, and A. Suter, "First Time Proof of sage's Tolerability and Efficacy in Menopausal Women With Hot Flushes," *Advances in Therapy*, vol. 28, no. 6, pp. 490–500, 2011.

Boots, A. W., G. R. Haenen, and A. Bast, "Health Effects of Quercetin: from Antioxidant to Nutraceutical," *European Journal of Pharmacology*, vol. 585, no. 2-3, pp. 325–337, 2008.

Borrelli, F., and E. Ernst, "Black Cohosh (Cimicifuga racemosa): A Systematic Review of Adverse Events," *American Journal of Obstetrics and Gynecology*, vol. 199, no. 5, pp. 455–466, 2008.

Boyle, N. B., C. Lawton, and L. Dye, "The Effects of Magnesium Supplementation on Subjective Anxiety and Stress—A Systematic Review," *Nutrients*, vol. 9, no. 5, p. 429, 2017.

Bramati, L., M. Minoggio, C. Gardana, et al. Quantitative Characterization of Flavonoid Compounds in Rooibos Tea (Aspalathus linearis) by LC–UV/DAD. *Journal of Agricultural and Food Chemistry*, vol. 50, no. 20, pp. 5513–5519, 2002.

Brien, S., G. T. Lewith, and G. McGregor, "Devil's Claw (*Harpagophytum procumbens*) as a Treatment for Osteoarthritis: A Review of Efficacy and Safety," *Journal of Alternative and Complementary Medicine*, vol. 12, no. 10, pp. 981–993, 2006.

Buhner, S. H., Herbal Antivirals: Natural Remedies for Emerging & Resistant Viral Infections, Storey Publishing, North Adams, MA, 2013.

Bundy, R., A. F. Walker, R. W. Middleton, G. Marakis, and J. C. Booth, "Artichoke Leaf Extract Reduces Symptoms of Irritable Bowel Syndrome and Improves Quality of Life in Otherwise Healthy Volunteers Suffering from Concomitant Dyspepsia: A Subset Analysis," *Journal of Alternative and Complementary Medicine*, vol. 10, no. 4, pp. 667–669, 2004.

Cai, H., F. Liu, P. Zuo, et al., "Practical Application of Antidiabetic Efficacy of Lycium barbarum Polysaccharide in Patients With Type 2 Diabetes," *MedChem*, vol. 11, no. 4, pp. 383–390, 2015.

Carneiro, D. M., R. C. Freire, T. C. Honorio, et al., "Randomized, Double-Blind Clinical Trial to Assess the Acute Diuretic Effect of *Equisetum arvense* (Field Horsetail) in Healthy Volunteers," *Evidence-Based Complementary and Alternative Medicine* vol. 2014, p. 760683, 2014.

Cases, J., A. Ibarra, N. Feuillere, M. Roller, and S. G. Sukkar, "Pilot Trial of Melissa officinalis L. Leaf Extract in the Treatment of Volunteers Suffering from Mild-to-Moderate Anxiety Disorders and Sleep Disturbances," *Mediterranean Journal of Nutrition and Metabolism*, vol. 4, no. 3, pp. 211–218, 2011.

Cavanagh, H. M., and J. M. Wilkinson, "Biological Activities of Lavender Essential Oil," *Phytotherapy Research*, vol. 16, no. 4, pp. 301–308, 2002.

Chevassus, H., J. B. Gaillard, A. Farret, et al., "A Fenugreek Seed Extract Selectively Reduces Spontaneous Fat Intake in Overweight Subjects," *The European Journal of Clinical Pharmacology*, vol. 66, no. 5, pp. 449–455, 2010.

Chithra, V., and S. Leelamma, "*Coriandrum sativum* – Effect on Lipid Metabolism in 1,2-Dimethyl Hydrazine Induced Colon Cancer," *Journal of Ethnopharmacology*, vol. 71, no. 1-2, pp. 457–63, 2000.

Chrubasik, J. E., B. D. Roufogalis, H. Wagner, S. A. Chrubasik, "A Comprehensive Review on the Stinging Nettle Effect and Efficacy Profiles. Part II: Urticae Radix," *Phytomedicine*, vol. 14, no. 7-8, pp. 568–579, 2007.

Chrubasik, S., J. Thanner, O. Künzel, C. Conradt, A. Black, S. Pollak, "Comparison of Outcome Measures During Treatment With the Proprietary Harpagophytum Extract Doloteffin in Patients With Pain in the Lower Back, Knee or Hip," *Phytomedicine*, vol. 9, no. 3, pp. 181–94, 2002.

Clare, B. A., R. S. Conroy, K. Spelman, "The Diuretic Effect in Human Subjects of an Extract of Taraxacum officinale folium Over a Single Day," *Journal of Alternative and Complementary Medicine*, vol. 15, no. 8, pp. 929–934, 2009.

Combs, G. F. Jr., The Vitamins: Fundamental Aspects in Nutrition and Health. 5th Edition. Academic Press, New York, NY, 2017.

Deng, G., H. Lin, A. Seidman, M. Fornier, G. D'Andrea, K. Wesa, S. Yeung, S. Cunningham-Rundles, A. J. Vickers, B. Cassileth, "A Phase I/II Trial of a Polysaccharide Extract from *Grifola frondosa* (Maitake Mushroom) in Breast Cancer Patients: Immunological Effects," *Journal of Cancer Research and Clinical Oncology*, vol. 135, no. 9, pp. 1215–1221, 2009.

Deng, R., and T. J. Chow, "Hypolipidemic, Antioxidant, and Anti-Inflammatory Activities of Microalgae Spirulina," *Cardiovascular Therapeutics*, vol. 28, no. 4, pp. e33–e45, 2010.

Domitrović, R., H. Jakovac, Z. Romic, D. Rahelić, Z. Tadić, "Antifibrotic Activity of Taraxacum officinale Root in Carbon Tetrachloride-Induced Liver Damage in Mice," *Journal of Ethnopharmacology*, vol. 130, no. 3, pp. 569–577, 2010.

Dvorakova, M., and P. Landa, "Anti-Inflammatory Activity of Natural Stilbenoids: A Review," *Pharmacological Research*, vol. 124, pp. 126–145, 2017.

Eidi, M., A. Eidi, A. Saeidi, S. Molanaei, A. Sadeghipour, M. Bahar, K. Bahar, "Effect of Coriander Seed (*Coriandrum sativum* L.) Ethanol Extract on Insulin Release from Pancreatic Beta Cells in Streptozotocin-Induced Diabetic Rats," *Phytotherapy Research*, vol. 23, no. 3, pp. 404–406, 2009.

Federico, A., M. Dallio, C. Loguercio, "Silymarin/Silybin and Chronic Liver Disease: A Marriage of Many Years," *Molecules*, vol. 22, no. 2, p. 191, 2017.

Ferlemi, A. V., and F. N. Lamari, "Rosemary Leaf Extract (*Rosmarinus officinalis* L.) – Containing Carnosic Acid and Carnosol as Main Bioactive Components – and Fruit Extracts Rich in Anthocyanins: Antioxidant Effects in Common Carp (*Cyprinus Carpio* L.) Hepatocytes," *European Journal of Nutrition*, vol. 55, no. 4, pp. 1613–1621, 2016.

Fiore, C., M. Eisenhut, R. Krausse, E. Ragazzi, D. Pellati, D. Armanini, J. Bielenberg, "Antiviral Effects of Glycyrrhiza Species," *Phytotherapy Research*, vol. 22, no. 2, pp. 141–148, 2008.

Fuangchan, A., P. Sonthisombat, T. Seubnukarn, et al., "Hypoglycemic Effect of Bitter Melon Compared With Metformin in Newly Diagnosed Type 2 Diabetes Patients," *Journal of Ethnopharmacology*, vol. 134, no. 2, pp. 422–428, 2011.

Gagnier, J. J., S. Chrubasik, and E. Manheimer, "*Harpgophytum procumbens* for Osteoarthritis and Low Back Pain: A Systematic Review," *BMC Complementary and Alternative Medicine*, vol. 4, p. 13, 2004.

Gambero, A., and M. L. Ribeiro, "The Positive Effects of Yerba Maté (Ilex paraguariensis) in Obesity," *Nutrients*, vol. 7, no. 2, pp. 730–750, 2015.

Gonzales, G. F., "Ethnobiology and Ethnopharmacology of *Lepidium meyenii* (Maca), a Plant from the Peruvian Highlands," *Evidence-Based Complementary and Alternative Medicine*, vol. 2012, p. 193496, 2012.

Grober, U., J. Schmidt, and K. Kisters, "Magnesium in Prevention and Therapy," *Nutrients*, vol. 7, no. 9, pp. 8199–8226, 2015.

Gupta, K., M. Y. Chou, A. Howell, C. Wobbe, R. Grady, and A. E. Stapleton, "Cranberry Products Inhibit Adherence of p-Fimbriated Escherichia Coli to Primary Cultured Bladder and Vaginal Epithelial Cells," *Journal of Urology*, vol. 177, no. 6, pp. 2357–2360, 2007.

Hamidpour, R., S. Hamidpour, M. Hamidpour, and M. Shahlari, "Chemistry, Pharmacology, and Medicinal Property of Sage (salvia) to Prevent and Cure Diseases Such as Obesity, Diabetes, Depression, Dementia, Lupus, Autism, Heart Disease, and Cancer," *Journal of Traditional and Complementary Medicine*, vol. 4, no. 2, pp. 82–88, 2014.

Hao, Q., B. R. Dong, and T. Wu, "Probiotics for Preventing Acute Upper Respiratory Tract Infections," *The Cochrane Database of Systematic Reviews*, vol. 2, p. CD006895, 2015. doi: 10.1002/14651858. CD006895.pub3.

Heck, C. I., and D. Mejia, "Yerba Mate Tea (Ilex paraguariensis): A Comprehensive Review on Chemistry, Health Implications, and Technological Considerations," *Journal of Food Science*, vol. 72, no. 9, pp. R138–R151, 2007.

Hempel, S., S. J. Newberry, A. R. Maher, Z. Wang, J. N. Miles, R. Shanman, and P. G. Shekelle, "Probiotics for the Prevention and Treatment of Antibiotic-Associated Diarrhea: A Systematic Review and Meta-Analysis," *JAMA*, vol. 307, no. 18, pp. 1959–1969, 2012.

Hernández-Camacho, J. D., M. Bernier, G. López-Lluch, and P. Navas, "Coenzyme Q10 Supplementation in Aging and Disease," *Frontiers in Physiology*, vol. 9, p. 44, 2018.

Hewlings, S. J., and D. S. Kalman, "Curcumin: A Review of Its' Effects on Human Health," *Foods*, vol. 6, no. 10, p. 92, 2017.

Hill, C., F. Guarner, G. Reid, G. R. Gibson, D. J. Merenstein, B. Pot, and P. C. Calder, "Expert Consensus Document: The International Scientific Association for Probiotics and Prebiotics Consensus Statement on the Scope and Appropriate Use of the Term Probiotic," *Nature Reviews Gastroenterology & Hepatology*, vol. 11, no. 8, pp. 506–514, 2014.

Ho, H. V., J. L. Sievenpiper, A. Zurbau, S. Blanco Mejia, E. Jovanovski, F. Au-Yeung, and V. Vuksan, "The Effect of Oat β-Glucan on LDL-Cholesterol, non-HDL-Cholesterol and apoB for CVD Risk Reduction: A Systematic Review and Meta-Analysis of Randomised-Controlled Trials," *British Journal of Nutrition*, vol. 116, no. 8, pp. 1369–1382, 2016.

Hooper, L., C. Kay, A. Abdelhamid, P. A. Kroon, J. S. Cohn, E. B. Rimm, and A. Cassidy, "Effects of Chocolate, Cocoa, and Flavan-3-Ols on Cardiovascular Health: A Systematic Review and Meta-Analysis of Randomized Trials," *The American Journal of Clinical Nutrition*, vol. 95, no. 3, pp. 740–751, 2012.

Hubbard, B. P., and D. A. Sinclair, "Small Molecule SIRT1 Activators for the Treatment of Aging and Age-Related Diseases," *Trends in Pharmacological Sciences*, vol. 35, no. 3, pp. 146–154, 2014.

Imenshahidi, M., and H. Hosseinzadeh, "Berberis Vulgaris and Berberine: An Update Review," *Phytotherapy Research*, vol. 30, no. 11, pp. 1745–1764, 2016.

Iravani, S., and B. Zolfaghari, "Pharmaceutical and Nutraceutical Effects of Pinus pinaster Bark Extract," *Research in Pharmaceutical Sciences*, vol. 6, no. 1, pp. 1–11, 2011.

Jaric, S., O. Kostic, Z. Mataruga, et al., "Traditional Wound-Healing Plants Used in the Balkan Region (Southeast Europe)," *Journal of Ethnopharmacology*, vol. 211, pp. 311–328, 2018.

Jepson, R. G., G. Williams, and J. C. Craig, "Cranberries for Preventing Urinary Tract Infections," *Cochrane Database of Systematic Reviews*, vol. 10, p. CD001321, 2012.

Jiménez, S., S. Gascon, A. Luquin, M. Laguna, C. Ancin-Azpilicueta, and M. J. Rodríguez-Yoldi, "*Rosa canina* Extracts Have Antiproliferative and Antioxidant Effects on Caco-2 Human Colon Cancer," *PLoS One*, vol. 11, no. 7, p. e0159136, 2016.

Juergens, U. R., M. Stöber, and H. Vetter, "The Anti-Inflammatory Activity of L-Menthol Compared to Mint Oil in Human Monocytes in Vitro: A Novel Perspective for Its Therapeutic Use in Inflammatory Diseases," *European Journal of Medical Research*, vol. 3, no. 12, pp. 539–545, 1998.

Kalt, W., A. Cassidy, L. R. Howard, R. Krikorian, A. J. Stull, F. Tremblay, and R. Zamora-Ros, "Recent Research on the Health Benefits of Blueberries and Their Anthocyanins," *Advances in Nutrition*, vol. 11, no. 2, pp. 224–236, 2020.

Kalt, W., A. Hanneken, P. Milbury, and F. Tremblay, "Recent Research on the Health Benefits of Blueberries and Their Anthocyanins," *Advances in Nutrition*, vol. 11, no. 2, pp. 224–236, 2020.

Kapoor, S., and S. Saraf, "Assessment of Viscoelasticity and Hydration Effect of Herbal Moisturizers Using Bioengineering Techniques," *Pharmacognosy Magazine*, vol. 6, no. 24, pp. 298–304, 2010.

Katz, D. L., K. Doughty, and A. Ali, "Cocoa and Chocolate in Human Health and Disease," *Antioxidants & Redox Signaling*, vol. 15, no. 10, pp. 2779–2811, 2011.

Kennedy, D. O., "B Vitamins and the Brain: Mechanisms, Dose and Efficacy – A Review," *Nutrients*, vol. 8, no. 2, p. 68, 2016.

Khan, N., and H. Mukhtar, "Tea and Health: Studies in Humans," *Current Pharmaceutical Design*, vol. 19, no. 34, pp. 6141–6147, 2013.

Khanna, R., J. K. MacDonald, and B. G. Levesque, "Peppermint Oil for the Treatment of Irritable Bowel Syndrome: A Systematic Review and Meta-Analysis," *Journal of Clinical Gastroenterology*, vol. 48, no. 6, pp. 505–512, 2014.

Kong, W., J. Wei, P. Abidi, M. Lin, S. Inaba, C. Li, and Y. Wang, "Berberine Is a Novel Cholesterol-Lowering Drug Working Through a Unique Mechanism Distinct from Statins," *Nature Medicine*, vol. 10, no. 12, pp. 1344–1351, 2004.

Koshak, A., L. Wei, E. Koshak, S. Wali, O. Alamoudi, A. Demerdash, M. Qutub, P. N. Pushparaj, and M. Heinrich, "*Nigella sativa* Supplementation Improves Asthma Control and Biomarkers: A Randomized, Double-Blind, Placebo-Controlled Trial," *Phytotherapy Research*, vol. 31, no. 3, pp. 403–409, 2017. doi:10.1002/ptr.5761.

Kreydiyyeh, S. I., J. Usta, and R. Copti, "Effect of Diosgenin on Urinary and Plasma Electrolytes in Rats Fed a High Sodium Diet," *Plant Foods for Human Nutrition*, vol. 56, no. 3, pp. 225–232, 2001.

Krikorian, R., M. D. Shidler, T. A. Nash, W. Kalt, M. R. Vinqvist-Tymchuk, B. Shukitt-Hale, and J. A. Joseph, "Blueberry Supplementation Improves Memory in Older Adults," *Journal of Agricultural and Food Chemistry*, vol. 58, no. 7, pp. 3996–4000, 2010.

Lei, L., and Y. Liu, "Efficacy of Coenzyme Q10 in Patients With Cardiac Failure: A Meta-Analysis of Clinical Trials," *BMC Cardiovascular Disorders*, vol. 17, no. 1, pp. 1–8, 2017.

Lembo, A., and M. Camilleri, "Chronic Constipation," *New England Journal of Medicine*, vol. 349, no. 14, pp. 1360–1368, 2003.

Leung, L., R. Birtwhistle, J. Kotecha, S. Hannah, and S. Cuthbertson, "Anti-Diabetic and Hypoglycaemic Effects of *Momordica charantia* (Bitter Melon): A Mini Review," *British Journal of Nutrition*, vol. 102, no. 12, pp. 1703–1708, 2009.

Li, S. P., P. Li, T. T. Dong, and K. W. Tsim, "Anti-Oxidation Activity of Different Types of Natural Cordyceps sinensis and Cultured Cordyceps Mycelia," *Phytomedicine*, vol. 8, no. 3, pp. 207–212, 2001. doi:10.1078/0944-7113-00030. PMID: 11417914.

Li, Y., J. Yao, C. Han, J. Yang, M. T. Chaudhry, S. Wang, and Y. Yin, "Quercetin, Inflammation and Immunity," *Nutrients*, vol. 8, no. 3, p. 167, 2016.

Lin, Z. B., "Cellular and Molecular Mechanisms of Immuno-Modulation by Ganoderma lucidum," *Journal of Pharmacological Sciences*, vol. 99, no. 2, pp. 144–153, 2005.

Liu, X., J. Wei, F. Tan, S. Zhou, G. Würthwein, P. Rohdewald, and Pycnogenol, "French Maritime Pine Bark Extract, Improves Endothelial Function of Hypertensive Patients," *Life Sciences*, vol. 74, no. 7, pp. 855–862, 2004.

Lukas, S. E., D. Penetar, J. Berko, et al., "An Extract of the Chinese Herbal Root Kudzu Reduces Alcohol Drinking by Heavy Drinkers in a Naturalistic Setting," *Alcoholism: Clinical and Experimental Research*, vol. 29, no. 5, pp. 756–762, 2005.

MacKay, D., "Hemorrhoids and Varicose Veins: A Review of Treatment Options," *Alternative Medicine Review*, vol. 6, no. 2, pp. 126–140, 2001.

Maenthaisong, R., N. Chaiyakunapruk, S. Niruntraporn, and C. Kongkaew, "The Efficacy of Aloe vera Used for Burn Wound Healing: A Systematic Review," *Burns*, vol. 33, no. 6, pp. 713–718, 2007.

Mahady, G. B., S. L. Pendland, A. Stoia, et al., "In Vitro Susceptibility of Helicobacter Pylori to Botanical Extracts Used Traditionally for the Treatment of Gastrointestinal Disorders," *Phytotherapy Research*, vol. 19, no. 11, pp. 988–991, 2005.

Maizels, M., A. Blumenfeld, and R. Burchette, "A Combination of Riboflavin, Magnesium, and Feverfew for Migraine Prophylaxis: A Randomized Trial," *Headache*, vol. 44, no. 9, pp. 885–890, 2004.

McFarland, L. V., "Systematic Review and Meta-Analysis of *Saccharomyces boulardii* in Adult Patients," *World Journal of Gastroenterology*, vol. 16, no. 18, pp. 2202–2222, 2010.

Meyer, D., and M. Stasse-Wolthuis, "The Bifidogenic Effect of Inulin and Oligofructose and Its Consequences for Gut Health," *European Journal of Clinical Nutrition*, vol. 63, no. 11, pp. 1277–1289, 2009. doi:10.1038/ejcn.2009.64. PMID: 19690573.

Miller, P. E., M. Van Elswyk, and D. D. Alexander, "Long-Chain Omega-3 Fatty Acids Eicosapentaenoic Acid and Docosahexaenoic Acid and Blood Pressure: A Meta-Analysis of Randomized Controlled Trials," *American Journal of Hypertension*, vol. 27, no. 7, pp. 885–896, 2014.

Mlcek, J., T. Jurikova, S. Skrovankova, and J. Sochor, "Quercetin and Its Anti-Allergic Immune Response," *Molecules*, vol. 21, no. 5, p. 623, 2016.

Moayyedi, P., A. C. Ford, N. J. Talley, F. Cremonini, A. E. Foxx-Orenstein, L. J. Brandt, and E. M. Quigley, "The Efficacy of Probiotics in the Treatment of Irritable Bowel Syndrome: A Systematic Review," *Gut*, vol. 59, no. 3, pp. 325–332, 2010.

Morse, N. L., and P. M. Clough, "A Meta-Analysis of Randomized, Placebo-Controlled Clinical Trials of Efamol Evening Primrose Oil in Atopic Eczema. Where Do We Go from Here in Light of More Recent Discoveries?" *Current Pharmaceutical Biotechnology*, vol. 7, no. 6, pp. 503–524, 2006.

Ms., L., P. H. Koulivand, and A. Gorji, "Lemon Verbena, a Review of the Ethnopharmacology, Phytochemistry and Pharmacology," *Journal of Ethnopharmacology*, vol. 213, pp. 50–66, 2018.

Müller, W. E., "Current St. John's Wort Research from Mode of Action to Clinical Efficacy," *Pharmacological Research*, vol. 47, no. 2, pp. 101–109, 2003.

Muñoz, L. A., A. Cobos, O. Diaz, and J. M. Aguilera, "Chia Seed (Salvia Hispanica): An Ancient Grain and a New Functional Food," *Food Reviews International*, vol. 29, no. 4, pp. 394–408, 2013. doi:10.1080/8 7559129.2013.818014.

Nagpal, M., and S. Sood, "Role of Curcumin in Systemic and Oral Health: An Overview," *Journal of Natural Science, Biology and Medicine*, vol. 4, no. 1, pp. 3–7, 2013.

Neelakantan, N., M. Narayanan, R. J. de Souza, and R. M. van Dam, "Effect of Fenugreek (*Trigonella foenum-graecum* L.) Intake on Glycemia: A Meta-Analysis of Clinical Trials," *Nutrition Journal*, vol. 13, p. 7, 2014. doi:10.1186/1475-2891-13-7

Ngan, A., and R. Conduit, "A Double-Blind, Placebo-Controlled Investigation of the Effects of Passiflora incarnata (passionflower) Herbal Tea on Subjective Sleep Quality," *Phytotherapy Research*, vol. 25, no. 8, pp. 1153–1159, 2011.

Nicastro, H. L., S. A. Ross, and J. A. Milner, "Garlic and Onions: Their Cancer Prevention Properties," *Cancer Prevention Research*, vol. 8, no. 3, pp. 181–189, 2015.

Nosalova, G., A. Strapkova, A. Kardosova, P. Capek, L. Zathurecky, and E. Bukovska, "Cough Suppressive Effect of Polysaccharides from Marshmallow (*Althaea officinalis* L., var. robusta)," *Pharmacies*, vol. 47, no. 3, pp. 224–226, 1992.

Nostro, A., A. R. Blanco, M. A. Cannatelli, V. Enea, G. Flamini, I. Morelli, A. Sudano Roccaro, and V. Alonzo, "Susceptibility of Methicillin-Resistant Staphylococci to Oregano Essential Oil, Carvacrol and Thymol," *FEMS Microbiology Letters*, vol. 230, no. 2, pp. 191–195, 2004.

Ogawa, K., Y. Kuse, K. Tsuruma, S. Kobayashi, M. Shimazawa, and H. Hara, "Protective Effects of Bilberry and Lingonberry Extracts Against Blue Light-Emitting Diode Light-Induced Retinal Photoreceptor Cell Damage in Vitro," *BMC Complementary and Alternative Medicine*, vol. 14, p. 120, 2014.

Pal, S., A. Khossousi, C. Binns, S. Dhaliwal, and V. Ellis, "The Effect of a Fiber Supplement Compared to a Healthy Diet on Body Composition, Lipids, Glucose, Insulin and Other Metabolic Syndrome Risk Factors in Overweight and Obese Individuals," *British Journal of Nutrition*, vol. 105, no. 1, pp. 90–100, 2011.

Panossian, A., and G. Wikman, "Pharmacology of Schisandra chinensis Bail.: An Overview of Russian Research and Uses in Medicine," *Journal of Ethnopharmacology*, vol. 118, no. 2, pp. 183–212, 2008.

Pareek, A., M. Suthar, G. S. Rathore, and V. Bansal, "Feverfew (*Tanacetum Parthenium* L.): A Systematic Review," *Pharmacognosy Reviews*, vol. 5, no. 9, pp. 103–110, 2011.

Pase, M. P., J. Kean, J. Sarris, C. Neale, A. B. Scholey, and C. Stough, "The Cognitive-Enhancing Effects of *Bacopa monnieri*: A Systematic Review of Randomized, Controlled Human Clinical Trials," *Journal of Alternative and Complementary Medicine*, vol. 18, no. 7, pp. 647–652, 2012.

Perrinjaquet-Moccetti, T., A. Busjahn, C. Schmidlin, A. Schmidt, B. Bradl, and C. Aydogan, "Food Supplementation With an Olive (*Olea europaea* L.) Leaf Extract Reduces Blood Pressure in Borderline Hypertensive Monozygotic Twins," *Phytotherapy Research*, vol. 22, no. 9, pp. 1239–1242, 2008.

Perry, R., K. Hunt, and E. Ernst, "Nutritional Supplements and Other Complementary Medicines for Infantile Colic: A Systematic Review," *Pediatrics*, vol. 127, no. 4, pp. 720–733, 2011.

Persson, I. A., K. Persson, S. Hagg, and R. G. Andersson, "Effects of Green Tea, Black Tea and Rooibos Tea on Angiotensin-Converting Enzyme and Nitric Oxide in Healthy Volunteers," *Public Health Nutrition*, vol. 13, no. 5, pp. 730–737, 2010.

Petropoulos, S., F. Di Gioia, G. Polizzi, M. Papademetriou, S. Sampaio, A. Alexopoulos, V. Gkoutzioulias, and K. Tzima, "Fenugreek (*Trigonella foenum-graecum* L.): An Overview of the Past and a Look Into the Future," *Food Reviews International*, vol. 37, no. 1, pp. 77–125, 2021. doi:10.1080/87559129.2020. 1743734

Pittler, M. H., and E. Ernst, "Horse Chestnut Seed Extract for Chronic Venous Insufficiency," *Cochrane Database of Systematic Reviews*, vol. 11, no. 11, p. CD003230, 2012.

Potgieter, M., E. Pretorius, and M. S. Pepper, "Primary and Secondary Coenzyme Q10 Deficiency: The Role of Therapeutic Supplementation," *Nutrition Reviews*, vol. 71, no. 3, pp. 180–188, 2013.

Prasad, A. S., "Zinc in Human Health: Effect of Zinc on Immune Cells," *Molecular Medicine*, vol. 14, no. 5-6, pp. 353–357, 2008.

Prasad, S., A. K. Tyagi, and B. B. Aggarwal, "Recent Developments in Delivery, Bioavailability, Absorption and Metabolism of Curcumin: The Golden Pigment from Golden Spice," *Cancer Research and Treatment: Official Journal of Korean Cancer Association*, vol. 46, no. 1, p. 2, 2014.

Prashant, G. M., A. R. Pradeep, and A. P. Manojkumar, "Clinical Efficacy of a Natural Dentifrice Based on Herbs for the Control of Plaque and Gingivitis: A Clinical Comparative Study," *Indian Journal of Dental Research*, vol. 21, no. 4, pp. 532–535, 2010.

Pratte, M. A., K. B. Nanavati, V. Young, and C. P. Morley. An Alternative Treatment for Anxiety: A Systematic Review of Human Trial Results Reported for the Ayurvedic Herb Ashwagandha (*Withania somnifera*). *Journal of Alternative and Complementary Medicine*, vol. 20, no. 12, pp. 901–908, 2014. doi:10.1089/acm.2014.0177. PMID: 25405876.

Rafieian-Kopaei, M., and M. Movahedi, "Systematic Review of Premenstrual, Postmenstrual and Infertility Disorders of Vitex Agnus Castus," *Electronic Physician*, vol. 9, no. 1, p. 3685, 2017.

Rahimikian, F., R. Rahimi, P. Golzareh, R. Bekhradi, and A. Mehran, "Effect of Foeniculum vulgare Mill. (Fennel) Ten Menopausal Symptoms in Postmenopausal Women: A Randomized, Triple-Blind, Placebo-Controlled Trial," *Menopause*, vol. 24, no. 9, pp. 1017–1021, 2017.

Raina, K., R. P. Singh, R. Agarwal, and C. Agarwal, "Oral Grape Seed Extract Inhibits Prostate Tumor Growth and Progression in TRAMP Mice," *Cancer Research*, vol. 67, no. 12, pp. 5976–5982, 2007.

Ramasamy, U. S., K. Venema, H. Gruppen, and H. A. Schols, "Effect of Soluble Dietary Fiber on in Vitro Digestion of Casein," *Food Chemistry*, vol. 153, pp. 90–97, 2014.

Randall, C., H. Randall, F. Dobbs, C. Hutton, and H. Sanders, "Randomized Controlled Trial of Nettle Sting for Treatment of Base-of-Thumb Pain," *Journal of the Royal Society of Medicine*, vol. 93, no. 6, pp. 305–309, 2000.

Reay, J. L., D. O. Kennedy, and A. B. Scholey, "Single Doses of Panax Ginseng (G115) Reduce Blood Glucose Levels and Improve Cognitive Performance During Sustained Mental Activity," *Journal of Psychopharmacology*, vol. 19, no. 4, pp. 357–365, 2005.

Reginster, J. Y., R. Deroisy, L. C. Rovati, R. L. Lee, E. Lejeune, O. Bruyere, and M. E. Lenz, "Long-Term Effects of Glucosamine Sulphate on Osteoarthritis Progression: A Randomised, Placebo-Controlled Clinical Trial," *The Lancet*, vol. 357, no. 9252, pp. 251–256, 2001.

Rehman, J., J. M. Dillow, S. M. Carter, et al., "Increased Production of Antigen-Specific Immunoglobulins G and M Following in Vivo Treatment With the Medicinal Plants *Echinacea angustifolia* and *Hydrastis canadensis*," *Immunology Letters*, vol. 68, no. 2-3, pp. 391–395, 1999.

Ried, K., C. Toben, and P. Fakler, "Effect of Garlic on serum Lipids: An Updated Meta-Analysis," *Nutrition Reviews*, vol. 71, no. 5, pp. 282–299, 2013.

Rizos, E. C., E. E. Ntzani, E. Bika, M. S. Kostapanos, and M. S. Elisaf, "Association Between Omega-3 Fatty Acid Supplementation and Risk of Major Cardiovascular Disease Events: A Systematic Review and Meta-Analysis," *JAMA*, vol. 308, no. 10, pp. 1024–1033, 2012.

Roberfroid, M., "Prebiotics: The Concept Revisited," *The Journal of Nutrition*, vol. 137, no. 3, pp. 830S–837S, 2007.

Rock, C. L., and M. E. Swendseid, "Plasma Beta-Carotene Response in Humans after Meals Supplemented With Dietary Pectin," *The American Journal of Clinical Nutrition*, vol. 55, no. 1, pp. 96–99, 1992.

Rodriguez-Leyva, D., C. M. Dupasquier, R. McCullough, and G. N. Pierce, "The Cardiovascular Effects of Flaxseed and Its Omega-3 Fatty Acid, Alpha-Linolenic Acid," *The Canadian Journal of Cardiology*, vol. 26, no. 9, pp. 489–496, 2010.

Rohdewald, P., "A Review of the French Maritime Pine Bark Extract (Pycnogenol), a Herbal Medication With a Diverse Clinical Pharmacology," *International Journal of Clinical Pharmacology and Therapeutics*, vol. 40, no. 4, pp. 158–168, 2002.

Roohani, N., R. Hurrell, R. Kelishadi, and R. Schulin, "Zinc and Its Importance for Human Health: An Integrative Review," *Journal of Research in Medical Sciences*, vol. 18, no. 2, pp. 144–157, 2013.

Rosanoff, A., and M. R. Plesset, "Oral Magnesium Supplements Decrease High Blood Pressure (SBP> 155 mmHg) in Hypertensive Subjects on Anti-Hypertensive Medications: A Targeted Meta-Analysis," *Magnesium Research*, vol. 26, no. 3, pp. 93–99, 2013.

Roschek, B. Jr., R. C. Fink, M. McMichael, and R. S. Alberte, "Nettle Extract (Urtica dioica) Affects Key Receptors and Enzymes Associated With Allergic Rhinitis," *Phytotherapy Research*, vol. 23, no. 7, pp. 920–926, 2009.

Ryan, J., K. Croft, T. Mori, K. Wesnes, J. Spong, L. Downey, C. Kure, J. Lloyd, and C. Stough, "An Examination of the Effects of the Antioxidant Pycnogenol on Cognitive Performance, Serum Lipid Profile, Endocrinological and Oxidative Stress Biomarkers in an Elderly Population," *Journal of Psychopharmacology*, vol. 22, no. 5, pp. 553–562, 2008.

Sanodiya, B. S., G. S. Thakur, R. K. Baghel, G. B. Prasad, and P. S. Bisen, "*Ganoderma lucidum*: A Potent Pharmacological Macrofungus," *Current Pharmaceutical Biotechnology*, vol. 10, no. 8, pp. 717–742, 2009.

Sarris, J., C. Stough, C. A. Bousman, Z. T. Wahid, G. Murray, R. Teschke, K. M. Savage, A. Dowell, C. Ng, and I. Schweitzer, "Kava in the Treatment of Generalized Anxiety Disorder: A Double-Blind, Randomized, Placebo-Controlled Study," *Journal of Clinical Psychopharmacology*, vol. 33, no. 5, pp. 643–648, 2013.

Sazawal, S., G. Hiremath, U. Dhingra, P. Malik, S. Deb, and R. E. Black, "Efficacy of Probiotics in Prevention of Acute Diarrhoea: A Meta-Analysis of Masked, Randomised, Placebo-Controlled Trials," *The Lancet Infectious Diseases*, vol. 6, no. 6, pp. 374–382, 2006.

Schilcher, H., S. Kammerer, and T. Wegener, Leitfaden Phytotherapie. 5th edition. Munich: Urban und Fischer Verlag/Elsevier GmbH; 2016.

Schneider, T., and H. Rübben, "Stinging Nettle Root Extract (Bazoton-Uno) in Long Term Treatment of Benign Prostatic Syndrome (BPS). Results of a Randomized, Double-Blind, Placebo-Controlled Multicenter Study After 12 Months," *Urologe A*, vol. 43, no. 3, pp. 302–306, 2004.

Selmi, C., P. S. Leung, L. Fischer, B. German, C. Y. Yang, T. P. Kenny, and M. E. Gershwin, "The Effects of Spirulina on Anemia and Immune Function in Senior Citizens," *Cellular & Molecular Immunology*, vol. 8, no. 3, pp. 248–254, 2011.

Senapati, S., S. Banerjee, and D. N. Gangopadhyay, "Evening Primrose Oil Is Effective in Atopic Dermatitis: A Randomized Placebo-Controlled Trial," *Indian J Dermatol Venereol Leprol*, vol. 74, no. 5, pp. 447–452, 2008.

Sforcin, J. M., "Propolis and the Immune System: A Review," *Journal of Ethnopharmacology*, vol. 113, no. 1, pp. 1–14, 2007. doi:10.1016/j.jep.2007.05.012. Epub 2007 May 22.

Shams, T., M. S. Setia, R. Hemmings, J. McCusker, M. Sewitch, and A. Ciampi, "Efficacy of Black Cohosh-Containing Preparations on Menopausal Symptoms: A Meta-Analysis," *Alternative Therapies in Health and Medicine*, vol. 16, no. 1, pp. 36–44, 2010.

Shara, M., and S. J. Stohs, "Efficacy and Safety of White Willow Bark (Salix alba) Extracts," *Phytotherapy Research*, vol. 29, no. 8, pp. 1112–1116, 2015.

Sienkiewicz, M., M. Łysakowska, J. Ciećwierz, P. Denys, and E. Kowalczyk, "The Antimicrobial Activity of Thyme Essential Oil Against Multidrug Resistant Clinical Bacterial Strains," *Microbial Drug Resistance*, vol. 18, no. 2, pp. 137–148, 2012.

Slavin, J., "Fiber and Prebiotics: Mechanisms and Health Benefits," *Nutrients*, vol. 5, no. 4, pp. 1417–1435, 2013. doi:10.3390/nu5041417

Soumyanath, A., Y. P. Zhong, S. A. Gold, et al., "Centella asiatica Accelerates Nerve Regeneration upon Oral Administration and Contains Multiple Active Fractions Increasing Neurite Elongation in-Vitro," *Journal of Pharmacy and Pharmacology*, vol. 57, no. 9, pp. 1221–1229, 2005.

Sowmya, P., and P. Rajyalakshmi, "Hypocholesterolemic Effect of Germinated Fenugreek Seeds in Human Subjects," *Plant Foods for Human Nutrition*, vol. 53, no. 4, pp. 359–365, 1999.

Surjushe, A., R. Vasani, and D. G. Saple, "Aloe vera: A Short Review," *Indian Journal of Dermatology*, vol. 53, no. 4, p. 163, 2008.

Swanson, D., R. Block, and S. A. Mousa, "Omega-3 Fatty Acids EPA and DHA: Health Benefits Throughout Life," *Advances in Nutrition*, vol. 3, no. 1, pp. 1–7, 2012.

Swathy, S. S., S. Panicker, R. S. Nithya, M. M. Anuja, S. Rejitha, and M. Indira, "Antiperoxidative and Antiinflammatory Effect of *Sida cordifolia* Linn. on Quinolinic Acid Induced Neurotoxicity," *Neurochemical Research*, vol. 35, no. 9, pp. 1361–1367, 2010.

Taavoni, S., N. Ekbatani, and M. Kashaniyan, "Effect of Valerian on Sleep Quality in Postmenopausal Women: A Randomized Placebo-Controlled Clinical Trial," *Menopause*, vol. 20, no. 9, pp. 991–995, 2013.

Tacklind, J., R. MacDonald, I. Rutks, J. U. Stanke, and T. J. Wilt, "*Serenoa repens* for Benign Prostatic Hyperplasia," *The Cochrane Database of Systematic Reviews*, vol. 2012, no. 12, p. CD001423, 2012.

Teas, J., M. E. Baldeón, D. E. Chiriboga, J. R. Davis, A. J. Sarries, and L. E. Braverman, "Could Dietary Seaweed Reverse the Metabolic Syndrome?" *Asia Pacific Journal of Clinical Nutrition*, vol. 18, no. 2, pp. 145–154, 2009.

Thring, T. S., P. Hili, and D. P. Naughton, "Anti-Collagenase, Anti-Elastase and Anti-Oxidant Activities of Extracts from 21 Plants," *BMC Complementary and Alternative Medicine*, vol. 11, no. 1, pp. 1–8, 2011.

Thring, T. S., P. Hili, and D. P. Naughton, "Antioxidant and Potential Anti-Inflammatory Activity of Extracts and Formulations of White Tea, Rose, and Witch Hazel on Primary Human Dermal Fibroblast Cells," *Journal of Inflammation (Lond)*, vol. 8, no. 1, p. 27, 2011.

Timmers, S., M. de Ligt, E. Phielix, T. van de Weijer, J. Hansen, E. Moonen-Kornips, G. Schaart, I. Kunz, M. K. Hesselink, V. B. Schrauwen-Hinderling, and P. Schrauwen, "Resveratrol as Add-on Therapy in Subjects With Well-Controlled Type 2 Diabetes: A Randomized Controlled Trial," *Diabetes Care*, vol. 39, no. 12, pp. 2211–2217, 2016.

Towheed, T. E., L. Maxwell, T. P. Anastassiades, B. Shea, J. Houpt, V. Robinson, and G. Wells, "Glucosamine Therapy for Treating Osteoarthritis," *Cochrane Database of Systematic Reviews*, vol. 2, p. CD002946, 2005.

Tsigos, C., V. Hainer, A. Basdevant, et al., "Management of Obesity in Adults: European Clinical Practice Guidelines," *Obese Facts*, vol. 1, no. 2, pp. 106–116, 2008.

Ullah, R., M. Nadeem, A. Khalique, et al., "Nutritional and Therapeutic Perspectives of Chia (*Salvia hispanica* L.): A Review," *Journal of Food Science and Technology*, vol. 53, no. 4, pp. 1750–1758, 2016. doi:10.1007/s13197-015-1967-0.

van Die, M. D., H. G. Burger, H. J. Teede, and K. M. Bone, "Vitex agnus-Castus Extracts for Female Reproductive Disorders: A Systematic Review of Clinical Trials," *Planta Medica*, vol. 79, no. 7, pp. 562–575, 2013.

Venables, M. C., C. J. Hulston, H. R. Cox, and A. E. Jeukendrup, "Green Tea Extract Ingestion, Fat Oxidation, and Glucose Tolerance in Healthy Humans," *The American Journal of Clinical Nutrition*, vol. 87, no. 3, pp. 778–784, 2008.

Vetvicka, V., and J. Vetvickova, "Beta-Glucans, History, and the Present: Immunomodulatory Aspects and Mechanisms of Action," *Journal of Immunotoxicology*, vol. 5, no. 1, pp. 47–57, 2007.

Viljoen, E., J. Visser, N. Koen, and A. Musekiwa, "A Systematic Review and Meta-Analysis of the Effect and Safety of Ginger in the Treatment of Pregnancy-Associated Nausea and Vomiting," *Nutrition Journal*, vol. 13, p. 20, 2014.

Vlad, S. C., M. P. LaValley, T. E. McAlindon, and D. T. Felson, "Glucosamine for Pain in Osteoarthritis: Why Do Trial Results Differ?" *Arthritis & Rheumatism: Official Journal of the American College of Rheumatology* vol. 56, no. 7, pp. 2267–2277, 2007.

Wachtel-Galor, S., J. Yuen, J. A. Buswell, and I. F. F. Benzie, *Ganoderma lucidum* (Lingzhi or Reishi): A Medicinal Mushroom. In Herbal Medicine: Biomolecular and Clinical Aspects, CRC Press, New York, NY, 2011.

Wattanathorn, J., L. Mator, S. Muchimapura, et al., "Positive Modulation of Cognition and Mood in the Healthy Elderly Volunteer Following the Administration of *Centella asiatica*," *Journal of Ethnopharmacology*, vol. 116, no. 2, pp. 325–332, 2008.

Whitehead, A., E. J. Beck, S. Tosh, and T. M. Wolever, "Cholesterol-Lowering Effects of Oat β-Glucan: A Meta-Analysis of Randomized Controlled Trials," *The American Journal of Clinical Nutrition*, vol. 100, no. 6, pp. 1413–1421, 2014.

Winther, K., J. Campbell-Tofte, and H. S. Hansen, "Bioactive Ingredients of Rose Hips (*Rosa canina* L.) With Special Reference to Antioxidative and Anti-Inflammatory Properties: in Vitro Studies," *Botanics*, vol. 6, pp. 11–23, 2016.

Yin, J., H. Xing, and J. Ye, "Efficacy of Berberine in Patients With Type 2 Diabetes," *Metabolism*, vol. 57, no. 5, pp. 712–717, 2008.

Zakay-Rones, Z., E. Thom, T. Wollan, and J. Wadstein, "Randomized Study of the Efficacy and Safety of Oral Elderberry Extract in the Treatment of Influenza A and B Virus Infections," *Journal of International Medical Research*, vol. 32, no. 2, pp. 132–140, 2004.

Zhang, Y., X. Li, D. Zou, W. Liu, J. Yang, N. Zhu, and Y. Zhu, "Treatment of Type 2 Diabetes and Dyslipidemia With the Natural Plant Alkaloid Berberine," *The Journal of Clinical Endocrinology & Metabolism*, vol. 93, no. 7, pp. 2559–2565, 2008.

Zong, G., A. Gao, F. B. Hu, and Q. Sun, "Whole Grain Intake and Mortality From All Causes, Cardiovascular Disease, and Cancer: A Meta-Analysis of Prospective Cohort Studies," *Circulation*, vol. 133, no. 24, pp. 2370–2380, 2016. doi:10.1161/CIRCULATIONAHA.115.021101.

7 The Future of Natural Health Sciences

Natural Health Sciences is a constantly developing and growing field with scientific and technological advances as well as the ever-increasing health awareness of society. This sector is expanding people's capabilities to protect and improve their health while offering new and effective treatments.

7.1 PERSONALIZED MEDICINE

Personalized medicine (also known as precision medicine) is a healthcare approach based on the development of individualized treatment and preventive strategies, taking into account a patient's genetic, environmental, and lifestyle factors. This approach aims to create more accurate and effective strategies to prevent, diagnose, and treat diseases [1–3].

Personalized medicine provides customized healthcare solutions for individual patients, taking into account genetic, environmental, and lifestyle factors. Natural health sciences can be used as part of personalized medicine. For example, the determination of the most appropriate herbal treatments for the genetic structure or lifestyle of a particular patient can be demonstrated.

With the proliferation of advanced genetic and genomic testing, personalized medicine is a rapidly evolving field. These tests determine a patient's genetic makeup, allowing them to determine the most appropriate treatment specific to their genetic makeup and better predict disease risks.

In the natural health sciences, personalized medicine often involves recommending specific diets, exercise programs, herbal remedies, and other natural health practices in relation to genetic, environmental, and lifestyle factors. For example, a patient's genetic test results may indicate that a particular herbal remedy or dietary supplement may be more effective for him.

Additionally, based on a patient's lifestyle and environmental factors like their stress levels, diet, or exercise habits, a personalized health and wellness (also known as wellness) program can be created that is most effective for them. This holds great hope for the future of medicine and health care, aiming to achieve better health outcomes and a higher quality of life for patients. Personalized treatments include:

7.1.1 Personalized Herbal Treatment

Some herbal remedies can be customized according to the genetic makeup, lifestyle, and health status of the individual. For example, the effectiveness of ginseng and echinacea may vary from person to person, and this may be related to genetic and environmental factors [4].

7.1.2 Personalized Aromatherapy

Some people may be more sensitive to certain essential oils, and this may be due to genetic or environmental factors. Aromatherapy treatments can be customized according to an individual's needs and reactions [5].

7.1.3 Personalized Acupuncture

Acupuncture treatments can be customized based on an individual's energy (Qi) flow, overall health, and specific health issues. Different acupuncture points provide different therapeutic effects [6].

DOI: 10.1201/9781003520252-8

7.1.4 Personalized Diet and Nutrition

Customized nutrition recommendations can be made based on the individual's genetic makeup, life-style, and health status. This can be vitamin and mineral supplements, as well as diets that contain or exclude certain nutrients [7].

7.1.5 Personalized Mindfulness and Meditation

Mindfulness and meditation techniques can be tailored to suit the individual's personal needs and goals. For example, some individuals may respond better to calming techniques, while others may respond better to more active techniques [8].

7.1.6 Personalized Yoga

Yoga poses and breathing techniques can be tailored to an individual's flexibility, strength, and overall health. Yoga can also be customized to address specific health issues, such as low back pain or stress management [9].

7.1.7 Personalized Massage Therapy

Massage therapy can be customized according to an individual's health status, lifestyle, and specific health goals. For example, different techniques, such as deep tissue massage or Swedish massage, provide different therapeutic effects [10].

7.1.8 Personalized Ayurveda

Ayurvedic medicine offers customized treatment strategies based on an individual's *dosha* (body type) and overall health status. This can include both nutritional recommendations and herbal remedies [11].

7.1.9 Personalized Homeopathy

Homeopathic medicine offers customized treatment based on an individual's overall health status, symptoms, and lifestyle. How an individual will respond to a particular homeopathic remedy can vary greatly from person to person [12].

7.1.10 Personalized Reiki

Reiki energy healing can be tailored to an individual's energy levels and health status. Reiki prac-titioners may focus on specific *chakras* or energy centers to dissolve energy blocks and promote overall well-being [13].

7.2 INTEGRATIVE HEALTH APPROACHES

This approach combines natural health practices with traditional medical treatments. For example, a patient may also use holistic practices such as yoga or meditation while undergoing cancer treat-ment. Integrative health aims to enable patients to play a more active role in the treatment process and improve their overall quality of life [14–16].

Integrative health is an approach that combines traditional and complementary health practices. This approach focuses on promoting the physical, mental, and emotional health of the individual as a whole and is patient-centered. Integrative health encourages the active participation of patients and includes self-care and prevention strategies.

One of the important features of the integrative health approach is the personalization of treatment. This is based on the understanding that each individual's genetic, environmental, and lifestyle factors have an impact on their own health status and treatment responses. Hence, integrative health practitioners can customize treatments to meet each patient's unique needs and goals.

The integrative health approach can combine many different treatment modules. These often combine conventional medicine (e.g., medications and surgery) with complementary therapies (e.g., herbal medicine, acupuncture, massage, yoga, and meditation). The treatment plan is usually based on a holistic assessment of the patient and can include both physical and emotional, mental, and social health goals.

Another important feature of the integrative health approach is that it emphasizes prevention. This is accomplished by encouraging lifestyle changes (e.g., healthy eating, regular exercise, and stress management techniques) and encouraging patients to take active steps to improve their health and prevent disease.

This approach has become increasingly popular in recent years, and many health institutions have established private clinics and centers that provide integrative health services. In addition, many medical schools and nursing schools have also incorporated integrative health practices into their curricula.

More research is still needed to evaluate the efficacy and safety of the integrative health approach. However, current evidence suggests that this approach can improve the quality of life of patients with chronic diseases and lower the cost of health care.

Some medical centers that adopt an integrative health approach are listed below:

1. Duke Integrative Medicine: The Duke University Health System is home to an integrative medicine center that serves the holistic health and recovery needs of patients. Duke Integrative Medicine takes a personalized medicine approach and provides its patients with a treatment plan tailored to their individual needs. This is an approach that combines traditional medicine practices with complementary and alternative medicine practices [17].

2. Cleveland Clinic's Center for Integrative and Lifestyle Medicine: The Cleveland Clinic has established a center for integrative and lifestyle medicine. This center offers stress management, nutrition, movement, and complementary medicine practices to its patients. The center adopts an approach that combines traditional medicine practices with complementary and alternative medicine practices [18].

3. Mayo Clinic's Complementary and Integrative Medicine Program: The Mayo Clinic offers a variety of services to its patients through its complementary and integrative medicine program. These services include acupuncture, massage therapy, meditation, stress management, and more. With these services, Mayo Clinic aims to improve patients' general health, manage diseases, and improve their quality of life [19].

4. The Osher Center for Integrative Medicine: Major institutions such as the University of California, San Francisco (UCSF), and Harvard Medical School have established centers for integrative medicine. These centers offer a range of services designed to meet individual needs. Services often include acupuncture, yoga, meditation, massage therapy, nutritional counseling, and more [20].

5. MD Anderson Cancer Center's Integrative Medicine Program: MD Anderson Cancer Center offers an integrative medicine program that aims to improve patients' quality of life during and after cancer treatments. This program includes services such as acupuncture, massage therapy, meditation, physical therapy, energy therapy, and nutritional counseling [21].

7.3 DIGITAL HEALTH AND TELEMEDICINE: APPLICATIONS TO NATURAL HEALTH SCIENCES

Digital health and telemedicine are changing the delivery of health care through the use of digital technologies. These technologies are increasingly used in the practice of natural health sciences and holistic medicine, as well as in the practice of general medicine. Thus, natural health sciences can reach a wider audience by using digital technologies. For example, a naturopath or dietitian may meet with patients through telemedicine or offer health and wellness courses on an online platform.

7.3.1 Digital Health and Natural Health Sciences

Digital health technologies can expand and deepen the practices and principles of the natural health sciences. Mobile health ("mHealth") applications, such as helping users track nutrition, sleep, stress management, exercise, and other health-related behaviors. This type of personal information allows individuals to better understand their health status and adjust their natural approach to health to their individual needs [22].

Furthermore, digital health platforms allow users to obtain health information, nutrition and lifestyle guidance, and information about natural therapies. These platforms can help users feel informed and confident when making health-related decisions [23].

7.3.2 Telemedicine and Natural Health Sciences

Telemedicine plays an important role in overcoming barriers to access between natural health science practitioners and patients. In many cases, access to natural health care can be difficult due to geographical restrictions. Telemedicine enables specialists to provide services to patients from their homes. This provides a significant advantage, especially for individuals living in rural and remote areas [24].

Telemedicine can also be used to support a variety of applications of natural health sciences. For example, services such as acupuncture, massage therapy, physiotherapy, dietetic counseling, and psychological counseling may be offered through video conferencing or other digital means [25].

However, the use of digital health and telemedicine in the natural health sciences depends on a number of factors, including access to technology, digital literacy, data privacy and security concerns, regulatory frameworks, and reimbursement policies.

7.4 INNOVATIVE RESEARCH AND PRODUCT DEVELOPMENT

Scientific and technological advances are constantly creating new opportunities in the development of natural health products and services to improve existing practices and treatments. These processes help build up scientific evidence on the effectiveness and safety of natural health approaches while also offering more treatment options for patients and healthcare professionals. For example, genetic engineering and biotechnology can be used in the development and customization of herbal medicines.

7.4.1 Innovative Research

Innovative research expands the existing knowledge base on efficacy and safety in the natural health sciences. For example, the sciences of genetics and epigenetics can help us better understand how a person's genetic makeup and lifestyle factors (such as diet, exercise, and stress) interact and affect health status [26]. This knowledge supports the development of personalized natural health strategies.

Another important area of research is microbiota research. In recent years, research on the effects of the human gut microbiota on health and disease has led to the development and use of probiotic and prebiotic products [27].

7.4.2 Product Development

Innovative research is also driving the development of natural health products. For example, some research shows that herbal remedies, vitamins, minerals, and other natural ingredients may be effective in managing specific health conditions [28]. This information can lead to the development of new natural health products and the improvement of existing ones.

However, these developments highlight the importance of scientific rigor and regulatory oversight of high standards in the natural health sciences. Solid scientific evidence must be provided for the effectiveness and safety of products, and regulatory frameworks must ensure that consumers are safe and that dishonest and non-misleading information is used when advertising products [29].

7.5 SUSTAINABLE AND ETHICAL PRACTICES

In the future, natural health sciences are expected to promote sustainable and ethical practices. This includes issues such as the protection of natural resources, the adoption of fair-trade practices, and the protection of animal rights.

The natural health sciences are developing rapidly as a field that has the potential to expand the ways we maintain and improve health. The combination of science and technology and the power of nature can lead to more effective and personalized health solutions [30].

The applications of natural health sciences have an impact not only on the health of people, but also on the health of the planet. Therefore, sustainability and ethics should be at the heart of practices, research, and policies in this area.

7.5.1 Sustainability

Sustainability is directly related to the management and conservation of natural resources. For example, some herbal remedies contain ingredients derived from endangered species. This requires the conservation of biodiversity and the promotion of sustainable collection practices [31].

At the same time, the production and distribution of herbal remedies and other natural health products can use significant amounts of energy and water and cause greenhouse gas emissions. Therefore, the environmental impact of these processes must be minimized through the reduction of the carbon footprint and the use of sustainable packaging solutions [32].

7.5.2 Ethics

Ethics in the natural health sciences includes the responsibility to ensure that products and services are used safely, effectively, and fairly. This means honestly presenting scientific evidence, avoiding misleading or exaggerated claims, and enforcing ethical principles such as informed consent and patient confidentiality [33].

In addition, research and practice in this area should protect the rights and interests of consumers, local communities, and indigenous peoples. For example, it is important that local and indigenous knowledge and practices are used fairly and ethically, without biopiracy [34].

7.6 TECHNOLOGICAL ADVANCES AND THEIR IMPACT

Technological advances are influencing all aspects of the natural health sciences. Information access, data analysis, personalized treatments, and public health improvements are a few examples of these changes.

Technological advances have triggered a number of evolutions in the health field, but in the natural health sciences, these effects are particularly pronounced. Technology has significantly expanded access to information, the development of personalized treatments, and the ability to improve general public health.

7.6.1 Access to Advanced Information

Digitalization has significantly expanded the public's access to information on natural health sciences. The internet, social media, and mobile apps have enabled people to learn more about health care and alternative treatment options [35]. These technological advances have also encouraged faster and wider knowledge sharing, which has paved the way for more research and awareness in the natural health sciences.

7.6.2 Development of Personalized Therapies

Technology has enabled the development of personalized treatments based on genetic information. Genomic information can help determine how certain genetic variations contribute to susceptibility to diseases and how they respond to certain treatments. This allows healthcare professionals to create more effective and personalized treatment protocols that take into account each patient's unique genetic makeup [36].

7.6.3 Public Health Improvements

Telemedicine and other digital health care play an important role in overcoming barriers to accessing health care. Thanks to these technological advances, people have access to a wider range of healthcare services, regardless of their geographical location. This represents a great opportunity, especially for individuals living in rural or remote areas [37].

7.6.4 Examples of Developing Personalized Treatments

1. 23andMe: 23andMe uses technology to provide genetic information to consumers. Clients can use the genetic test results to determine health risks, genetic characteristics, and ancestry information. Based on this genetic information, natural health products and lifestyle changes can be personalized [38].
2. Fitbit: Fitbit is a wearable technology that allows users to track their health and wellness data. Users can track a range of data, from sleep quality to heart rate. This information can be used to make personalized recommendations for a healthier lifestyle within the framework of natural health sciences [39].
3. Headspace: This mobile app focuses on meditation and mental health. Users have access to personalized meditation and mental health programs to reduce stress, improve sleep quality, and support overall mental health [40].
4. Teladoc: Teladoc offers telemedicine services so that patients can access healthcare services regardless of their geographic location. This is especially important for individuals who live in rural areas or have limited mobility [41].

5. MyFitnessPal: This app helps users track their nutrition and exercise data. This can help choose the right nutritional and exercise options, allowing for a personalized approach to the natural health sciences [42].

7.6.5 Information Retrieval and Data Analysis

The Internet and digital technologies have facilitated access to information in the field of natural health sciences. This has enabled the general public, health professionals, and researchers to learn more about the effectiveness of alternative and complementary treatment methods [30].

Big data analytics and artificial intelligence also support research in the natural health sciences. Computerized analysis extracts meaningful information from large data sets and, for example, is used to analyze the effectiveness of herbal remedies.

Technological advances are transforming information access and data analysis in the natural health sciences and contributing on a large scale. The combination of science, medicine, and technology greatly increases the potential to improve the quality of health care and provide personalized health care.

7.6.5.1 *Information Retrieval*

Technological innovations in patient information access enable individuals to learn more about their own health status and make more informed decisions. For example, genetic testing kits allow individuals to identify genetic risk factors and select healthier lifestyle choices based on this information [38].

In addition, web-based health information platforms and mobile health applications offer users access to health information anytime and anywhere. These platforms and apps can help users control symptoms, learn about illnesses, and search for healthcare services [42, 43].

7.6.5.2 *Data Analysis*

In the natural health sciences, data analysis can help better understand diseases, improve treatment methods, and predict patients' health outcomes. For example, big data analytics and machine learning techniques can be used to discover patterns and relationships in health data. These techniques can be used in disease diagnosis, treatment planning, and disease risk prediction [44, 45].

In addition, analysis of genetic and genomic data can help identify genetic diseases and genetic risk factors. Genetic testing and genomic analyses could shape the future of personalized medicine because genetic information can improve the ability of individuals to predict health outcomes and treatment responses [46, 47]. The following are concrete examples of information retrieval and data analysis:

7.6.5.2.1 *Information Access*

1. Genetic Testing Kits: Companies like 23andMe offer users the ability to understand genetic risk factors and the geography of their ancestors. This information is usually analyzed through a saliva sample collected from the home and made available to users online [38].
2. Web-Based Health Information Platforms: WebMD is a popular health information website that offers information on a wide range of health topics. This site allows users to get detailed information about specific diseases, conditions, and treatments [43].
3. Mobile Health Apps: Apps like MyFitnessPal help users track calorie intake and physical activity. It also makes recommendations for users to achieve their goals [42].

7.6.5.2.2 *Data Analysis*

1. Big Data Analysis: Big data analysis can extract meaningful information from complex and large data sets. For example, healthcare providers can evaluate the outcomes of certain

treatments by analyzing patient data or predicting patients' risk of developing a particular disease [44].
2. Machine Learning: Machine learning can help diagnose diseases and plan treatment. For example, a machine learning model can predict a patient's risk of developing a particular disease using a patient's medical history, lab test results, and other data [45].
3. Genetic and Genomic Data Analysis: Genetic testing and genomic analysis can help identify genetic diseases and genetic risk factors. For example, a genetic test can determine whether an individual has a particular genetic disease or condition [46, 47].

7.6.6   Personalized Treatments

Technological advances have enabled the development of personalized treatments in the natural health sciences. Genetic and non-genetic biomarkers are used to determine how a person will respond to a particular treatment. This information can help create more effective and personalized treatment protocols.

Personalized treatments are an approach that considers a combination of genetic, environmental, and lifestyle factors. This acknowledges the idea that each individual is unique and therefore each patient needs a unique treatment. Some examples of natural medicine and personalized treatments are listed below:

1. Personalized Nutrition Plans: Every person's body is different, and this brings with it different nutritional needs. Natural health professionals can create a customized nutrition plan for each individual, taking into account genetics, lifestyle, and current health status [48].
2. Herbal Remedies: Some herbal remedies can be customized based on an individual's genetic makeup, lifestyle, and current health status. For example, for some individuals, valerian root may be effective for insomnia, while for others it may be less effective [49].
3. Customized Detox Plans: Detoxification can help cleanse the body of toxins. However, each person's detox needs may be different, so a natural health professional can create a customized detox plan for each individual [50].
4. Personalized Physical Activity Plans: Each person's physical activity needs and abilities are different. A natural health professional can create a customized exercise plan that takes into account an individual's lifestyle, current health status, and personal goals [51].
5. Customized Stress Management Techniques: Stress can contribute negatively to many health problems. A natural health professional can recommend customized stress management techniques that take into account an individual's lifestyle, stress levels, and personal preferences [52].

7.6.7   Public Health Improvements

Finally, technological advances have also influenced the application of natural health sciences aimed at improving the overall level of public health. Digital health technologies, such as telemedicine and mobile health apps, have expanded access to health care. This is especially important for individuals living in rural or remote areas [53].

Public health is about implementing prevention strategies and health services to improve and protect the health of communities. In the field of natural health, public health can be improved in several ways:

1. Herbal Remedies and Public Health: Various herbal remedies can improve public health in specific communities as they are often more cost-effective and easily accessible. For example, the use of the Artemisia Annua plant in the treatment of malaria is an important public health development in the fight against malaria [54].

2. Natural Nutrition Education: Teaching proper eating habits plays an important role, especially in preventing chronic diseases such as obesity and heart disease. Therefore, natural nutrition education programs can improve public health [55].

3. Use of Traditional and Complementary Medicine: The World Health Organization has stated that Traditional and Complementary Medicine plays an important role in improving public health. For example, systems such as Ayurveda and traditional Chinese medicine can improve the overall health of individuals and prevent disease [56, 57].

4. Mental Health and Natural Treatments: Natural treatments such as meditation, yoga, and acupuncture can help manage mental health issues such as depression and anxiety. These approaches may be particularly helpful for people who don't have access to medications or want to avoid the side effects of medications [58].

5. Natural Cures and Chronic Diseases: Natural health practices can play an important role in managing chronic diseases such as diabetes, hypertension, and asthma. For example, special diets, herbal remedies, and physical exercises can be used in addition to standard treatment methods in the management of these diseases [59].

7.7   THE ROLE OF NATURAL HEALTH SCIENCES IN GLOBAL HEALTH CARE

The role of the natural health sciences in global health care is based on a wide range of factors. These include public health needs, existing health services and treatment protocols, cultural practices and priorities, and the organization and financing of general health services. The potential contributions of natural health sciences and their role in global health care can be summarized as follows:

1. Accessibility: Natural health sciences can play a critical role in providing access to health care, especially in developing countries and rural areas. Traditional medical practices often involve natural treatments that are adopted and practiced by local communities and are often low-cost. These treatments provide broader access to public health services and increase the sustainability of services [53].

2. Holistic Approach: Most of the natural health sciences take a holistic approach to health and disease issues. This focuses on the overall health and well-being of the individual and includes not only the treatment of symptoms of the disease, but also lifestyle, nutrition, stress management, and more. This approach is particularly useful for the prevention and management of chronic diseases [60].

3. Role of Patients: Natural health sciences encourage the active participation of patients in health care. This includes making informed decisions, lifestyle changes, and taking more responsibility for your own health care. This approach has the potential to improve health outcomes and reduce the cost of health care [61].

4. Cultural Relevance: Many natural health practices are deeply linked to specific cultural contexts. This can increase the cultural relevance and therefore acceptance of these treatments. Cultural relevance is an important factor in improving the effectiveness and sustainability of health services [62].

5. Sustainability: Natural health sciences are often based on natural and renewable resources. This can improve environmental sustainability and strengthen its capacity to respond to global environmental challenges such as climate change [63].

REFERENCES

1. The Personalized Medicine Coalition, "What is Personalized Medicine?" 2021. [Online]. Available: https://www.personalizedmedicinecoalition.org/Userfiles/PMC-Corporate/file/pmc_age_of_pmc_factsheet.pdf.

2. National Institutes of Health, "What is precision medicine?" 2021. [Online]. Available: https://ghr.nlm. nih.gov/primer/precisionmedicine/definition.

3. World Health Organization, "Genomics," [Online]. Available: https://www.genome.gov/genetics-glossary/ Personalized-Medicine.

4. P. Herman, "Characteristics of Patients Using Different Patient-Provider Communication Modes in a U.S. Population With Musculoskeletal Pain," *Patient Education and Counseling*, vol. 101, no. 8, pp. 1393–1401, 2018.

5. S. S. Hwang, "The Effects of Aromatherapy on Sleep Improvement: A Systematic Literature Review and Meta-Analysis," *Journal of Alternative and Complementary Medicine*, vol. 21, no. 2, pp. 61–68, 2015.

6. H. MacPherson, A. Vickers, M. Bland, D. Torgerson, M. Corbett, E. Spackman, P. Saramago, B. Woods, H. Weatherly, M. Sculpher, A. Manca, S. Richmond, A. Hopton, J. Eldred and I. Watt, "Acupuncture for Chronic Pain and Depression in Primary Care: A Programme of Research," *Programme Grants for Applied Research*, vol. 5. No. 3, Southampton (UK): NIHR Journals Library, 2017.

7. M. Müller and C. Bock, "Precision Nutrition: A Review of Personalized Nutritional Approaches for the Prevention and Management of Metabolic Syndrome," *Nutrients*, vol. 9, no. 8, p. 913, 2017.

8. F. Zeidan and D. Vago, "Mindfulness Meditation-Based Pain Relief: A Mechanistic Account," *Annals of the New York Academy of Sciences*, vol. 1373, no. 1, pp. 114–127, 2016.

9. T. Field, "Yoga Research Review," *Complementary Therapies in Clinical Practice*, vol. 24, pp. 145–161, 2016.

10. A. Furlan, "Massage for Low-Back Pain," *Cochrane Database of Systematic Reviews*, vol. 2015, no. 9, 2015.

11. B. Patwardhan, "Bridging Ayurveda With Evidence-Based Scientific Approaches in Medicine," *The EPMA Journal*, vol. 5, no. 1, p. 19, 2014.

12. M. Teixeira, "Homeopathic Use of Modern Medicines: Utilization of the Curative Rebound Effect," *Medical Hypotheses*, vol. 99, pp. 52–57, 2017.

13. A. Baldwin, "Reiki Improves Heart Rate Homeostasis in Laboratory Rats," *Journal of Alternative and Complementary Medicine*, vol. 23, no. 5, pp. 368–377, 2017.

14. V. Maizes, D. Rakel and C. Niemiec, "Integrative Medicine and Patient-Centered Care," *Explore (NY)*, vol. 5, no. 5, pp. 277–289, 2009.

15. C. Witt, D. Chiaramonte and S. Berman, "Defining Health in a Comprehensive Context: A New Definition of Integrative Health," *American Journal of Preventive Medicine*, vol. 53, no. 1, pp. 134–137, 2017.

16. B. Kligler, V. Maizes and S. Schachter, "Core Competencies in Integrative Medicine for Medical School Curricula: a Proposal," *Academic Medicine*, vol. 79, no. 6, pp. 521–531, 2004.

17. Duke Integrative Medicine, "About Us," [Online]. Available: https://www.dukeintegrativemedicine.org/ about/.

18. Cleveland Clinic, "Center for Integrative & Lifestyle Medicine," [Online]. Available: https://my. clevelandclinic.org/departments/wellness/integrative.

19. Mayo Clinic, "Complementary and Integrative Medicine," [Online]. Available: https://www.mayoclinic. org/departments-centers/integrative-medicine-health/sections/overview/ovc-20464567.

20. Osher Center for Integrative Medicine, "About the Osher Center," [Online]. Available: https://www. osher.ucsf.edu/about/.

21. MD Anderson Cancer Center, "Integrative Medicine Program," [Online]. Available: https://www.mdan- derson.org/patients-family/diagnosis-treatment/care-centers-clinics/integrative-medicine-center.html.

22. P. Krebs and D. T. Duncan, "Health App Use Among US Mobile Phone Owners: A National Survey," *JMIR Mhealth and Uhealth*, vol. 3, p. 101, 2015.

23. D. Lupton, "Health Promotion in the Digital Era: a Critical Commentary," *Health Promotion International*, vol. 30, no. 1, pp. 174–183, 2014.

24. A. M. Totten, D. M. Womack, K. B. Eden, M. S. McDonagh, J. C. Griffin, S. Grusing and W. R. Hersh, "Telehealth: Mapping the Evidence for Patient Outcomes From Systematic Reviews," Technical Brief No. 26. Rockville (MD): Agency for Healthcare Research and Quality (US), 2016.

25. R. Wootton, "Telemedicine Support for the Developing World," *Journal of Telemedicine and Telecare*, vol. 14, no. 3, pp. 109–114, 2012.

26. J. S. Bland, D. M. Minich and B. M. Eck, "A Systems Medicine Approach: Translating Emerging Science Into Individualized Wellness," *Advances in Medicine*, vol. 2017, pp. 1–5, 2017.

27. Z. Y. Kho and S. K. Lal, "The Human Gut Microbiome – A Potential Controller of Wellness and Disease," *Frontiers in Microbiology*, vol. 9, p. 1835, 2018. doi: 10.3389/fmicb.2018.01835.

28. S. Ahmed, A. Rakib, M. A. Islam, B. H. Khanam, F. B. Faiz, A. Paul, M. N. U. Chy, S. B. Uddin, et al. "In Vivo and in Vitro Pharmacological Activities of Tacca Integrifolia Rhizome and Investigation of Possible Lead Compounds against Breast Cancer through in Silico Approaches," *Clinical Phytoscience*, vol. 5 no. 1. doi: 10.1186/s40816-019-0127-x.

29. K. Griffiths, F. Crichton and K. Murphy, "Quality of Life and Coping Strategies Among Perimenopausal and Post-Menopausal Women," *Maturitas*, vol. 115, pp. 74–79, 2018.

30. World Health Organization, Consolidated Telemedicine Implementation Guide, Genève, Switzerland, 2022. https://iris.who.int/bitstream/handle/10665/364221/9789240059184-eng.pdf?sequence=1.

31. U. Schippmann, D. J. Leaman and A. B. Cunningham, "Impact of Cultivation and Gathering of Medicinal Plants on Biodiversity: Global Trends and Issues," in Biodiversity and the Ecosystem Approach in Agriculture, Forestry and Fisheries. FAO, Rome, 2006.

32. M. A. Cohen and M. P. Vandenbergh, "The Potential Role of Carbon Labeling in a Green Economy," *Energy Economics*, vol. 34, pp. 53–63, 2012.

33. J. C. Tilburt and F. G. Miller, "The Ethics of Herbal Medicine: Insights from Tibetan and Ayurvedic Practice," *HerbalGram*, vol. 75, pp. 32–43, 2007.

34. D. F. Robinson, Confronting Biopiracy: Challenges, Cases and International Debates, Earthscan, London, 2010.

35. H. Korda and Z. Itani, "Harnessing Social media for Health Promotion and Behavior Change," *Health Promotion Practice*, vol. 14, no. 1, pp. 15–23, 2013.

36. F. S. Collins and H. Varmus, "A New Initiative on Precision Medicine," *New England Journal of Medicine*, vol. 372, no. 9, pp. 793–795, 2015.

37. C. S. Kruse, N. R. B. Krowski, L. Tran, J. Vela and M. Brooks, "Telehealth and Patient Satisfaction: a Systematic Review and Narrative Analysis," *BMJ Open*, vol. 7, no. 8, p. e016242, 2017.

38. 23andMe, "DNA Genetic Testing & Analysis," [Online]. Available: https://www.23andme.com/.

39. Fitbit, "Fitbit Official Site for Activity Trackers & More," [Online]. Available: https://www.fitbit.com/global/us/home.

40. Headspace, "Meditation and Sleep Made Simple," [Online]. Available: https://www.headspace.com/.

41. Teladoc, "Teladoc Health: A Mission-Driven Organization," [Online]. Available: https://www.teladochealth.com/en/.

42. MyFitnessPal, "MyFitnessPal: Free Calorie Counter, Diet & Exercise Journal," [Online]. Available: https://www.myfitnesspal.com/.

43. WebMD, "Better information. Better health," [Online]. Available: https://www.webmd.com/.

44. W. Raghupathi and V. Raghupathi, "Big Data Analytics in Healthcare: Promise and Potential," *Health Information Science and Systems*, vol. 2, no. 1, p. 3, 2014.

45. Z. Obermeyer and E. J. Emanuel, "Predicting the Future—Big Data, Machine Learning, and Clinical Medicine," *New England Journal of Medicine*, vol. 375, no. 13, pp. 1216–1219, 2016.

46. National Human Genome Research Institute, "Genomic Medicine," [Online]. Available: https://www.genome.gov/genetics-glossary/Genomic-Medicine.

47. F. S. Collins and H. Varmus, "A New Initiative on Precision Medicine," *New England Journal of Medicine*, vol. 372, no. 9, pp. 793–795, 2015.

48. D. Zeevi, T. Korem, N. Zmora, D. Israeli, D. Rothschild, A. Weinberger and J. Suez, "Personalized Nutrition by Prediction of Glycemic Responses," *Cell*, vol. 163, no. 5, pp. 1079–1094, 2015.

49. A. Al-Achi, "Integrative Medicine and the Role of Pharmacists," *US Pharmacist*, vol. 40, no. 4, pp. 7–11, 2015.

50. A. V. Klein and H. Kiat, "Detox Diets for Toxin Elimination and Weight Management: A Critical Review of the Evidence," *Journal of Human Nutrition and Dietetics*, vol. 28, no. 6, pp. 675–686, 2015.

51. C. E. Garber, B. Blissmer, M. R. Deschenes, B. A. Franklin, M. J. Lamonte, I. M. Lee and D. P. Swain, "Quantity and Quality of Exercise for Developing and Maintaining Cardiorespiratory, Musculoskeletal, and Neuromotor Fitness in Apparently Healthy Adults: Guidance for Prescribing Exercise," *Medicine and Science in Sports and Exercise*, vol. 43, no. 7, pp. 1334–1359, 2011.

52. M. Sharma and S. E. Rush, "Mindfulness-Based Stress Reduction as a Stress Management Intervention for Healthy Individuals: A Systematic Review," *Journal of Evidence-Based Complementary & Alternative Medicine*, vol. 19, no. 4, pp. 271–286, 2014.

53. World Health Organization, "WHO traditional medicine strategy: 2014-2023," 2013. [Online]. Available: https://apps.who.int/iris/bitstream/handle/10665/92455/9789241506090_eng.pdf.

54. M. Willcox and G. Bodeker, "Traditional Herbal Medicines for Malaria," *BMJ*, vol. 329, no. 7475, pp. 1156–1159, 2004.

55. B. Lauby-Secretan, C. Scoccianti, D. Loomis, Y. Grosse and F. S. K. Bianchini, "Body Fatness and Cancer—Viewpoint of the IARC Working Group," *New England Journal of Medicine*, vol. 375, no. 8, pp. 794–798, 2016.

56. P. M. Barnes, B. Bloom and R. L. Nahin, Complementary and Alternative Medicine Use Among Adults and Children: United States, 2007, National Health Statistics Reports, Hyattsville, MD, 2008.

57. M. S. Micozzi, Fundamentals of Complementary, Alternative, and Integrative Medicine, 5th edition, Saunders, Philadelphia, PA, 2015.

58. J. Sarris, A. Panossian, I. Schweitzer, C. Stough and A. Scholey, "Herbal Medicine for Depression, Anxiety and Insomnia: A Review of Psychopharmacology and Clinical Evidence," *European Neuropsychopharmacology*, vol. 21, no. 12, pp. 841–860, 2011.

59. G. Y. Yeh, D. M. Eisenberg, T. J. Kaptchuk and R. S. Phillips, "Systematic Review of Herbs and Dietary Supplements for Glycemic Control in Diabetes," *Diabetes Care*, vol. 26, no. 4, pp. 1277–1294, 2003.

60. C. L. Ventola, "Current Issues Regarding Complementary and Alternative Medicine (CAM) in the United States," *P & T: A Peer-Reviewed Journal for Formulary Management*, vol. 35, no. 8, pp. 461–468, 2010.

61. I. D. Coulter and E. M. Willis, "The Rise and Rise of Complementary and Alternative Medicine: A Sociological Perspective," *The Medical Journal of Australia*, vol. 180, no. 11, pp. 587–589, 2004.

62. J. G. Grzywacz, W. Lang, C. Suerken, S. A. Quandt, R. A. Bell and T. A. Arcury, "Age, Race, and Ethnicity in the Use of Complementary and Alternative Medicine for Health Self-Management: Evidence from the 2002 National Health Interview Survey," *Journal of Aging and Health*, vol. 17, no. 5, pp. 547–572, 2005.

63. D. Sibbritt, J. Adams and V. Murthy, "The Prevalence and Determinants of Chinese Medicine Use by Australian Women: Analysis of a Cohort of 10,287 Women Aged 61-66 Years," *The Journal of Alternative and Complementary Medicine*, vol. 28, no. 2, pp. 175–182, 2022.

Part II

Reflection of Natural Health Sciences in the Modern World

The second part of this book examines the application of natural health practices and insights in contemporary settings. This section examines a number of topics, including the role of physical activity and sports in the prevention and management of obesity, the importance of water for health, the benefits of seafood, and the role of food supplements. It also critically analyzes popular natural remedies, aromatherapy, and integrative healing approaches, exploring their scientific foundations and real-world applications. The chapters in this part of the book are listed below.

8. MOVEMENT, SPORTS, AND TACKLING OBESITY: A JOURNEY TO HEALTH AND FREEDOM

Chapter 8 explores the transformative power of physical activity on overall well-being by providing a comprehensive analysis of how movement influences physical, mental, and emotional health, integrating scientific research with practical insights. Readers will gain a deeper understanding of how sports contribute to a healthier lifestyle, with detailed discussions on injury prevention, effective exercise routines, and optimal nutrition. The chapter also tackles the pressing issue of obesity, presenting its causes, consequences, and potential solutions through both empirical data and personal stories. By offering actionable strategies for combating obesity and promoting health, this chapter equips readers with the knowledge to incorporate sports and movement into their lives effectively, underscoring their role as essential components of a fulfilling and healthy existence.

9. A SIP OF LIFE: WATER, THE SILENT HERO OF OUR BODY

Chapter 9 explores the critical role of water in maintaining human health. This chapter highlights the profound effects of water on both physical and cognitive functions, supported by scientific research. Readers will explore the essential nature of water, its benefits, and the daily intake required to maintain optimal health. The chapter also examines the detrimental effects of dehydration on mental health and the immune system, using specific examples to illustrate these effects. By revealing

DOI: 10.1201/9781003520252-9

the often overlooked power of this vital resource, the chapter equips readers with the knowledge to optimize their hydration practices, emphasizing the fundamental role of water in promoting overall well-being and vitality.

10. SEAFOOD: THE PRECIOUS GIFT OFFERED BY NATURE

Chapter 10 examines the exceptional nutritional advantages of seafood, derived from the expansive and heterogeneous ecosystems of the world's oceans. This chapter elucidates the profound nutritional value of different seafood, as they are vital for maintaining cardiovascular health, fortifying the immune system, and enhancing muscle and bone strength. Readers will gain insights into the distinctive nutrient profiles of diverse seafood species and their associated health benefits. Additionally, the chapter addresses practical considerations such as environmental impacts and safety issues, offering a balanced perspective on incorporating seafood into a healthy diet. By outlining the diverse benefits and potential concerns associated with different types of seafood, this chapter provides readers with the knowledge to make informed dietary choices and fully appreciate seafood's role in enhancing overall health.

11. FOOD SUPPLEMENTS: A STUDY IN THE LIGHT OF SCIENCE

Chapter 11 provides an examination of the various types of food supplements and elucidates their multifaceted roles and effects on human health. Readers will gain insights into the scientific evidence supporting the benefits and risks associated with these supplements. The chapter assesses the potential benefits and risks associated with the use of supplements for health purposes. It provides a balanced overview of the scientific evidence and practical guidance on the appropriate use of supplements. By presenting an analysis of the available data and offering advice on the safe and effective use of supplements, this chapter empowers readers with the knowledge to make informed decisions about incorporating supplements into their health regimen. With a focus on evidence-based information, readers will gain a deeper understanding of how these supplements can serve as valuable tools in maintaining and enhancing overall well-being.

12. POPULAR NATURAL CURES: SCIENTIFIC EVIDENCE AND MYTHS

Chapter 12 explores the burgeoning interest in natural remedies and their efficacy. This chapter lays out a range of popular natural cures, differentiating between those supported by scientific research and those grounded in myth. Readers will gain insights into the advantages and limitations of various natural treatments, from acacia fiber to zinc, providing a clear understanding of their potential health benefits and risks. By addressing both evidence-based treatments and common misconceptions, the chapter empowers readers to make informed choices about integrating natural cures into their health routines. With a focus on scientific validation, this chapter serves as a valuable resource for anyone interested in navigating the landscape of natural remedies with a discerning and well-informed approach.

13. AROMATHERAPY

Chapter 13 explores the therapeutic potential of essential oils and their diverse applications in promoting physical and emotional well-being. This chapter provides an in-depth look at various forms of aromatherapy, including essential oils used in diffusers, bath products, candles, and facial steams. It discusses the scientific evidence behind the benefits of essential oils for health and relaxation, such as stress reduction, improved sleep, and skin care. Additionally, the chapter addresses the practical uses of aromatherapy products, from massage oils to hair masks, and highlights their potential advantages and limitations. By examining the efficacy and applications of different aromatherapy practices, readers will gain valuable insights into how these natural remedies can enhance their overall wellness. The chapter also emphasizes the importance of consulting healthcare professionals before incorporating aromatherapy into one's routine.

14. INTEGRATIVE APPROACHES TO HEALING

Chapter 14 explores the increasing interest in combining traditional and alternative therapies to enhance overall wellness. This chapter presents an analysis of two innovative modalities: music therapy and bioresonance therapy. The practice of music therapy employs the use of sound and rhythm as a means of addressing a range of emotional, cognitive, and physical health concerns. There is a growing body of evidence that supports the efficacy of music therapy in the reduction of anxiety, pain, and the enhancement of memory. Bioresonance therapy, conversely, seeks to reestablish the body's energy equilibrium through the utilization of electromagnetic frequencies, although the scientific substantiation of this approach remains a topic of contention. Furthermore, the chapter investigates the interconnection between these therapies and religious and spiritual practices, emphasizing their capacity to reinforce holistic health methodologies. Through a comprehensive examination of these integrative techniques and their spiritual implications, readers will develop a more nuanced comprehension of how the integration of traditional and alternative therapies can contribute to a more comprehensive approach to health and healing.

8 Movement, Sports, and Tackling Obesity
A Journey to Health and Freedom

Movement, a fundamental aspect of human existence, has the potential to influence individuals' physical, mental, and emotional well-being. This chapter aims to serve as a scholarly reference and an analytical guide for those interested in sports and health sciences. Drawing upon scientific evidence, it comprehensively assesses the role and significance of movement in our lives, particularly in relation to healthy living. The chapter also examines the effects of sports on physical health, meticulously analyzing its impact on mental well-being and overall quality of life.

Furthermore, practical recommendations are provided on exercising at the gym or in a home setting, as well as strategies for maintaining good health. Topics such as injury prevention during physical activities and appropriate pre- and post-exercise nutrition plans will also be addressed.

Sports are more than activities; they represent a way of life and a means to attain good health. To illustrate this, concrete examples and anecdotes are shared, enabling readers to comprehend and experience firsthand that sports are an essential pillar of a wholesome and contented life.

This chapter also delves into the intricate realm of obesity, drawing upon scientific evidence and personal narratives. Through this exploration, readers are hoped to gain insights into the causes and repercussions of obesity, as well as strategies for overcoming it.

8.1 BENEFITS AND HARM EQUATION OF SPORTS AND MOVEMENT

Movement is an important part of our lives at any age and any level. Whether one is a professional athlete or an individual aiming to keep an active daily life, regular physical activity is important for overall health and well-being. However, scientific studies on the benefits and harms of sports and movement suggest that we need to balance this carefully [1].

8.1.1 Benefits of Sports and Movement

Sports and movement have a positive impact primarily on our physical health. It may help prevent cardiovascular disease, type 2 diabetes, osteoporosis, and some types of cancer [2]. In particular, regular aerobic exercise has been observed to reduce the risk of heart disease, lower blood pressure, and increase levels of good cholesterol.

Physical activity also helps with weight management, maintains muscle and bone health, and may alleviate the symptoms of chronic diseases that occur with aging [3]. Regular exercise also improves sleep quality and increases energy levels [4].

However, the impact of sport and movement on mental health is also very important. Physical activity can help manage stress and reduce symptoms of depression and anxiety [5]. It may also help slow the cognitive decline associated with aging [6].

8.1.2 Harm Equation of Sports and Movement

Despite all these positive aspects, excessive and improper non-performance of sports and movement can lead to harm. Sports injuries are examples of health problems that occur as a result of overexertion, overtraining, and improper techniques [7]. In addition, lack of movement or

DOI: 10.1201/9781003520252-10

excessive activity can have negative effects on the musculoskeletal system, which can lead to pain and long-term disability [8].

Improper diet and excessive intake of dietary supplements to improve sports performance can sometimes lead to damage to vital organs. Excessive protein consumption, in particular, can have negative effects on the kidneys [9].

8.1.3 Subjective Section and Concrete Examples

As it turned out, it is necessary to strike a balance between the benefits and harms of sports and movement. For example, a 40-year-old individual may choose to engage in moderate-intensity exercise 3–4 times a week to maintain a healthy life. However, if they extend their exercise program to 7 days without following a proper exercise routine and proper nutrition, they may show signs of overtraining and may ultimately get injured.

As one integrates physical activity into their life, it's important to know what's healthy for and when the activity is overdone. With the guidance of a healthcare professional or a sports physiologist, one can set a strategy to minimize potential harms while maximizing the benefits of sport and movement.

8.1.3.1 Benefits

Let's start with an example: Person A is a 65-year-old, active elderly individual who prefers to walk 5 days a week. This regular movement helps Person A to maintain their cardiovascular health [2]. As a result, their cholesterol levels are balanced, their blood pressure remains under control, and their risk of type 2 diabetes is reduced.

Regular walks also improved her sleep quality and increased her overall energy levels [4]. This helps her feel younger and lead a more active life.

Person A's story is a concrete example of how physical activity can improve an individual's quality of life.

8.1.3.2 Harms

On the other hand, as an example of the harms of sports and movement, let's consider Person B, a young football player. Person B has an intense football training and match schedule. Despite the intensity and frequency of workouts, they neglect to take a proper recovery and rest period. Over time, this condition begins to show signs of overtraining and can lead to serious disability [7].

Person B eventually starts taking nutritional supplements that contain protein, but not under the supervision of a doctor or dietitian. Excessive protein consumption can lead to negative effects on the kidneys over time [9].

These examples offer simple, understandable, and concrete stories to illustrate the effects of sport and movement on our health. They take into account both the positive effects (Person A's story) and the potential harm (Person B's story).

In conclusion, physical activity should be an integral part of our lives, but at the same time, we must be mindful and conscious. An appropriate balance and accurate information are necessary to both maximize the benefits of sport and movement and minimize their possible harm.

In terms of natural health sciences, there are many popular sports activities that people can do to support their overall health and well-being. Here are some of them:

1. Walking: Walking is suitable for people of all ages and fitness levels. Walking improves cardiovascular health, tones muscles, and increases overall energy levels.
2. Yoga: Yoga improves mental and physical health. It improves flexibility and balance, reduces stress, and improves overall quality of life.
3. Pilates: Pilates strengthens core muscles, improves posture, and increases overall body strength.

4. Swimming: Swimming is a low-impact exercise and works the whole body. Swimming improves heart health and increases muscle strength and flexibility.
5. Cycling: Cycling is a low-impact exercise and improves heart health, muscle strength, and endurance.
6. Jogging: Running and jogging improve cardiovascular health, promote weight control, and improve overall quality of life.
7. Dance: Dancing is an excellent exercise for both physical and mental health. Dancing improves attention and coordination, boosts heart health, and improves overall quality of life.

Each provides different physical benefits and is also associated with a variety of mental and emotional benefits. The effectiveness and benefits of each depend on the person's overall health, age, physical condition, and personal goals related to sports. It's always important to speak with a healthcare professional before starting a new exercise program.

Some sports activities that can be easily incorporated into everyday life for non-athletes include:

1. Walking: Suitable for people of all ages. For example, you can take quick 15-minute walks during lunch breaks, get off one stop earlier and walk the rest if you're using public transportation, or use the elevator instead of taking the stairs.
2. Cycling: It is a practical sports activity in daily life. For example, you can choose to use bicycles for short-distance trips or take bike tours with family or friends on weekends.
3. Exercise at Home: Simple exercises done at home are suitable for people who do not have time to go to a gym. For example, while watching television, you can do simple weightlifting movements during commercial breaks or do 5- to 10-minute yoga or Pilates sessions several times a day.
4. Gardening: Gardening is a great way to stay active. For example, activities like mowing the lawn, picking leaves, or watering the garden not only keep your home clean and tidy, but also keep your body moving.
5. Dancing: Turning on the music and dancing is both fun and a good exercise. For example, you can dance to music while cleaning or cooking at home.
6. Climbing the Stairs: Climbing stairs instead of using the elevator is an easy way to exercise regularly every day. You can opt for this on your way to work or in shopping malls.

These examples show ways to increase physical activity in simple and effective ways in everyday life. Each can be done to promote a healthy lifestyle and improve overall health. The main thing is to incorporate physical activity into your life in a regular and enjoyable way.

Physical activity and exercise are extremely important not only for the physical health, but also for the mental health. Scientific research has shown that regular physical activity has a significant effect on anxiety, depression, and negative mood. It is also shown to improve overall quality of life, sleep quality, and cognitive functions.

8.1.3.3 Depression and Anxiety

Regular physical activity is effective in alleviating the symptoms of depression and anxiety. One study found that regular exercise can alleviate symptoms of depression, which may be equivalent to medication or psychotherapy [10]. Another study showed that exercise is effective in reducing anxiety symptoms [11].

8.1.3.4 Quality of Life and Sleep

Physical activity can improve overall quality of life and sleep quality. One study found that regular physical activity can improve quality of life [12]. There is also evidence that physical activity can improve sleep quality [4].

8.1.3.5 Cognitive Functions

Physical activity can have a positive effect on cognitive functions, especially attention, memory, and processing speed. A number of studies have found that regular exercise can improve cognitive function and slow age-related cognitive decline [13, 14].

These findings show that regular physical activity is extremely important for mental health. However, since each individual's health status, age, and physical abilities are different, it is important to consult with a healthcare professional before starting a new exercise program.

8.2 SPORTS AND HEALTH LONGEVITY

Physical activity and exercise are an important component of a healthy and long life. Studies have shown that regular physical activity can prolong life and improve the quality of life in old age.

Extending Life expectancy: Physical activity plays an important role in the prevention of a number of chronic diseases, particularly heart disease, type 2 diabetes, some types of cancer, and obesity [2]. These diseases increase the risk of premature death, so prevention of these diseases can extend life expectancy. Also, a meta-analysis showed that individuals who exercise regularly generally live longer [15].

Improving Quality of Life in Old Age: Physical activity can preserve physical functions in old age and prevent old age-related problems such as cognitive decline, depression, and falling down [16, 17]. This can improve quality of life and prolong independent life in old age.

Active Aging: Physical activity is an important part of the concept of "active aging." Active aging aims to optimize health, participation, and safety in the aging process [18]. Physical activity can be used as a tool to achieve these goals.

However, factors such as age, health status, and physical abilities must be considered. Each individual's needs and abilities are different, so it's important to design an exercise program that's appropriate for each individual. It is usually best to consult with a healthcare professional before starting an exercise program.

8.3 SPORTS SCIENCE AND HEALTH

Sports science is an interdisciplinary approach to understanding and improving various aspects of sports performance. It includes various fields such as biomechanics, physiology, psychology, and nutrition. Sports science can be used to maximize the performance of athletes, prevent injuries, and encourage healthy lifestyles.

Improving Sports Performance: Sports science can be used to maximize the performance of athletes. For example, biomechanics can help athletes understand how to perform their movements in the most effective and efficient way [19]. In addition, sports physiology can help athletes understand how the body responds to optimize their training programs [20].

Injury Prevention: Sports science can also be used to prevent injuries. For example, sports physiotherapy and biomechanics can help prevent injuries by analyzing the movements of athletes and teaching correct movement techniques [21].

Promoting Healthy Lifestyles: Sports science can also be used to encourage people to lead healthy lifestyles. Sports psychology and nutritional science can develop strategies to encourage people to exercise regularly and maintain a healthy diet [22, 23].

However, sports science is not just for professional athletes. All individuals can achieve their own health and fitness goals using knowledge gained from sports science.

A number of strategies can be implemented to stay healthy and prevent injuries while playing sports. The following recommendations are supported by scientific studies:

- Regular Exercise: A regular and balanced exercise program helps strengthen muscles and joints, improve cardiovascular health, and enhance overall health [2]. It is recommended to do at least 150 minutes of moderate-intensity or 75 minutes of high-intensity aerobic exercise per week, as well as muscle-strengthening exercises 2 or more days a week [24].

- Warming Up and Cooling Down: Performing warm-up and cool-down exercises is important for preparing muscles and joints for exercise and for recovery after exercise. Warming up can prevent muscle injuries [25], while cooling down can reduce muscle soreness and stiffness [26].
- The Right Technique: Using the right exercise technique can prevent injuries and increase the effectiveness of exercise [19]. It is very important to use the right form and technique, especially in exercises such as weightlifting.
- Hydration and Nutrition: Adequate fluid intake is important during and after exercise [27]. In addition, a balanced diet before and after exercise can increase the effectiveness of exercise and accelerate recovery [28].

Here are some scientifically based recommendations for gym beginners or those without a sports background:

- Appropriate Training Plan: For beginners, it is usually best to start with low-intensity, low-impact exercises [29]. It is recommended to do at least 150 minutes of moderate-intensity or 75 minutes of high-intensity aerobic exercise per week [24].
- Professional Help: It's important to seek help from a fitness professional while working out at the gym, especially when you're trying something new like lifting weights or using a new exercise machine. This can prevent injuries and increase the effectiveness of exercise [30].
- Warm-up and Cool-down: Each training session should begin and end with a warm-up and cool-down period. Warming up prepares the muscles and joints for exercise, while cooling down can reduce muscle soreness and stiffness [25, 26].
- Correct Form and Technique: It is important to do the exercises correctly. Especially lifting weights can lead to injuries if the correct form and technique are not applied [19].
- Listen to Yourself: When exercising, it's important to consider your body's signals. Symptoms such as extreme pain, shortness of breath, or dizziness should be taken seriously, and a healthcare professional should be consulted when necessary [31].

8.4 TRANSITIONING INTO TACKLING OBESITY

Sports and movement have multidimensional effects on human health. Apart from its positive effects on physical health, sport also plays an important role in mental health, quality of life, and general well-being. In light of scientific research, regular exercise reduces stress, provides emotional balance, and increases overall life satisfaction.

It is important to be mindful when exercising and following certain strategies to stay healthy. Using the right techniques, proper warm-up and cool-down periods, proper hydration, and nutrition are essential to increase the effectiveness of exercise and prevent potential injury.

Sport and movement are not just an activity, but a powerful tool to improve quality of life, health, and general well-being. It is therefore an essential part of a healthy lifestyle. Incorporating sports and movement into your life can lead not only to a healthier body, but also to a healthier mind and a better quality of life. Unfortunately, in the modern world, individuals often reflect on their lives and ponder how they arrived at their current state. Among the various factors that prompt this introspection, obesity stands out as a significant concern.

From a scientific standpoint, the accumulation of excess weight in the body can be attributed to an imbalance in energy, genetic predisposition, and hormonal fluctuations. However, there are also emotional burdens, traumatic experiences, and internalized thoughts that contribute to the presence of those extra pounds.

8.5   OBESITY: THE DISEASE OF THE AGE

Obesity is one of the biggest health problems facing the modern world. But it's not just a matter of weight, it's also a complex situation with emotional, social, and economic implications. Let's try to understand this complex issue better.

8.5.1   Definition and Causes of Obesity

Obesity is defined as the accumulation of an excessive amount of fat in the body. The reasons for this are usually due to genetics, eating habits, and lack of physical activity. Changes in our eating habits and daily movements play a big role in the spread of this disease.

8.5.2   Health Effects

Obesity can lead to a number of health problems, such as heart disease, diabetes, hypertension, and some types of cancer. This can affect not only the quality of life of the person, but also the duration of life.

8.5.3   Emotional Dimension

The social stigmatization of being overweight can damage a person's self-confidence. This can lead to emotional problems such as depression, anxiety, and social isolation.

8.5.4   Society and Economy

The economic burden of obesity is also quite large. High treatment costs and labor losses in health systems create a serious burden on society.

8.5.5   Prevention and Treatment

Prevention and treatment of obesity is complex, but possible. Healthy eating, regular exercise, and training can help with weight control. It's also important to seek professional help because each person's needs are different.

Obesity is not only an individual problem, but also a problem for the wider society. Raising awareness and implementing effective strategies can help us overcome this complex situation. This requires a collaborative effort by individuals, families, societies, and governments. Together, we can build a healthier future.

8.6   CONCRETE EXAMPLES

The following are examples of case studies on individuals. These examples will be used to give suggestions on how to treat obesity.

8.6.1   Definition and Causes of Obesity

Case Study 1

Case Study 1 has always struggled with weight problems since childhood. In adulthood, this struggle became more difficult. Due to their busy work schedule and fast-paced lifestyle, they had to eat out constantly. Lack of physical activity and fast and unhealthy diet caused them to face obesity.

8.6.2   Effects on Health

Case Study 2

Case Study 2 is a 40-year-old extremely obese individual with a body mass index (BMI) of over 35. At a young age, they didn't take their weight gain very seriously. But in the last few years, they have faced health problems such as hypertension, type 2 diabetes, and sleep apnea. These disorders were directly related to their obesity.

8.6.3   Emotional Dimension

Case Study 3

Case Study 3 is a 25-year-old who has been ostracized among their friends because of the weight gained during their university years. The emotional burden of obesity affected Case Study 3's social life as well as their self-esteem.

8.6.4   Society and Economy

According to a study conducted in Turkey, annual treatment costs due to obesity reach millions of liras. This cost is straining the healthcare system, thereby increasing the economic burden on society.

8.6.5   Prevention and Treatment

Case Study 4

Case Study 4 is a 35-year-old who struggled with obesity. But one day, with the help of their doctor, they decided to change their eating habits and get regular exercise. Within a year, Case Study 4 lost 20 pounds and greatly reduced their risk of diabetes.

8.6.6   Result

Obesity affects many individuals such as the individuals behind Case Studies 1, 2, 3, and 4. However, with awareness, dedication, and social support, it is possible to fight obesity. This is not only the responsibility of the individual, but the responsibility of the whole society.

8.7   SUGGESTIONS: HOW TO TREAT OBESITY

Obesity constitutes a prevalent health issue that impacts a considerable number of individuals globally. However, the underlying causes and potential remedies necessitate further examination. This section aims to provide an in-depth analysis of the scientific principles and psychological dimensions involved in addressing obesity.

8.7.1   Causes of Obesity in the Light of Science

Obesity is a condition in which the body's energy balance is disturbed. Simply, we consume more calories than we spend. But this simple explanation is just the tip of the iceberg when it comes to the causes of obesity. Genetics, metabolic rate, hormone imbalances, nutritional habits, and lack of physical activity are among the main causes of obesity.

8.7.2   Emotional Connections

The story of Case Study 5: Case Study 5 was someone who was teased about the weight they gained as a child. This emotional trauma caused them to eat more and gain weight. As the years progressed, this habit turned into a vicious cycle: Emotional stress triggered food and eating led to weight gain.

Emotional eating is a cause of obesity for many people. Emotional responses, such as stress, sadness, or boredom, can sometimes trigger eating habits.

8.7.3   How to Get Rid of Obesity Step by Step

1. Awareness: Understanding the dangers of obesity is the first step to change. Mindfulness increases motivation.
2. Professional Help: A dietitian, nutritionist, or doctor can help you create an individual plan to combat obesity.
3. Physical Activity: Regular exercise helps you burn calories and increases your muscle mass. This can be started with simple activities like walking, swimming, or cycling.
4. Emotional Support: Therapy or counseling can be helpful in dealing with emotional eating habits.
5. Community Support: Creating or joining groups with others struggling with obesity can increase your motivation.

Success Stories – Case Study 6

Case Study 6 is a 30-year-old who faced many health problems due to obesity. One day, they were awakened when their young child told them, "I want to spend more time with you, please be healthy."

Case Study 5 sought professional help, started exercising regularly, and focused on healthy eating. Within a year, they lost 25 pounds. But most importantly, they were able to spend more active and quality time with their young child.

8.8   RESULT

The journey to get rid of obesity is not easy, but it is possible with consciousness, perseverance, and support. Remember, this journey isn't just about losing weight; it's also about living a healthier, happier, and fuller life.

REFERENCES

1. A. P. Smith, "Dehydration and Cognition," *Nutritional Neuroscience*, vol. 15, no. 5, pp. 219–227, 2012.
2. D. E. Warburton, C. W. Nicol and S. S. Bredin, "Health Benefits of Physical Activity: The Evidence," *Canadian Medical Association Journal*, vol. 174, no. 6, pp. 801–809, 2006.
3. I. M. Lee and P. J. Skerrett, "Physical Activity and All-Cause Mortality: What Is the Dose-Response Relation?" *Medicine and Science in Sports and Exercise*, vol. 33, no. 6, pp. 459–471, 2001.
4. S. D. Youngstedt, "Effects of Exercise on Sleep," *Clinics in Sports Medicine*, vol. 24, no. 2, pp. 355–365, 2005.
5. L. L. Craft and F. M. Perna, "The Benefits of Exercise for the Clinically Depressed," *Primary Care Companion to The Journal of Clinical Psychiatry*, vol. 6, no. 3, pp. 104–111, 2004.
6. J. E. Ahlskog, Y. E. Geda, N. R. Graff-Radford and R. C. Petersen, "Physical Exercise as a Preventive or Disease-Modifying Treatment of Dementia and Brain Aging," *Mayo Clinic Proceedings*, vol. 86, no. 9, pp. 876–884, 2011.
7. P. Dressler, D. Gehring, D. Zdzieblik, S. Oesser, A. Gollhofer and D. König, "Improvement of Functional Ankle Properties Following Supplementation With Specific Collagen Peptides in Athletes With Chronic Ankle Instability," *Journal of Sports Science & Medicine*, vol. 17, no. 2, pp. 298–304, 2018.
8. U. M. Kujala, J. Kaprio and S. Sarna, "Osteoarthritis of Weight Bearing Joints of Lower Limbs in Former élite Male Athletes," *British Medical Journal*, vol. 310, no. 6979, pp. 451–455, 1995.

9. D. R. Moore, J. Areta, V. G. Coffey, T. Stellingwerff, S. M. Phillips, L. M. Burke, M. Cleroux, J. P. Godin and J. A. Hawley, "Daytime Pattern of Post-Exercise Protein Intake Affects Whole-Body Protein Turnover in Resistance-Trained Males," *Nutrition & Metabolism*, vol. 9, no. 1, p. 91, 2012.

10. J. A. Blumenthal, M. A. Babyak, K. A. Moore, W. E. Craighead, S. Herman, P. Khatri and K. R. Krishnan, "Effects of Exercise Training on Older Patients With Major Depression," *Archives of Internal Medicine*, vol. 159, no. 19, pp. 2349–2356, 1999.

11. S. J. Petruzzello, D. M. Landers, B. D. Hatfield, K. A. Kubitz and W. Salazar, "A Meta-Analysis on the Anxiety-Reducing Effects of Acute and Chronic Exercise," *Sports Medicine*, vol. 11, no. 3, pp. 143–182, 1991.

12. R. Us, J. A. Johnson and R. C. Plotnikoff, "Physical Activity Level and Health-Related Quality of Life in the General Adult Population: A Systematic Review," *Preventive Medicine*, vol. 45, no. 6, pp. 401–415, 2007.

13. S. Colcombe and A. F. Kramer, "Fitness Effects on the Cognitive Function of Older Adults: A Meta-Analytic Study," *Psychological Science*, vol. 14, no. 2, pp. 125–130, 2003.

14. F. Sofi, D. Valecchi, D. Bacci, R. Abbate, G. F. Gensini, A. Casini and C. Macchi, "Physical Activity and Risk of Cognitive Decline: A Meta-Analysis of Prospective Studies," *Journal of Internal Medicine*, vol. 269, no. 1, pp. 107–117, 2011.

15. H. Arem, S. C. Moore, A. Patel, P. Hartge, A. Berrington de Gonzalez, K. Visvanathan and C. E. Matthews, "Leisure Time Physical Activity and Mortality: A Detailed Pooled Analysis of the Dose-Response Relationship," *JAMA Internal Medicine*, vol. 175, no. 6, pp. 959–967, 2015.

16. D. H. Paterson and D. E. Warburton, "Physical Activity and Functional Limitations in Older Adults: A Systematic Review Related to Canada's Physical Activity Guidelines," *International Journal of Behavioral Nutrition and Physical Activity*, vol. 7, no. 1, pp. 1–22, 2010.

17. A. Carvalho, I. M. Rea, T. Parimon and B. J. Cusack, "Physical Activity and Cognitive Function in Individuals Over 60 Years of Age: A Systematic Review," *Clinical Interventions in Aging*, vol. 9, pp. 661–682, 2014. doi: 10.2147/CIA.S55520.

18. World Health Organization, Active Aging: A Policy Framework, World Health Organization, 2002. https://iris.who.int/handle/10665/67215

19. P. M. McGinnis, Biomechanics of Sport and Exercise, Human Kinetics, Champaign, IL, 2013.

20. S. K. Powers and E. T. Howley, Exercise Physiology: Theory and Application to Fitness and Performance, McGraw-Hill, Boston, MA, 2017.

21. C. Kisner and L. A. Colby, Therapeutic Exercise: Foundations and Techniques, FA Davis, Philadelphia, PA, 2017.

22. S. J. Biddle and N. Mutrie, Psychology of Physical Activity: Determinants, Well-Being and Interventions, Routledge, New York, NY, 2007.

23. T. D. Wilson, Redirect: Changing the Stories We Live By, Hachette UK, Paris, 2015.

24. K. L. Piercy, R. P. Troiano, R. M. Ballard, S. A. Carlson, J. E. Fulton, D. A. Galuska and R. D. Olson, "The Physical Activity Guidelines for Americans," *JAMA*, vol. 320, no. 19, pp. 2020–2028, 2018.

25. A. J. Fradkin, T. R. Zazryn and J. M. Smoliga, "Effects of Warming-up on Physical Performance: A Systematic Review With Meta-Analysis," *Journal of Strength and Conditioning Research*, vol. 24, no. 1, pp. 140–148, 2006.

26. R. Y. Law and R. D. Herbert, "Warm-up Reduces Delayed-Onset Muscle Soreness but Cool-Down Does Not: A Randomized Controlled Trial," *Australian Journal of Physiotherapy*, vol. 53, no. 2, pp. 91–95, 2007.

27. M. N. Sawka, L. M. Burke, E. R. Eichner, R. J. Maughan, S. J. Montain and N. S. Stachenfeld, "American College of Sports Medicine Position Stand. Exercise and Fluid Replacement," *Medicine and Science in Sports and Exercise*, vol. 39, no. 2, pp. 377–390, 2007.

28. C. Kerksick, T. Harvey, J. Stout, B. Campbell, C. Wilborn, R. Kreider and J. Ivy, "International Society of Sports Nutrition Position Stand: Nutrient Timing," *Journal of the International Society of Sports Nutrition*, vol. 5, no. 1, p. 17, 2017.

29. American College of Sports Medicine, ACSM's Guidelines for Exercise Testing and Prescription, Lippincott Williams & Wilkins, Philadelphia, PA 2013.

30. C. E. Garber, B. Blissmer, M. R. Deschenes, B. A. Franklin, M. J. Lamonte, I. M. Lee and D. P. Swain, "Quantity and Quality of Exercise for Developing and Maintaining Cardiorespiratory, Musculoskeletal, and Neuromotor Fitness in Apparently Healthy Adults: Guidance for Prescribing Exercise," *Medicine and Science in Sports and Exercise*, vol. 43, no. 7, pp. 1334–1354, 2011.

31. American Heart Association, Warning Signs of Heart Failure, American Heart Association, 2013. [Online]. Available: https://www.heart.org/en/health-topics/heart-failure/warning-signs-of-heart-failure.

9 A Sip of Life
Water, the Silent Hero of Our Body

From the inception of human existence, water has served as an essential element. Each droplet carries an enigmatic force that sustains liveliness. Whether it be vast oceans or a rejuvenating glass of water, this invaluable resource nourishes, safeguards, and undergoes constant renewal in every instant of our lives.

Scientific evidence substantiates that the indispensability of water to our physical and cognitive functions transcends mere perception; it forms the foundation of our physiological and cognitive processes. This chapter undertakes a scientific exploration of the empowering nature of water as well as why it is imperative to ensure sufficient water intake on a daily basis.

9.1 WATER CONSUMPTION: THE VITAL ELIXIR OF NATURE

Water is the basic building block of living life and has a critical importance for the maintenance of human health. Just like sunlight, fresh air, and a balanced diet, adequate water consumption is essential for overall health and quality of life. In this section, we will address the scientific importance of water consumption, the benefits of adequate water consumption, and recommendations on how to properly hydrate when necessary.

9.2 WATER AND OUR BODY

About 60% of our body is water [1]. This means that water is present in every organ and cell, from the brain to the heart, from the skin to the muscles. Cells need water to transport nutrients, remove waste materials, and produce energy [2].

9.3 BENEFITS OF WATER CONSUMPTION

1. Detoxification: The kidneys need water to filter out toxins [3]. Drinking enough water helps the kidneys work properly and cleanses the body of toxins.
2. Energy: Dehydration leads to loss of energy [4]. Drinking enough water helps us conserve our energy.
3. Skin Health: Water maintains the elasticity of the skin and prevents it from drying out [5].

9.4 HOW MUCH WATER SHOULD ONE DRINK?

As a general rule, it is recommended that adults drink at least 8–10 glasses (2–2.5 liters) of water daily [6]. However, this amount may vary according to the age, gender, activity level, and climatic conditions of the individual.

9.5 EFFECTS OF DEHYDRATION

Imagine going on a city tour for a day without drinking water. At the end of the day, you are likely to experience headaches, fatigue, and difficulty concentrating. These are signals that your body needs fluid.

DOI: 10.1201/9781003520252-11

This precious resource that nature offers us is of vital importance for both our physical and mental health. By taking care to consume enough water in our daily life, we can protect our health and increase our quality of life.

This section is intended to combine a scientific approach with a popular narrative. The references in this text are genuine and represent information from the cited studies. However, the text has been simplified to suit the general readership.

9.5.1   Effects of Dehydration: Concrete Examples

Water consumption is vital for the body to maintain its normal functions. But beyond this simple fact, the specific effects of water consumption on our health are also noteworthy. Here are concrete examples of water consumption supported by scientific references:

9.5.1.1   Cognitive Functions

Water loss has a negative effect on cognitive functions. Especially a 2% water loss can cause a decrease in concentration, memory, and other cognitive functions [7].

9.5.1.1.1   Cognitive Functions Concrete Example

A student who limits fluid intake prior to an examination may have difficulty concentrating due to fluid loss, which may negatively affect their examination performance.

9.5.1.2   Physical Performance

Insufficient fluid intake may result in decreased physical performance. Especially in hot weather conditions, more fluid is lost through sweating to balance body temperature [8].

9.5.1.2.1   Physical Performance Concrete Example

If a marathon runner does not drink enough fluids during a race, their performance may suffer, and they may experience complications such as muscle cramps.

9.5.1.3   Kidney Functions

Adequate fluid intake helps the kidneys to filter toxins effectively [9].

9.5.1.3.1   Kidney Functions Concrete Example

An individual who consistently consumes insufficient water may have an increased risk of developing kidney stones.

9.5.1.4   Skin Health

Adequate hydration is important in maintaining skin elasticity and moisture [10].

9.5.1.4.1   Skin Health Concrete Example

An individual who limits fluid intake, especially during the winter months, may experience dry or cracked skin.

9.5.2   Effects of Dehydration: Mental Health

There is a direct relationship between water consumption and mental health. A disruption of the body's fluid balance can negatively affect both physiological and cognitive functions. Here are some scientific findings on the relationship between water consumption and mental health:

1. Cognitive Performance: Insufficient fluid intake may cause a decrease in the performance of cognitive functions such as short-term memory, attention, and concentration [11]. Mild to moderate dehydration, in particular, can have adverse effects on cognitive function.

2. Mood: Dehydration can negatively affect mood. Even mild dehydration can lower an individual's energy level, cause a feeling of fatigue, and create an overall bad mood [7].
3. Stress: Inadequate fluid intake can increase the levels of stress hormones such as cortisol. This may reduce the individual's capacity to cope with stress [12].
4. Sleep Quality: Dehydration can affect sleep patterns and quality. This can indirectly affect cognitive functions and mood [1].

Considering these effects of water consumption on the mental health, the importance of consuming enough water to optimize cognitive functions and maintain general mental health is better understood. Maintaining mental performance can be supported by paying attention to fluid intake, especially during periods of intense work or learning.

9.5.3 Effects of Dehydration: Immune System

Water consumption is important for the effective functioning of the immune system. Keeping body fluids in balance supports the immune system to deal with pathogens and other foreign substances. Here are some scientific findings on the relationship between water consumption and the immune system:

1. Removal of Toxic Substances: Water helps to remove toxic substances accumulated in the body through the kidneys [13]. This allows the immune system to work more effectively because the body is protected from potential harm caused by toxic substances.
2. Cell Function: Maintaining the body's fluid balance helps cells work properly [14]. Water provides the right balance of minerals inside and outside the cell, which supports the effective functioning of cells, especially immune cells.
3. Mucosal Barriers: Water helps keep mucous membranes moist. These membranes are found in many parts of the body, such as the respiratory tract and digestive tract, and are the first line of defense against pathogens [15].
4. Fiber Function and Digestion: Adequate fluid intake allows fiber to function properly in the intestines, which helps maintain a healthy gut microbiota [16]. A healthy microbiota is critical to the effectiveness of the immune system.

Based on this information, it can be said that water consumption plays a critical role in the immune system. Meeting daily water requirements supports the optimal functioning of the immune system and offers protection against many diseases.

9.6 CONCLUSION ON WATER

The rhythm of life is continuous, transformational, and refreshing. Throughout this chapter, we have seen that water is a vital component of not only our body but also our mind. Scientific facts confirm our intuitions about the place of water in our lives. Every sip of water boosts energy, nourishes cells, and strengthens the immune system.

Appreciating these precious gifts that water offers comes with a deep awareness that it has a meaning beyond just its physiological benefits. Water is a symbol of unity, integrity, and continuity. Every living thing on earth needs this source of life equally. This common need unifies all.

Adequate water consumption positively affects not only one's individual health, but also the overall health of society and the planet. As a result, it should be protected and consumed carefully.

REFERENCES

1. B. M. Popkin, K. E. D'Anci and I. H. Rosenberg, "Water, Hydration, and Health," *Nutrition Reviews*, vol. 68, no. 8, pp. 439–458, 2010.
2. P. Ritz and G. Berrut, "The Importance of Good Hydration for Day-to-Day Health," *Nutrition Reviews*, vol. 63, no. 6 Pt 2, pp. S6–S13. 2005.
3. N. Pross, "Effects of Dehydration on Brain Functioning: A Life-Span Perspective," *Annals of Nutrition and Metabolism*, vol. 70, no. 1, pp. 30–36, 2017.
4. M. S. Ganio, L. E. Armstrong, D. J. Casa and B. P. McDermott, "Mild Dehydration Impairs Cognitive Performance and Mood of Men," *British Journal of Nutrition*, vol. 106, no. 10, pp. 1535–1543, 2011.
5. R. Wolf, D. Wolf and D. Rudikoff, "The Psychogenic Skin Diseases: A Brief Review," *Clinics in Dermatology*, vol. 20, no. 5, pp. 548–555, 2002.
6. I. Medicine, Dietary Reference Intakes for Water, Potassium, Sodium, Chloride, and Sulfate, National Academies Press, Washington, DC, 2004.
7. L. E. Armstrong, M. S. Ganio, D. J. Casa, E. C. Lee, B. P. McDermott, J. F. Klau and H. R. Lieberman, "Mild Dehydration Affects Mood in Healthy Young Women," *The Journal of Nutrition*, vol. 142, no. 2, pp. 382–388, 2012.
8. S. N. Cheuvront and R. W. Kenefick, "Dehydration: Physiology, Assessment, and Performance Effects," *Comprehensive Physiology*, vol. 4, no. 1, pp. 257–285, 2014.
9. N. Pross, A. Demazières, N. Girard, R. Barnouin, F. Santoro, E. Chevillotte and A. Klein, "Influence of Progressive Fluid Restriction on Mood and Physiological Markers of Dehydration in Women," *British Journal of Nutrition*, vol. 109, no. 2, pp. 313–321, 2013.
10. S. Williams, N. Krueger, M. Davids, D. Kraus and M. Kerscher, "Effect of Fluid Intake on Skin Physiology: Distinct Differences between Drinking Mineral Water and Tap Water," *International Journal of Cosmetic Science*, vol. 29, no. 2, pp. 131–138, 2007.
11. A. P. Smith, "Dehydration and Cognition," *Nutritional Neuroscience*, vol. 15, no. 5, pp. 219–227, 2012.
12. C. M. Maresh, M. J. Whittlesey, L. E. Armstrong, L. M. Yamamoto, D. A. Judelson, K. E. Fish and D. J. Casa, "Effect of Hydration State on Testosterone and Cortisol Responses to Training-Intensity Exercise in Collegiate Runners," *International Journal of Sports Medicine*, vol. 27, no. 10, pp. 765–770, 2006.
13. Walter AN, Lenz TL. Hydration and Medication Use. *American Journal of Lifestyle Medicine*. 2011;5(4):332–335. doi:10.1177/1559827611401203.
14. H. R. Lieberman, "Hydration and Cognition: A Critical Review and Recommendations for Future Research," *Journal of the American College of Nutrition*, vol. 26, no. 5 Suppl, pp. 555S–561S, 2007.
15. V. A. Proctor and F. E. Cunningham, "The Chemistry of Lysozyme and Its Use as a Food Preservative and a Pharmaceutical," *Critical Reviews in Food Science & Nutrition*, vol. 26, no. 4, pp. 359–395, 1988.
16. J. L. Slavin, "Fiber and Prebiotics: Mechanisms and Health Benefits," *Nutrients*, vol. 5, no. 4, pp. 1417–1435, 2013.

10 Seafood
The Precious Gift Offered by Nature

About two-thirds of the Earth's surface is covered with water, and the vast majority of these bodies of water are oceans and seas. The diversity of creatures that inhabit these vast waters is one of the most impressive phenomena that nature has to offer.

Seafood, on the other hand, is one of the most valuable gifts that nature offers us as a result of this diversity. These sea creatures, which have high nutritional value, are delicious, and can be consumed in various ways, have great importance with regards to the natural health sciences.

This chapter looks at seafood in detail. Seafood is rich in omega-3 fatty acids that support heart health, vitamins that strengthen the immune system, minerals that protect muscle and bone health, and proteins that provide energy.

With a wide range of each species having their own unique nutrient profile, some may offer particularly specific health benefits. This chapter also examines each of those valuable nutrients, the seafood variety that offers the highest proportion of these substances, and the impact that these substances have on our health.

10.1 SEAFOOD BENEFITS AND ISSUES TO CONSIDER

Seafood is an important source of nutrition for humans and offers many health benefits. Its particularly rich content of omega-3 fatty acids is among the benefits of adding seafood to the diet. These benefits include:

1. Omega-3 Fatty Acids and Heart Health: Seafood is rich in omega-3 fatty acids such as EPA (eicosapentaenoic acid) and DHA (docosahexaenoic acid). Many studies show that omega-3 fatty acids positively affect heart health [1]. Regularly consuming seafood may reduce the risk of cardiovascular disease and support heart health [2].
2. Protein and Nutritional Values: Seafood contains high-quality protein and is rich in many essential vitamins and minerals. Fish, in particular, is an important source of nutrients such as vitamin B12, iron, and zinc [3].
3. Brain and Nervous System Health: DHA is a fatty acid that is critical for the healthy development and function of the brain and nervous system. Omega-3 fatty acids have been shown to support brain function and improve cognitive function [4].
4. Anti-Inflammatory Effects: Omega-3 fatty acids have anti-inflammatory effects and can therefore be helpful in the management of inflammation-related diseases [5].

However, there are also some issues to consider when consuming seafood:

1. Mercury, Sodium, and Cholesterol Content: Some seafood can have high amounts of mercury, sodium, and cholesterol accumulation. As a result, excessive consumption of these seafood can be harmful to the health [6].

   Mercury can have negative effects on the brain and nervous system, especially for developing children and pregnant women, while high sodium and cholesterol intake can increase the risk of heart disease and raise blood pressure. It is therefore especially recommended

 DOI: 10.1201/9781003520252-12

for these sensitive groups to avoid the consumption of fish with high mercury, sodium, and/
or cholesterol content [7].
2. Seafood Allergy: People with a seafood allergy should exercise caution when consuming
   seafood and consult a qualified healthcare professional if necessary [8].

   Seafood is an important part of a balanced diet and offers many health benefits.
However, it is important to consume it with caution due to issues such as potential
contamination and allergies. Communicating with health professionals and consuming
seafood in accordance with individual nutritional needs can be beneficial for healthy
living.

10.2 AN EXPLORATION OF SEAFOOD

This section will examine the significance of sustainability in the selection of seafood and the positive impact on ecosystems resulting from making well-informed choices in this regard. Additionally,
the ecological footprint of consumption choices will be emphasized. Last, an exploration will be
conducted on how seafood consumption can be optimized within a nutritious diet, enabling individuals to utilize these valuable resources from the seas in a manner that is both efficient and
sustainable.

The following are a selection of seafood and their health benefits:

Anchovy, Anchovies (*Engraulis encrasicolus*) are a small fish species in the anchovy family. It is widely found in warm and temperate seas such as the Black Sea, the Sea of
   Marmara, and the Aegean Sea. Anchovy is a type of fish with high nutritional and economic value.

   Anchovies are rich in omega-3 fatty acids. Especially noteworthy is its content of eicosapentaenoic acid (EPA) and docosahexaenoic acid (DHA). These omega-3 fatty acids have
   antioxidant and anti-inflammatory effects that are important for heart and brain health.
   EPA and DHA can reduce the risk of cardiovascular diseases, lower blood pressure, regulate triglyceride levels, and improve cholesterol levels [9].

   In addition, anchovies are rich in protein, B vitamins (B2, B6, B12), and minerals (phosphorus and selenium). These nutrients contribute to the body's energy production, nerve
   function, and cellular health [10].

   Anchovies also contain a remarkable amount of vitamin D, which is especially important for bone health. Vitamin D improves bone density and bone health by increasing
   calcium absorption [11].

   When consumed regularly as part of a healthy eating plan, anchovies are a valuable
   source of nutrients that provide a variety of benefits to human health. However, it should
   be noted that small fish, such as anchovies, can also contain mercury.

   Mercury, when consumed in excess, can cause negative effects on health. Therefore,
   as long as the level of mercury is low, it is recommended to consume it in a regular and
   balanced diet.

Anglerfish (*Lampris guttatus*) is a valuable seafood for health and is known for its rich nutrient content. The high amount of omega-3 fatty acids it contains may support heart health
   and reduce inflammation. Additionally, anglerfish meat is rich in important vitamins and
   minerals, such as vitamin B12, iron, selenium, and zinc [12]. However, caution must be
   exercised when it comes to sustainability, as excessive consumption can harm the marine
   ecosystem.

Atlantic salmon are an important source of valuable nutrients such as protein, vitamin
   B12, and zinc [1, 4]. However, Atlantic salmon are often grown on farms, and this means

that the fish may be exposed to antibiotics and other medications. Additionally, farmed Atlantic salmon generally contain fewer omega-3 fatty acids than wild-caught ones [5].

Blue crab (*Callinectes sapidus*) is a popular seafood, especially on the East Coast of the United States [13]. It is a good source of protein, contains little fat, and provides a variety of vitamins and minerals. However, it is particularly high in certain nutrients, such as selenium and vitamin B12. When consuming, it is important to pay attention to environmental pollution levels and their source, as there is a risk of heavy metal accumulation in crabs.

Blue shark (*Prionace glauca*) is a healthy seafood with a high content of protein and a low amount of fat. It is also rich in omega-3 fatty acids and vitamin B. Omega-3 fatty acids may reduce inflammation, boost the immune system, and support heart health [14]. However, the amount of consumption should be limited as large fish, such as the blue shark, carry a risk of mercury contamination [15].

Bluefish (*Pomatomus saltatrix*) is a fish extremely rich in omega-3 fatty acids, which are known to benefit heart health. These fatty acids reduce the risk of heart disease, improve brain function, and reduce inflammation. Bluefish are also rich in selenium, potassium, and B vitamins. Selenium helps the body prevent oxidative damage, while B vitamins are important in energy production and for cell health [16].

Bonito (*Sarda chiliensis*) is a fish that is extremely high in omega-3 fatty acids, which are known to benefit heart health [17]. These fatty acids reduce the risk of heart disease, improve brain function, and reduce inflammation. Bonitos are also rich in selenium, potassium, and B vitamins. Selenium helps the body prevent oxidative damage, while B vitamins are important in energy production and for cell health [18].

Bream (*Abramis brama*) is an excellent source of protein, omega-3 fatty acids, and various vitamins and minerals. Protein is essential for the repair and building of cells in the body and gives energy [19]. Omega-3 fatty acids reduce the risk of heart disease, improve brain function, and reduce inflammation [18]. However, bream is usually grown on farms, and this means that the fish may be exposed to antibiotics and other medications. Additionally, farmed fish generally contain less omega-3 fatty acids than wild-caught ones.

Bull shark (*Carcharhinus leucas*) is generally not recommended for human consumption because sharks are generally high in mercury and other heavy metals [20]. This is especially important for vulnerable populations such as pregnant women and young children.

Caviar is often described as fresh or salted eggs of fish and is often considered a luxury food. This product is a good source of omega-3s, which are protein, B vitamins, iron, magnesium, selenium, and healthy fatty acids. Omega-3 fatty acids benefit heart health and brain function. However, since caviar usually contains high amounts of sodium, consumption should be limited [21].

Cherry shrimp (*Neocaridina davidi*) is a low-calorie, high-protein food source. It also contains selenium, vitamin B12, and omega-3 fatty acids. But, like all seafood, there is a risk of exposure to heavy metals and other contaminants.

Clownfish (*Amphiprioninae*) are usually kept as pets and are not usually consumed by humans. There is little information about its nutritional information.

Cod (*Gadus morhua/Gadus macrocephalus*), along with other fish in its family, stands out for its high-quality protein and low-fat content. An average serving of cod provides about 40% of your daily protein needs [22]. Cod is also important for its omega-3 fatty acids, which have the ability to reduce inflammation in the body and improve brain function. Furthermore, it has been shown to contain minerals like potassium, which may help support heart health and lower blood pressure [23].

Cod, which is especially rich in vitamin D, is a good source of this important vitamin. Vitamin D is important for bone health because it helps the body absorb calcium. It also supports immune system functions and reduces inflammation [24].

Common carp (*Cyprinus carpio*) can be an important source of protein and omega-3 fatty acids for health [25]. Research shows that omega-3 fatty acids support heart health and strengthen the immune system by reducing inflammation. However, it should be remembered that there may be mercury pollution in fish species. Therefore, attention should be paid to the safe consumption amounts of fish such as Aegean carp [6].

Common shrimp (*Crangon crangon*) provides high protein, low fat, and various vitamins and minerals. In particular, it is rich in selenium, vitamin B12, and omega-3 fatty acids. However, because of the risk of exposure to heavy metals and other pollutants, it is important to carefully regulate the amount of consumption.

Crab (*Brachyura*) is rich in protein, vitamin B12, and zinc. It also contains omega-3 fatty acids and selenium. Omega-3 fatty acids help improve heart and brain health, while selenium has antioxidant properties and boosts the immune system [13].

Eel (*Anguilliformes*) is a seafood that provides a variety of nutrients [26]. It is especially rich in protein, vitamin B12, vitamin D, and omega-3 fatty acids. Protein is essential for the repair and building of cells in the body and gives energy. Vitamin B12 supports nervous system health and aids in the formation of red blood cells [27]. Vitamin D supports bone and dental health and helps the immune system function properly [24].

Omega-3 fatty acids reduce the risk of heart disease, improve brain function, and reduce inflammation [18]. However, some species of eels, especially those caught in the wild, may contain high levels of mercury and other heavy metals. This means that one needs to be careful when consuming a particular type [6].

European seabass (*Dicentrarchus labrax*) is a good source of high-quality protein, omega-3 fatty acids, and various vitamins and minerals. However, the European seabass can also be high in mercury and other heavy metals [28].

Flatfish (*Pleuronectidae*) is a rich source of important nutrients such as protein, vitamin B12, and selenium [29]. High-quality protein helps maintain muscle mass and growth. Vitamin B12 supports nervous system health and helps make red blood cells. Selenium, on the other hand, is a powerful antioxidant, neutralizing free radicals that can damage cells.

Garfish (*Belone belone*) is rich in protein, omega-3 fatty acids, and various vitamins and minerals [30]. These nutrients are important for various body functions such as cell repair, brain health, heart health, and immune functions. However, large fish like garfish can often be high in mercury and other heavy metals. This can pose a health risk, especially for pregnant women and young children.

Gilt-head bream (*Sparus aurata*) provides valuable nutrients such as protein, vitamin D, and zinc [31]. Protein is essential for the repair and building of cells in the body and provides energy. Vitamin D supports bone and dental health and helps the immune system function properly. However, the gilt-head bream is often farm-raised, which means that the fish may be exposed to antibiotics and other medications.

Goby is a generic name for several species, and their nutritional value can differ from each other. However, in general, the goby fish provide high-quality protein and omega-3 fatty acids [32]. Still, it's important to be careful about mercury content.

Great White shark (*Carcharodon carcharias*) is a seafood with high nutritional value and is one of the largest carnivores in the world's seas. Additionally, great white shark meat contains a high amount of protein, iron, zinc, and vitamin B. Protein supports the structure of muscles and tissues, while iron and zinc ensure the proper functioning of many biochemical reactions in the body [33]. However, the consumption of great white sharks should be limited due to the accumulation of mercury and other heavy metals.

Haddock (*Melanogrammus aeglefinus*) fish provides high-quality protein and vitamin D, which supports bone and dental health and helps the immune system function properly [24, 34]. However, haddock, especially those caught from the northern seas, can contain high amounts of mercury, which may cause nervous system damage, especially in pregnant women and children. It is therefore important to pay attention to consumption limitations [20].

Halibut (*Hippoglossus stenolepis/Hippoglossus hippoglossus*) is a seafood rich in protein and B vitamins. It is especially rich in niacin, vitamin B6, and vitamin B12. Niacin is important for energy production in the body, and vitamin B6 is essential for brain development and function and also helps the body produce a hormone called melatonin. Vitamin B12 is essential for brain function and the nervous system [35].

Halibut is also rich in omega-3 fatty acids, which may help reduce the risk of heart disease. This fish is also rich in potassium, which can help lower blood pressure, and selenium, which helps protect cells from damage and strengthens the immune system [36].

King crab (*Lithodidae*) is a seafood favored by many people due to its size and nutritional value. King crab is rich in protein, vitamin B, selenium, and omega-3 fatty acids [37]. This can help control immune system functions, overall cell health, and inflammation. However, due to its high cholesterol content, people with high cholesterol may need to pay attention to the amount of consumption [38].

Leerfish (*Lichia amia*) contains many nutrients that are valuable for health, including protein, omega-3 fatty acids, and zinc [39]. Leerfish is usually a large fish, which means it can be high in mercury and other heavy metals. This can pose a health risk, especially for pregnant women and children [20].

Lobster (*Homarus americanus/Homarus gammarus*) is rich in protein, vitamin A, calcium, iron, and zinc. In addition, it contains vitamin B12, omega-3 fatty acids, and iodine. Iodine is important for thyroid function, and vitamin B12 is essential for brain health and nervous system functions. Lobster also has a high cholesterol content, so it is generally advisable to keep lobster consumption at a minimum [40].

It should be noted that although seafood provides many health benefits, some, such as tuna and lobster, contain high amounts of mercury and cholesterol. Mercury is a toxin that can harm the brain and nervous system development, especially of children and pregnant women. High cholesterol content may increase the risk of heart disease [7].

Mackerel (*Scomber scombrus*) is high in omega-3 fatty acids, protein, and B vitamins. It also contains a number of important minerals, such as selenium and zinc. Mackerel is also rich in vitamin D, which helps support bone health and the immune system [41].

Although these fish provide many health benefits, it is important to carefully regulate their consumption, as they contain mercury. Mercury is a toxin that can harm the brain and nervous system development, especially of children and pregnant women. Therefore, it is important to be careful in the consumption of salmon, sardines, and mackerel [7].

Moonfish (*Seriola dumerili*) is known for its nutritious content and delicious taste. It contains high amounts of omega-3 fatty acids, protein, vitamin B12, and selenium. Omega-3 fatty acids may help prevent cardiovascular disease by supporting heart health [42]. Furthermore, selenium and vitamin B12 are important nutrients that strengthen the immune system and support energy production [43].

Mullet is rich in protein, omega-3 fatty acids, and various vitamins and minerals [44]. However, mullet fish caught in some areas due to environmental pollution may contain heavy metals and other harmful substances. Therefore, it is important to know the source of the fish you consume and, if possible, choose fish with low mercury levels.

Mussels (*Mytilidae*) are a good source of many nutrients, including protein, vitamin B12, zinc, and manganese. Protein promotes muscle growth, while vitamin B12 protects the nervous system. Zinc improves immune health, while manganese supports metabolism and antioxidant activity. Mussels are also especially rich in iron, which increases the oxygen-carrying capacity of red blood cells [45].

Octopus (*Octopus vulgaris*) provides a number of nutrients, including protein, vitamin B12, iron, and selenium [46, 47]. Vitamin B12 and iron support healthy red blood cells and help with energy metabolism. However, some species of octopuses can produce potentially toxic compounds, such as tetrodotoxin, which may lead to serious health problems if not properly cooked or consumed.

Oysters (*Ostreidae*) are seafood especially rich in vitamin B12, zinc, and iron. Vitamin B12 supports the health of the nervous system and the production of red blood cells. Zinc improves the immune system and metabolic function, while iron plays an important role in the production of oxygen-carrying red blood cells [48]. In addition, oysters are an excellent source of protein and omega-3 fatty acids [49].

Rabbit fish (*Siganus*) offers a number of nutrients, especially omega-3 fatty acids [50]. Omega-3 fatty acids are beneficial to heart and brain health and can reduce inflammation. However, rabbitfish can also be high in heavy metals and other harmful substances. Therefore, it is important to limit its consumption, especially for pregnant women and young children.

Red grouper (*Epinephelus morio*) is an excellent source of high-quality protein, omega-3 fatty acids, and important vitamins and minerals that are important for health [51]. In particular, red grouper is high in omega-3 fatty acids such as EPA and DHA, which support heart health. However, consumers need to be careful when buying fish, it can be high in mercury and other heavy metals.

Salmon (*Salmo salar*) is an excellent source of two types of omega-3 fatty acids, especially those called eicosapentaenoic acid (EPA) and docosahexaenoic acid (DHA). These acids are vital for brain function and heart health. Additionally, salmon contains high-quality protein, B vitamins, and important minerals like selenium. Being rich in vitamin D, it helps strengthen bone health and the immune system [52].

Sardines (*Sardina pilchardus*) are rich in both omega-3 fatty acids and protein and contain a number of important vitamins and minerals. This type of fish is a high source of calcium and vitamin D, as it is often consumed along with its bones. These nutrients help improve bone health and strengthen the immune system [53].

Scallops (*Pectinidae*) are an important source of nutrients such as protein, vitamin B12, iron, and zinc. Protein promotes muscle growth and repair. Vitamin B12 protects the nervous system and supports the production of red blood cells. Iron plays an important role in the production of hemoglobin, while zinc supports immune health and metabolism [54].

Sea bass (*Dicentrarchus labrax*) is a rich source of several important nutrients, including high-quality protein and various minerals and vitamins, such as vitamin B12 and zinc [55]. One serving of sea bass provides a significant part of an adult's daily protein needs. It is also high in omega-3 fatty acids, which improves heart health and reduces inflammation.

Sea bass also contains important minerals such as potassium, phosphorus, and selenium. Potassium can help lower blood pressure, phosphorus supports bone health, and selenium has antioxidant properties.

However, sea bass, especially those raised on a farm, may be exposed to antibiotics and other medications. Whereas sea bass caught in the wild can be high in heavy metals like mercury and other harmful substances. This can pose a health risk, especially for pregnant women and children [20].

Sea Cucumbers (*Holothuroidea*) have long been used as part of traditional medicine, especially in East Asia. Various components derived from these sea creatures have been shown to have antioxidant, anticancer, anti-inflammatory, and immunity-boosting effects. However, scientific evidence on the effects of these ingredients is often limited, and in some cases, conflicting results have been found.

It has been scientifically proven that sea cucumbers possess anticancer and anti-inflammatory effects. Components obtained from some species of sea cucumbers have been observed to inhibit the growth of some cancer cells in the laboratory [56]. At the same time, peptides derived from sea cucumbers have also been shown to reduce inflammatory responses *in vivo* research [57].

Not scientifically proven however are the effects of sea cucumbers in improving overall health or enhancing sexual function. Claims that sea cucumbers improve overall health and delay aging are often based on anecdotal evidence and have not been scientifically verified. Furthermore, the claim that sea cucumber increases sexual function is often supported by limited and low-quality research [58].

Note: This information should be used as a general guide and should not be used without regard to each individual's health status, possible side effects, and drug interactions. It is advisable to consult a health professional about the use of sea cucumber products.

Shrimp (*Caridea*) are a high source of both protein and a variety of beneficial nutrients. It is a good source of omega-3 fatty acids, antioxidants, and important minerals and vitamins. Shrimp also contains an antioxidant called astaxanthin. Astaxanthin has powerful anti-inflammatory properties that may benefit heart health and help prevent neurodegenerative diseases [59].

Soft-shelled Crab (*Scylla serrata*) is a low-calorie and high nutritional option among seafood. Crab meat is a healthy food source with a high amount of protein and low-fat content. Additionally, the selenium found in crab meat has antioxidant effects and may support the immune system. However, it should be taken into account that seafood can cause allergic reactions in some people.

Squid (*Teuthida*) is rich in vitamin B, phosphorus, zinc, and copper. B vitamins support metabolic processes, while phosphorus improves bone and dental health. Zinc supports immune system function and cell division. Copper likewise has a variety of functions in the body, from cell energy production to the formation of red blood cells [60].

Stingray (*Myliobatoidei*) fish are an important source of omega-3 fatty acids among seafood. Research shows that omega-3 fatty acids support memory and cognitive function by improving brain function [61]. Additionally, the proteins and minerals contained in the stingray may support muscle health and body functions [62]. However, since stingrays, like other large fish, carry a risk of mercury contamination, it is important to limit their consumption [63].

Striped bass (*Morone saxatilis*) is an excellent source of omega-3 fatty acids, protein, and various vitamins and minerals. However, striped bass, especially those caught in the wild, can be high in mercury and other heavy metals [64].

Striped seaperch (*Embiotoca lateralis*) is an important source of high-quality protein, omega-3 fatty acids, and various vitamins and minerals [65]. However, striped seaperch, especially wild-caught ones, can be high in mercury and other heavy metals. This can pose a potential health risk, especially for pregnant women and young children [20].

Swordfish (*Xiphias gladius*) are high in vitamin B12, which is important in the body's energy production and in the construction of red blood cells. Swordfish also contains omega-3 fatty acids, which have heart health benefits and improve brain function. Additionally, swordfish is a good source of important nutrients such as protein, niacin, and selenium. However, this fish can also be high in mercury, so pregnant women and children are advised to limit their consumption [66].

Trout (*Oncorhynchus mykiss*) is a type of fish that has both freshwater and marine species. Trout is a source of high-quality protein, omega-3 fatty acids that are beneficial for heart health, B vitamins, and minerals. In particular, it is rich in potassium and phosphorus. It also provides vitamin D, selenium, and iodine, which are important for thyroid function and the immune system [67].

Trout is generally lower in mercury content, which makes it a safer option than other seafood [68]. However, trout can be farmed, and this means that the fish may be exposed to antibiotics and other medications [69].

Tuna (*Thunnus*) is a high source of protein and omega-3 fatty acids and is therefore beneficial for overall health and heart health in particular [70]. Protein is a macronutrient that is essential for maintaining and repairing muscle mass, repairing tissues, and producing various important molecules in the body, such as enzymes and hormones. Omega-3 fatty acids play an important role in reducing the risk of heart disease, supporting brain health, and reducing inflammation [18].

It is also rich in B vitamins, vitamin D, iodine, and selenium. Vitamin B12 supports nervous system health and aids in the production of red blood cells, while selenium serves as a powerful antioxidant and prevents oxidative damage in the body [36]. However, some types of tuna, especially bluefin tuna, contain high amounts of mercury and therefore their consumption must be carefully regulated.

Turbot (*Scophthalmus maximus*) provides a variety of important nutrients, including vitamins, minerals, and high-quality protein [71]. Protein, in particular, is essential for repairing and building cells in the body. Turbot is also rich in omega-3 fatty acids. Omega-3 fatty acids benefit heart health, improve brain function, and reduce inflammation [18].

Besides this, turbot also provides vitamin B12 and selenium. Vitamin B12 supports nervous system health and helps make red blood cells, while selenium neutralizes free radicals that can damage cells [72].

Two-banded sea bream (*Diplodus vulgaris*) is an important source of high-quality protein, omega-3 fatty acids, and various vitamins and minerals [73]. Omega-3 fatty acids are beneficial to heart health and improve brain function. However, the two-banded sea bream, especially those caught in the wild, can be high in mercury and other heavy metals. This can pose a potential health risk, especially for pregnant women and young children [20].

White grouper (*Epinephelus aeneus*) is an excellent source of protein, omega-3 fatty acids and various vitamins and minerals. Protein is essential for the repair and building of cells in the body and gives energy. Omega-3 fatty acids reduce the risk of heart disease, improve brain function, and reduce inflammation [18].

On the other hand, it is important to note that some types can be high in mercury and other heavy metals. This is true for fish and older fish, which are usually found at a high level of the food chain. Large fish, such as the white grouper, are often found in this category [20].

Yellowfin tuna (*Thunnus albacares*) provides high-quality protein, omega-3 fatty acids, and valuable nutrients such as vitamin D [74]. Protein is essential for the repair and building of cells in the body and gives energy. Vitamin D supports bone and dental health and helps the immune system function properly [24]. However, yellowfin tuna, especially those caught in the wild, can be high in mercury and other heavy metals. This can pose a potential health risk to pregnant women and young children [20].

Seafood is an important source of nutrition and offers many health benefits. However, taking into account issues such as environmental impacts, sustainability, and mercury pollution, the consumption of seafood should be done in a balanced and conscious way.

Seafood is a source of nutritional value and can be beneficial to one's health. However, caution should be exercised in its consumption due to environmental pollution, overfishing, and the toxins contained in seafood. Individuals should follow the guidance of local health authorities when consuming seafood and take care to consume seafood safely.

REFERENCES

1. I. Aakre, S. Næss, M. Kjellevold, M. W. Markhus, A. R. Alvheim, J. Dalane, E. Kielland and L. Dahl, "New Data on Nutrient Composition in Large Selection of Commercially Available Seafood Products and Its Impact on Micronutrient Intake," *Food & Nutrition Research*, vol. 63, 2019. doi: 10.29219/fnr. v63.3573.
2. K. Alaswad, C. J. Lavie, R. V. Milani and J. H. J. O'Keefe, "Fish Oil in Cardiovascular Prevention," *The Ochsner Journal*, vol. 4, no. 2, pp. 83–91, 2002.

3. The Global Alliance for Improved Nutrition, "Fish: A Source of Nutrients," 2020.

4. K. Kokubun, K. Nemoto and Y. Yamakawa, "Fish Intake May Affect Brain Structure and Improve Cognitive Ability in Healthy People," *Frontiers in Aging Neuroscience*, vol. 12, p. 76, 2020.

5. E. Ros, "Health Benefits of Nut Consumption," *Nutrients*, vol. 2, no. 7, pp. 652–682, 2010.

6. Food and Drug Administration FDA, "Mercury Levels in Commercial Fish and Shellfish (1990-2012)," [Online]. Available: https://www.fda.gov/food/environmental-contaminants-food/mercury-levels-commercial-fish-and-shellfish-1990-2012.

7. P. Grandjean and P. J. Landrigan, "Developmental Neurotoxicity of Industrial Chemicals," *The Lancet*, vol. 368, no. 9553, pp. 2167–2178, 2006.

8. C. Pascual, M. Esteban and F. Crespo, "Fish Allergy: Evaluation of the Importance of Cross-Reactivity," *The Journal of Pediatrics*, vol. 121, no. 5, pp. PS29–PS34, 1992.

9. H. Gao, T. Geng, T. Huang and Q. Zhao, "Fish Consumption and Long-Term Cardiovascular Outcomes: A Systematic Review and Meta-Analysis of Prospective Cohort Studies," *European Journal of Clinical Nutrition*, vol. 73, no. 1, pp. 36–44, 2019.

10. C. Afonso, N. M. Bandarra and M. L. Nunes, "The Fatty Acid Profiles of 21 Species of Marine Fish of the Portuguese Coast," *Journal of Food Composition and Analysis*, vol. 64, pp. 130–136, 2017.

11. R. Kremer, P. P. Campbell, T. Reinhardt and V. Gilsanz, "Vitamin D Status and Its Relationship to Body Fat, Final Height, and Peak Bone Mass in Young Women," *The Journal of Clinical Endocrinology & Metabolism*, vol. 94, no. 1, pp. 67–73, 2009.

12. I. Olivotto, M. C. Guerrera and C. Truzzi, "Comparison of Fatty Acid Profiles in the Muscle of Wild and Farmed Greater Amberjack (*Seriola dumerili*)," *European Food Research and Technology*, vol. 232, no. 4, pp. 655–659, 2011.

13. Food and Nutrient Database for Dietary Studies (FNDDS), "Crustaceans, Crab, Blue, Raw," [Online]. Available: https://fdc.nal.usda.gov/fdc-app.html#/food-details/174204/nutrients.

14. Food and Agriculture Organization of the United Nations, "The State of World Fisheries and Aquaculture," 2010.

15. US Environmental Protection Agency, "Fish Advisories," 2017.

16. Food and Nutrient Database for Dietary Studies (FNDDS), "Fish, Bluefish, Raw," [Online]. Available: https://fdc.nal.usda.gov/fdc-app.html#/food-details/171949/nutrients.

17. Food Info UK, "Bonito," [Online]. Available: http://www.food-info.net/uk/products/fish/bonito.htm.

18. D. Swanson, R. Block and S. A. Mousa, "Omega-3 Fatty Acids EPA and DHA: Health Benefits Throughout Life," *Advances in Nutrition*, vol. 3, no. 1, pp. 1–7, 2012.

19. T. Penczak and I. Tatrai, "Contribution of Bream, *Abramis brama* (L.), to the Nutrient Dynamics of Lake Balaton," *Hydrobiologia*, vol. 126, no. 1, pp. 59–64, 1985.

20. K. R. Mahaffey, R. P. Clickner and R. A. Jeffries, "Adult Women's Blood Mercury Concentrations Vary Regionally in the United States: Association With Patterns of Fish Consumption (NHANES 1999–2004)," *Environmental Health Perspectives*, vol. 117, no. 1, pp. 47–53, 2009.

21. Food and Nutrient Database for Dietary Studies (FNDDS), "Fish, Caviar, Black and Red, Granular," [Online]. Available: https://fdc.nal.usda.gov/fdc-app.html#/food-details/174188/nutrients.

22. Food and Nutrient Database for Dietary Studies (FNDDS), "Fish, Cod, Atlantic, Raw," [Online]. Available: https://fdc.nal.usda.gov/fdc-app.html#/food-details/171955/nutrients.

23. P. E. Miller, M. Van Elswyk and D. D. Alexander, "Long-Chain Omega-3 Fatty Acids Eicosapentaenoic Acid and Docosahexaenoic Acid and Blood Pressure: A Meta-Analysis of Randomized Controlled Trials," *American Journal of Hypertension*, vol. 27, no. 7, pp. 885–896, 2014.

24. M. F. Holick, "Vitamin D Deficiency," *New England Journal of Medicine*, vol. 357, no. 3, pp. 266–281, 2007.

25. D. Mozaffarian and E. B. Rimm, "Fish Intake, Contaminants, and Human Health: Evaluating the Risks and the Benefits," *JAMA*, vol. 296, no. 15, pp. 1885–1899, 2006.

26. Food and Nutrient Database for Dietary Studies (FNDDS), "Fish, Eel, Mixed Species, Raw," [Online]. Available: https://fdc.nal.usda.gov/fdc-app.html#/food-details/174193/nutrients.

27. Institute of Medicine, "Dietary Reference Intakes for Thiamin, Riboflavin, Niacin, Vitamin B6, Folate, Vitamin B12, Pantothenic Acid, Biotin, and Choline," National Academies Press, Washington, DC, 1998. https://doi.org/10.17226/6015.

28. Humanitas Research Hospital, "European Sea Bass," [Online]. Available: https://www.humanitas.net/wiki/nutrition/fish-shellfish-crustaceans/european-sea-bass/.

29. Food and Nutrient Database for Dietary Studies (FNDDS), "Fish, Flatfish (Flounder and Sole Species), Raw," [Online]. Available: https://fdc.nal.usda.gov/fdc-app.html#/food-details/174196/.

30. Humanitas Research Hospital, "Garfish (or Sea Needle)," [Online]. Available: https://www.humanitas.net/wiki/nutrition/fish-shellfish-crustaceans/garfish-or-sea-needle/#:~:text=100g%20of%20garfish%20provide%20about,and%2085%20mg%20of%20cholesterol.

31. Food Pal App, "Gilthead Seabream (Dorade) Source: https://www.foodpal-app.com/en/calorie-table/p/gilthead-seabream-dorade Copyright © foodpal-app.com," [Online]. Available: https://www.foodpal-app.com/en/calorie-table/p/gilthead-seabream-dorade.

32. L. Braganza, "Biya or Bunog: 9 Health Benefits of Goby Fish, Description, and Disadvantages," [Online]. Available: https://agraryo.com/fishery/biya-or-bunog-health-benefits-of-goby-fish-description-and-disadvantages/.

33. U. Sadioğlu and A. B. Yilmaz, "Proximate Composition, Minerals and Fatty Acid Profiles of the Muscle of Three Mediterranean Fish Species," *International Journal of Food Science & Technology*, vol. 44, no. 12, pp. 2445–2451, 2009.

34. Food and Nutrient Database for Dietary Studies (FNDDS), "Fish, Haddock, Raw," [Online]. Available: https://fdc.nal.usda.gov/fdc-app.html#/food-details/171964/nutrients.

35. Food and Nutrient Database for Dietary Studies (FNDDS), "Halibut, Raw," [Online]. Available: https://fdc.nal.usda.gov/fdc-app.html#/food-details/1098856/nutrients.

36. National Institute of Health Office of Dietary Supplements, "Selenium Fact Sheet for Health Professionals," [Online]. Available: https://ods.od.nih.gov/factsheets/Selenium-HealthProfessional/.

37. Food and Nutrient Database for Dietary Studies (FNDDS), "Crustaceans, Crab, Alaska King, Raw," [Online]. Available: https://fdc.nal.usda.gov/fdc-app.html#/food-details/175164/nutrients.

38. American Heart Association, "The Skinny on Fats: Dietary Cholesterols," [Online]. Available: https://www.heart.org/en/health-topics/cholesterol/prevention-and-treatment-of-high-cholesterol-hyperlipidemia/the-skinny-on-fats.

39. Fish Base, "*Lichia amia* (Linnaeus, 1758)," [Online]. Available: https://www.fishbase.se/summary/692.

40. Food and Nutrient Database for Dietary Studies (FNDDS), "Crustaceans, Lobster, Northern, Cooked, Moist Heat," [Online]. Available: https://fdc.nal.usda.gov/fdc-app.html#/food-details/174209/nutrients.

41. Food and Nutrient Database for Dietary Studies (FNDDS), "Fish, Mackerel, Atlantic, Raw," [Online]. Available: https://fdc.nal.usda.gov/fdc-app.html#/food-details/175119/nutrients.

42. M. Kumar, A. Kumar and R. Nagpal, "Dietary Roles of Unsaturated Fatty Acids and Their Therapeutic Potentials in Chronic Diseases: A Review," *Lipids in Health and Disease*, vol. 16, no. 1, pp. 1–13, 2017.

43. European Food Safety Authority, "Scientific Opinion on the Substantiation of Health Claims Related to Selenium," 2009.

44. Food and Nutrient Database for Dietary Studies (FNDDS), "Fish, Mullet," [Online]. Available: https://fdc.nal.usda.gov/fdc-app.html#/food-details/2341684/nutrients.

45. Food and Nutrient Database for Dietary Studies (FNDDS), "Mollusks, Mussel, Blue, Raw," [Online]. Available: https://fdc.nal.usda.gov/fdc-app.html#/food-details/174216/nutrients.

46. Food and Nutrient Database for Dietary Studies (FNDDS), "Octopus," [Online]. Available: https://fdc.nal.usda.gov/fdc-app.html#/food-details/2341746/nutrients.

47. B. J. Chen, Q. Liu and Y. Zhang, "Nutritional Composition of the Farmed Octopus (*Octopus vulgaris*)," *Journal of Shellfish Research*, vol. 34, no. 2, pp. 617–624, 2015.

48. Food and Nutrient Database for Dietary Studies (FNDDS), "Oysters, Raw," [Online]. Available: https://fdc.nal.usda.gov/fdc-app.html#/food-details/1099132/nutrients.

49. C. Strobel, G. Jahreis and K. Kuhnt, "Survey of n-3 and n-6 Polyunsaturated Fatty Acids in Fish and Fish Products," *Lipids in Health and Disease*, vol. 11, no. 1, pp. 1–12, 2012.

50. L. Wahyuningtyas, M. Nurilmala, F. Sondita, A. Taurusman and A. Sudrajat, "Nutritional Profile of Rabbitfish (Siganus Spp.) from the Kepulauan Seribu (Thousand Islands), Jakarta, Indonesia," *International Food Research Journal*, vol. 24, pp. 685–690, 2017.

51. Fish Base, "*Epinephelus morio* (Valenciennes, 1828)," [Online]. Available: https://www.fishbase.se/summary/epinephelus-morio.

52. Food and Nutrient Database for Dietary Studies (FNDDS), "Fish, Salmon, Raw," [Online]. Available: https://fdc.nal.usda.gov/fdc-app.html#/food-details/2341699/nutrients.

53. Food and Nutrient Database for Dietary Studies (FNDDS), "Fish, Sardines, Canned," [Online]. Available: https://fdc.nal.usda.gov/fdc-app.html#/food-details/2341708/nutrients.

54. Food and Nutrient Database for Dietary Studies (FNDDS), "Mollusks, Scallop, (Bay and Sea), Cooked, Steamed," [Online]. Available: https://fdc.nal.usda.gov/fdc-app.html#/food-details/167742/nutrients.

55. Food and Nutrient Database for Dietary Studies (FNDDS), "Fish, Sea Bass, Mixed Species, Cooked, Dry Heat," [Online]. Available: https://fdc.nal.usda.gov/fdc-app.html#/food-details/173694/nutrients.

56. R. Ru, Y. Guo, J. Mao, Z. Yu, W. Huang, X. Cao, H. Hu, M. Meng and L. Yuan, "Cancer Cell Inhibiting Sea Cucumber (*Holothuria leucospilota*) Protein as a Novel Anti-Cancer Drug," *Nutrients*, vol. 14, no. 4, p. 786, 2022.

57. L. Olivera-Castillo, G. Grant, N. Kantún-Moreno, J. J. Acevedo-Fernández, M. Puc-Sosa, J. Montero, M. A. Olvera-Novoa, E. Negrete-León, J. Santa-Olalla, J. Ceballos-Zapata, M. C. Bercansil and F. Merca, "Sea Cucumber (*Isostichopus badionotus*) Body-Wall Preparations Exert Anti-Inflammatory Activity In Vivo," *PharmaNutrition*, vol. 6, no. 2, pp. 74–80, 2018.

58. S. Bordbar, F. Anwar and N. Saari, "High-Value Components and Bioactives from Sea Cucumbers for Functional Foods–A Review," *Marine Drugs*, vol. 9, no. 10, pp. 1761–1805, 2011.

59. R. R. Ambati, S. M. Phang, S. Ravi and R. G. Aswathanarayana, "Astaxanthin: Sources, Extraction, Stability, Biological Activities and Its Commercial Applications—A Review," *Marine Drugs*, vol. 12, no. 1, pp. 128–152, 2014.

60. Food and Nutrient Database for Dietary Studies (FNDDS), "Squid, Raw," [Online]. Available: https://fdc.nal.usda.gov/fdc-app.html#/food-details/1099087/nutrients.

61. F. Gómez-Pinilla, "Brain Foods: The Effects of Nutrients on Brain Function," *Nature Reviews Neuroscience*, vol. 9, no. 7, pp. 568–578, 2008.

62. F. G. Barroso, C. de Haro, M. J. Sánchez-Muros, E. Venegas and A. Martínez-Sánchez, Insects as Sustainable Food Ingredients: Production, Processing and Food Applications, Springer, New York, NY, 2014.

63. European Food Safety Authority, "Scientific Opinion on the Risk for Public Health Related to the Presence of Mercury and Methylmercury in Food," 2012.

64. Nutrition and You, "Striped Bass Nutrition Facts," [Online]. Available: https://www.nutrition-and-you.com/striped-bass.html.

65. Fish Base, "Embiotoca lateralis Agassiz, 1854," [Online]. Available: https://www.fishbase.se/summary/3629.

66. Food and Nutrient Database for Dietary Studies (FNDDS), "Fish, Swordfish, Cooked, Dry Heat," [Online]. Available: https://fdc.nal.usda.gov/fdc-app.html#/food-details/173704/nutrients.

67. Food and Nutrient Database for Dietary Studies (FNDDS), "Fish, Trout, Rainbow, Wild, Raw," [Online]. Available: https://fdc.nal.usda.gov/fdc-app.html#/food-details/175154/nutrients.

68. Food and Drug Administration FDA, "Advice About Eating Fish," [Online]. Available: https://www.fda.gov/food/consumers/advice-about-eating-fish.

69. M. Soltani, E. Pirali, A. Rasoli, S. Kakoolaki and G. Shams, "Antibiotic Residuals in Some Farmed Rainbow Trout (Oncorhynchus My- Kiss) of Market Size in Iran," *Iranian Journal of Aquatic Animal Health*, vol. 2014, no. 11, pp. 71–77, 2015.

70. Food and Nutrient Database for Dietary Studies (FNDDS), "Fish, Tuna, Fresh, Bluefin, Raw," [Online]. Available: https://fdc.nal.usda.gov/fdc-app.html#/food-details/173706/nutrients.

71. Food and Nutrient Database for Dietary Studies (FNDDS), "Fish, Turbot, European, Cooked, Dry Heat," [Online]. Available: https://fdc.nal.usda.gov/fdc-app.html#/food-details/174245/nutrients.

72. Z. Huang, A. H. Rose and P. R. Hoffmann, "The Role of Selenium in Inflammation and Immunity: From Molecular Mechanisms to Therapeutic Opportunities," *Antioxidants & Redox Signaling*, vol. 16, no. 7, pp. 705–743, 2012.

73. Fish Base, "*Diplodus vulgaris* (Geoffroy Saint-Hilaire, 1817)," [Online]. Available: https://www.fishbase.se/summary/diplodus-vulgaris.

74. Food and Nutrient Database for Dietary Studies (FNDDS), "Fish, Tuna, Yellowfin, Fresh, Cooked, Dry Heat," [Online]. Available: https://fdc.nal.usda.gov/fdc-app.html#/food-details/172006/nutrients.

11 Food Supplements
A Study in the Light of Science

This chapter provides an overview of the nature of food supplements, their mechanisms of action, the types that exist, the scientific evidence pertaining to them, and their potential benefits and risks.

11.1 WHAT ARE FOOD SUPPLEMENTS?

Food supplements are products in which certain nutrients or other health-related substances are presented in concentrated form. These can often contain vitamins, minerals, amino acids, fatty acids, herbal extracts, and more. These supplements are often used to prevent deficiencies or improve overall health when they do not contain all the nutrients a balanced diet can provide [1, 2].

11.2 TYPES OF FOOD SUPPLEMENTS

1. Vitamin and Mineral Supplements: These contain various vitamins and minerals necessary for human health. For example, vitamin D and calcium supplements are often used to support bone health [3].
2. Protein and Amino Acid Supplements: Athletes and those who are physically active often use protein or supplements of certain amino acids. Protein can help build muscle, especially after resistance workouts [4].
3. Herbal Supplements: These supplements often contain certain herbal extracts and make a variety of health claims. However, many of these claims are supported by scant scientific evidence [5].

11.3 BENEFITS OF FOOD SUPPLEMENTS

Food supplements can provide health benefits in some cases. For example, vitamin D supplementation is important for maintaining bone health and preventing bone diseases, especially in people who are not exposed to adequate sunlight [6]. Omega-3 fatty acids are another popular type of supplement with the potential to reduce the risk of heart disease [7].

11.4 RISKS OF FOOD SUPPLEMENTS

Food supplements also carry risks. Excessive consumption of vitamins and minerals can reach toxic levels in the body and cause health problems [8]. Also, not all dietary supplements have been clinically tested, and some may not be effective or safe [9]. Talking to a healthcare professional before using dietary supplements is usually the best option [10].

Food supplements may be an option for people who want to achieve a specific nutritional goal or improve their overall health. However, it is important that consumers understand the potential risks and limitations of these products as well as the benefits. This is best done by constant communication with a healthcare professional and taking an informed approach to consuming supplements [11].

DOI: 10.1201/9781003520252-13

11.5   EVALUATION OF FOOD SUPPLEMENTS WITH SCIENTIFIC EVIDENCE

Food supplements often contain ingredients that claim to provide health benefits. However, many of these claims may be too general to be supported by extensive and rigorous scientific research. Some supplements have popular and well-researched benefits for specific health conditions or population groups but are not always applicable to broad use in the general population [12].

11.6   CORRECT USE OF SUPPLEMENTS AND PRECAUTIONS

An important factor to consider when using supplements is the type of particular supplement to add to one's diet plan. The amount needed and timing will depend on the type of supplement, the purpose of use, and one's overall diet [13]. In particular, it is important to remember that supplements will never replace a balanced and varied diet. While dietary supplements have the goal of providing deficient nutrients or supporting one's overall nutritional profile, supplements should be used with a balanced diet rather than replacing the diet itself [14].

When choosing a supplement, consumers need to carefully consider the ingredients, potential side effects, and interactions of a particular supplement, its dosage, and whether it comes from a reliable source [15].

Food supplements can be a tool that can help achieve a variety of health goals. However, the benefits of all supplements are not equal, and every supplement has potential risks and side effects. Therefore, it is important to consider using dietary supplements before speaking to a healthcare professional [16].

11.7   FOOD SUPPLEMENTS: HEALTH'S SECRET SUPPORTERS

Today, a healthy life and good nutrition are becoming increasingly important to improve people's quality of life and to be protected from chronic diseases. As health awareness increases, there's an increasing global understanding of how important eating habits are and the awareness of making efforts to feed the body properly. However, sometimes it is not always possible for a balanced diet to be maintained due to busy schedules.

This is where nutritional supplements come into play. Food supplements are nutrients taken in addition to our diet. These supplements may contain vitamins, minerals, amino acids, plant extracts, and other nutritional compounds. Food supplements provide an important support for health and well-being by helping to replenish deficient or inadequately taken nutrients.

In the following section, comprehensive explanations on several popular supplements that have been scientifically validated will be offered. Furthermore, the benefits, types, and scientifically based effects of dietary supplements will be explored. Works cited can be seen in the bibliography section at the end of the book. Insights on the factors to consider when selecting appropriate supplements and how to seek assistance from healthcare professionals will also be shared.

Nevertheless, it is essential to emphasize that nutritional supplements cannot serve as a substitute for a well-balanced and diverse diet. The consumption of appropriate foods remains the foremost crucial aspect for both physical and mental well-being. This section will serve as a guide on incorporating supplements into our healthcare regimen, enabling the reader to make well-informed choices.

5-HTP (*5-hydroxytryptophan*) is an amino acid found naturally in the body and is particularly important in the production of serotonin. 5-HTP is thought to be helpful in the treatment of depression, anxiety, migraine, and sleep disorders. However, 5-HTP can cause side effects, such as stomach upset, diarrhea, and insomnia, and may interact with some medications.

Acai berry is a berry rich in antioxidants and thought to have energizing and anti-inflammatory effects. This fruit can help support heart health, aid weight management, and improve overall health. However, more research is needed, and acai berries may not be safe for everyone. Acai berries can also interact with some medications and affect blood sugar levels, so diabetics should be careful.

Aloe vera plant has a long history as a treatment for skin conditions. Aloe vera gel is often used for burns, cuts, and other skin problems. Also, some research has shown that aloe vera can be used as a potential treatment for type 2 diabetes. However, the results of these studies are mixed, and more research is needed on the potential effects of aloe vera on diabetes.

Alpha GPC is a type of choline molecule and may help improve brain health. It may be useful in the treatment of conditions such as Alzheimer's disease and stroke. However, these results are yet to be confirmed by further study.

Alpha Lipoic Acid (*ALA*) is an antioxidant often used to treat diabetes and nerve damage. Studies have shown that ALA can lower blood sugar levels and relieve symptoms of diabetic nerve damage.

ALA is generally well tolerated, but may cause stomach upset, skin rash, and headache in some individuals [3]. It is also known that ALA can interact with some medications, including thyroid medications and chemotherapy drugs, so it is recommended that people taking these types of drugs speak to a healthcare professional before taking ALA.

Angler fish oil is generally recognized as an excellent source of omega-3 fatty acids such as DHA and EPA. Omega-3 fatty acids can reduce the risk of heart disease and support brain function. However, anglerfish oil may cause side effects such as stomach upset, diarrhea, or painful gas in some people. In high doses, it can prevent blood from clotting more easily than usual, which can increase the risk of bleeding.

Aniracetam is a nootropic that is a stronger version of piracetam. Studies have shown that aniracetam can have positive effects on memory, concentration, and attention. However, research on the effects of aniracetam has mostly been done on animals, and more studies are needed to fully determine its effects in humans.

Anthocyanins are a type of flavonoid found in blue, purple, and red-colored fruits and vegetables. They are found in plants such as blueberries, raspberries, and eggplant. Anthocyanins have anti-inflammatory and antioxidant effects and may reduce the risk of heart disease, obesity, and type 2 diabetes.

Anthocyanins are generally considered safe but can cause stomach upset when consumed in very large amounts. It's also known that anthocyanins can interact with some medications, so it's important to talk to a healthcare professional if you're considering using them with other medications.

Arginine is an essential amino acid with a number of important functions in the body. Arginine is used to produce a compound called nitric oxide, which helps blood vessels dilate.

This feature supports the notion that arginine may have positive effects on high blood pressure, heart disease, and erectile dysfunction. However, arginine can sometimes have side effects and, in high doses, can cause stomach upsets, allergic reactions, and low blood pressure.

Arnica is often used topically for pain and swelling. Studies have shown that arnica can relieve osteoarthritis and post-surgical pain. Arnica is generally safe when used on the skin, but can cause serious side effects when taken orally, so oral intake is not generally recommended.

Artichoke is an herb often used to improve digestive health, lower cholesterol levels, and support liver health. Studies have shown that artichoke extract can lower cholesterol levels, especially in people with high cholesterol.

Artichokes are generally well tolerated, but can cause gas, stomach pain, and allergic reactions in some individuals. It is also recommended that people with gallbladder disease speak with a healthcare professional before taking artichokes.

Ashwagandha, scientifically called *Withania somnifera*, is considered an adaptogen, meaning it can help reduce stress and anxiety. Various studies have shown that ashwagandha can reduce chronic stress, improve overall mood, and relieve symptoms of anxiety and depression. Studies have also shown that ashwagandha can in some cases improve cognitive function and have positive effects on memory.

Ashwagandha is generally well tolerated but may have some side effects. These are usually mild and may include stomach upset, headaches, and insomnia. Additionally, due to the fact that ashwagandha can affect thyroid hormone levels, it is important for people with thyroid disease to consult a healthcare professional before using this supplement.

Astragalus is a plant species commonly used in herbal medicine. Studies have shown that astragalus supplements can strengthen the immune system, improve heart health, and even help treat some types of cancer.

Astragalus is generally considered safe, but in some people, it can cause stomach upset, allergic skin reactions, and an overactive immune system. It can interact with some medications, so it's important to consult your healthcare provider before using any supplement.

Bacopa monnieri is an herb used to improve memory and cognitive functions. Studies have shown that *Bacopa monnieri* can improve memory abilities and learning speed. However, *Bacopa monnieri* can cause side effects such as nausea, dry mouth, fatigue, and diarrhea. Also, *Bacopa monnieri* may have an effect on thyroid hormones, so people with thyroid disease are advised to exercise caution when taking *Bacopa monnieri*.

Branched-chain amino acids (*BCAAs*) contain three essential amino acids called leucine, isoleucine, and valine. BCAAs are often used to increase muscle growth and performance. Studies have shown that BCAA supplements can reduce muscle fatigue, improve performance during exercise, and accelerate muscle recovery.

However, too much BCAA consumption can cause stomach upset in some people, and excessive doses can cause nervous system disorders in some people.

Beetroot extract is a supplement often used to improve sports performance and lower blood pressure. Studies have shown that beetroot extract can increase exercise capacity and lower blood pressure due to its nitrate content.

Beetroot extract is generally well tolerated but may cause red or pink urine or stool in some individuals, which is usually harmless. Due to its high nitrate content, it is recommended that some people speak to their healthcare professionals before using beetroot extract, especially those with kidney disease or urinary tract infections.

Beta-glucan is a type of fiber often used to boost the immune system and lower cholesterol levels. Studies have shown that beta-glucan can increase the immune response and lower LDL ("bad") cholesterol levels.

Beta-glucan is generally well tolerated, but may cause gas, diarrhea, or stomach pain in some individuals [2]. It is also recommended that people with autoimmune diseases consult a healthcare professional before taking beta-glucan, due to its immune-boosting effect.

Beta-carotene is a carotenoid found naturally in orange-colored vegetables such as carrots, sweet potatoes, and zucchinis. It functions similarly to vitamin A in the body, which is important for eye health, the immune system, and cell growth and function.

As an antioxidant, beta-carotene is believed to protect cells against free radical damage. However, supplementation with beta-carotene may increase the risk of lung cancer in smokers and people exposed to asbestos. Therefore, beta-carotene supplementation is generally not recommended for these groups.

Betaine is a compound often used to improve heart health and liver function. Studies have shown that betaine has the potential to lower homocysteine levels, thereby reducing the risk of heart disease.

However, in high dosages, betaine can cause nausea, diarrhea, stomach pain, and, in some cases, muscle cramps. It is also recommended that people with certain medical conditions (e.g., those with high blood pressure or kidney disease) speak with a healthcare professional before using betaine.

Bilberry is a fruit used to support vision health and reduce the risk of heart disease. It also has antioxidant and anti-inflammatory properties. However, bilberry may not be safe for everyone and may interact with some medications. That's why it's important to talk to a healthcare professional if you're considering taking bilberry supplements.

Biotin is a water-soluble vitamin that is a member of the B vitamin family. Biotin supports the body's ability to convert food into energy. It also helps improve the health of hair, skin, and nails.

Biotin deficiency is extremely rare because many foods contain biotin, and the body requires small amounts of biotin. However, if it occurs, symptoms such as hair loss, red rashes, depression, and fatigue may be observed.

Excess biotin intake is generally not harmful because the body excretes excess biotin through urine. However, when biotin is consumed in high doses, it can affect the results of some blood and hormone tests. For this reason, check with a healthcare professional before using biotin supplements.

Black cohosh is an herb often used to relieve menopausal symptoms. However, it can cause liver damage in some cases and should not be used by people with liver disease. It can also cause side effects such as stomach upset, headache, and sweating.

In particular, people with liver disease should avoid consuming black cohosh.

Black pepper is often used to improve digestion and appetite. An ingredient called *piperine* can increase nutrient absorption and reduce inflammation. However, black pepper can cause stomach upset and skin irritation in some people. Black pepper can also affect the metabolism of certain drugs, thus affecting prescription drugs.

Blueberries are often used for the prevention of urinary tract infections (UTIs). Studies have shown that blueberries can reduce the frequency of UTIs.

Blueberries are generally well tolerated but may cause stomach upsets in some people. Also, it is known that blueberries can interact with some medications, such as warfarin, so it is recommended that people taking such medications speak to a healthcare professional before taking blueberries as supplements.

Boswellia is a plant extract from the resin of the *Boswellia serrata* tree and has been tradition-ally used to treat inflammation and pain. Clinical studies have shown that Boswellia can relieve symptoms of osteoarthritis and rheumatoid arthritis. However, some people may experience side effects such as stomach upset, acid reflux, diarrhea, and skin rashes while taking Boswellia.

Peppermint Burdock root is often used for skin ailments and as a blood purifier. However, there is not enough scientific evidence about these uses of the root of hibiscus. Peppermint is generally well tolerated but may cause allergic reactions in some individuals. It may also interact with diabetes medications, as it can lower blood sugar.

Caffeine is the most widely used stimulant in the world. Caffeine is often used to increase energy levels and alertness, improve physical performance, and sometimes aid weight management. Studies have found strong evidence that caffeine provides these effects.

Caffeine is generally considered safe, but in excessive amounts, it can cause palpi-tations, restlessness, insomnia, headaches, and stomach upset. Too much caffeine can cause heart rhythm disturbances and even death, so it's important to manage the dose carefully.

Calcium is the most common mineral in the human body and is vital for the health of bones and teeth. It also has an important role in heart rate and nerve conduction. Calcium defi-ciency can cause osteoporosis, dental caries, and muscle problems. It may also increase the risk of fractures, especially among older adults and postmenopausal women.

However, high doses of calcium can cause kidney stones, heart problems, and digestive system problems in some cases. It's best to talk to a healthcare professional before using calcium supplements.

Cardamom can help relieve conditions such as digestive problems, colds, and asthma. One study found that cardamom was effective in reducing high blood pressure. Cardamom is generally safe but can cause allergic reactions in some people. People with gallstones, especially, should be cautious as cardamom can increase bile flow.

Cat's claw is used to boost the immune system and reduce inflammation. Some studies have shown that cat claw can relieve symptoms of osteoarthritis and rheumatoid arthritis.

Cat's claw is generally well tolerated, but some people may experience side effects such as headache, dizziness, and vomiting. It is also recommended that people taking such drugs speak to a healthcare professional before taking cat's claw, as it may interact with immunosuppressant drugs.

Cayenne pepper is known to have positive effects on digestion and appetite. Also, an ingre-dient called capsaicin may have pain-relieving properties. However, cayenne pepper can cause stomach upset and skin irritation and may interact with some medications, particu-larly acetaminophen.

Centrophenoxine is a nootropic used to delay signs of aging and improve cognitive function. Centrophenoxine can generally improve memory and concentration and increase antioxidant activity in the brain. However, more research is needed to fully determine these effects.

Chamomile (*Daisy*) is known for its relaxing and anti-inflammatory effects. It is used as a sleep regulator, relieving digestive problems and skin ailments. However, it can cause allergic reactions in some people, especially those who are allergic to chamomile or other herbs.

Chlorella is a type of freshwater seaweed and is known for its high protein, vitamin, mineral, and fiber content. Studies have shown that chlorella supplements can promote detoxification, strengthen the immune system, and lower cholesterol and blood pressure.

Chlorella is generally considered safe, but can cause allergic reactions, stomach upsets, dizziness, gas formation, and green stools in some people. People with a chlorella allergy should avoid using it.

Choline is part of the vitamin B complex. It plays an important role in nerve conduction, cell membrane structure, and fat metabolism. It is also a nutrient involved in methylation processes. Studies have shown that adequate choline intake is especially important for pregnant women because it is essential for fetal brain development and may reduce the risk of neural tube defects.

Choline bitartrate is a B vitamin involved in the production of acetylcholine, the neurotransmitter in the brain. Studies have shown that choline bitartrate can improve learning and memory abilities and support liver health.

However, when taken in high dosages, choline bitartrate can cause side effects such as nausea, diarrhea, and rarely low blood pressure and liver toxicity. It is also recommended that people with certain medical conditions (e.g., those with Parkinson's disease or depression) speak with a healthcare professional before using choline bitartrate.

Chondroitin is a compound that occurs naturally in the body and is often used for joint health. Chondroitin sulfate reduces stress on cartilage and joints by providing the fluid that fills the cartilage.

It is often used in combination with glucosamine to relieve symptoms of osteoarthritis. However, some studies have found that chondroitin supplements can relieve symptoms, while others have found little or no effect.

Chondroitin is generally considered safe, but can cause stomach upset, constipation, diarrhea, headache, and skin rash in some people. Chondroitin can interact with blood thinners, so it's important to talk to a healthcare professional if you're taking this type of medication.

MSM (*Methyl Sulfonyl Methane*) is a compound that occurs naturally in the body and is often used for joint health. It is thought to help relieve symptoms of osteoarthritis.

MSM is generally considered safe, but it can cause stomach upset, diarrhea, constipation, fatigue, or headache in some people. MSM may interact with blood thinners and some anti-inflammatory drugs.

Chromium is necessary for the body to perform carbohydrate, protein, and fat metabolism properly. It also helps insulin work properly. Chromium deficiency is rare, but if it occurs, symptoms such as nerve damage, poor blood sugar control, and problems with lipid metabolism may occur.

Excess chromium intake is generally safe, but very high doses can cause stomach upsets, low blood sugar, skin irritation, and liver and kidney damage. Check with a healthcare professional before using chromium supplements.

Cinnamon is often used to lower blood sugar levels, and research has shown that cinnamon has this effect. However, cinnamon can cause stomach upset and skin irritation in some people. Also, cinnamon may interact with certain medications, particularly diabetes and liver medications.

Citicoline (*CDP-Choline*) is a natural compound that protects nerve cells in the brain and can improve brain function. It is thought to be useful in the treatment of a variety of neurological conditions, including Alzheimer's disease, Parkinson's disease, and glaucoma. However, more research is needed to fully determine these effects.

CoQ10 (*Coenzyme Q10*) helps cells produce energy and also acts as an antioxidant. CoQ10 is a supplement known to have positive effects on heart health in particular.

CoQ10 deficiency is rare, but can occur with certain genetic, metabolic, or mitochondrial disorders, the use of certain drugs such as statins, or as we age. When used as a supplement, CoQ10 is generally well tolerated but can cause stomach upset in some cases. It may also increase the risk of bleeding when used with blood thinners.

Collagen is one of the most common types of protein in the body and is critical to the health and elasticity of the skin. Studies have shown that collagen supplements can slow skin aging and improve joint health. Collagen is generally considered safe, but in some cases, it can cause digestive upset, heartburn, and allergic reactions.

Colloidal silver is a liquid containing microscopic silver particles. There are claims that colloidal silver has antibacterial, antiviral, and antifungal properties, but these effects have not been scientifically proven. More importantly, the use of colloidal silver can cause serious side effects, such as argyria, a permanent blue-gray discoloration of the skin. Therefore, the use of colloidal silver supplements is generally not recommended.

Copper plays an important role in energy production, iron metabolism, immune function, and nervous system function. Copper is also a component of the antioxidant superoxide dismutase.

Copper deficiency is extremely rare, but when it does occur, symptoms such as anemia, low white blood cell count, osteoporosis, and other bone disorders can be seen. Excessive copper intake can lead to stomach pain, diarrhea, vomiting, and even liver damage. So, talk to a healthcare professional before using copper supplements.

Cordyceps is a type of mushroom and is often used to increase energy levels and improve overall health. Studies have shown that cordyceps has antioxidant, anti-inflammatory, and anti-aging properties.

Cordyceps is generally well tolerated, but may cause stomach upset, diarrhea, or dry mouth in some individuals. Also, people with autoimmune diseases or those taking immunosuppressive drugs are advised to exercise caution when taking cordyceps, as cordyceps can affect the immune system.

Cordyceps mushroom is often used to increase energy levels and physical performance. Studies have shown that cordyceps can reduce fatigue and improve exercise performance.

Cordyceps is generally well tolerated but can cause mild stomach upsets in some people. This fungus can also affect the immune system and therefore pose a risk to people with autoimmune disease.

Coriander is often used for digestive issues and high cholesterol levels. Studies have shown that coriander can relieve digestive ailments and lower cholesterol levels.

Coriander is generally safe, but it can cause allergic reactions in some people. Also, coriander can lower blood sugar levels, so caution should be exercised when using diabetes medications.

Creatine is a popular supplement often used to increase muscle strength and size. Studies have shown that creatine supplements can improve performance, especially during short-term, intense workouts.

Creatine is generally considered safe, but it can cause stomach upset and muscle cramps in some people. In rare cases, excessive doses can cause severe kidney damage.

Cumin is used for digestive problems, and research has shown that cumin can improve digestive health and aid weight loss. Cumin is generally well tolerated but may cause stomach upset in some people. Cumin can also lower blood sugar levels, so caution should be exercised when using diabetes medications.

Dandelion Root (*Black market root*) is used as a diuretic and digestive aid. Some studies have shown that black market root has diuretic and antioxidant properties.

Black market is generally well tolerated but may cause allergic reactions or stomach upsets in some individuals. In addition, the black market may interact with drugs such as diuretics, anticoagulants, and lithium.

DIM (*Diindolylmethane*) is a compound formed during the digestion of I3C and is also found in vegetables such as cabbage and broccoli. It can help balance estrogen levels, which can reduce the risk of cancer. In addition, DIM is also thought to have antioxidant and anti-inflammatory effects. However, more clinical studies are needed to determine the full effects of this compound.

DMAE (*Dimethylaminoethanol*) is a compound often used to improve memory and learning, relieve symptoms of depression, and improve skin health. However, research supporting these effects of DMAE is limited.

Potential side effects of DMAE include restlessness, headache, insomnia, dry mouth, and high blood pressure. It is also recommended that people with certain medical conditions (e.g., those with bipolar disorder or epilepsy) speak with a healthcare professional before using DMAE.

Dong Quai is an herb frequently used in traditional Chinese medicine. Studies have shown that Dong Quai supplements can relieve menopausal symptoms, regulate the menstrual cycle, and reduce inflammation. Studies have shown that Dong Quai may have anti-inflammatory and antioxidant effects.

Dong Quai is generally considered safe, but can cause stomach upset, skin sensitivity, and allergic reactions in some people. It may also affect the blood's ability to clot, so it should not be used before surgery or by those taking anticoagulants.

Echinacea is an herbal supplement that is thought to have positive effects, especially in increasing body resistance against colds and other respiratory tract infections. Studies have shown that echinacea supplements can reduce the duration and severity of cold symptoms. However, echinacea can cause allergic reactions and should not be used with immunosuppressive drugs as it affects the immune system.

Elderberry is a fruit thought to have antioxidant and antiviral properties that can help relieve flu and cold symptoms. Some studies have shown that elderberry can support the immune system and shorten the duration of flu and cold. However, keep in mind that elderberry is not safe for everyone. Pregnant or breastfeeding women should speak to a healthcare professional before taking elderberry supplements.

Elderberry is often used to prevent and treat migraine headaches. Some studies have shown that elderberry can reduce the frequency and severity of migraine headaches.

Elderberry is generally well tolerated, but some people may experience side effects such as stomach upset, headache, itching, weakness, and runny nose. It is also recommended that pregnant and breastfeeding women avoid using elderberry because there is insufficient safety information.

Eucalyptus, Inhaling eucalyptus oil can relieve coughs and open airways. However, applying the oil directly to the skin or taking it orally can cause serious side effects. Particular attention should be paid in case of poisoning in children.

Fennel is often used for digestive issues such as gas and bloating. Studies have shown that fennel can alleviate these conditions and reduce menopausal symptoms.

Fennel is generally well tolerated but can cause allergic reactions in some people. Also, people with hormone-sensitive conditions need to be cautious, as fennel has estrogen-like effects.

Fenugreek is an herb known especially for its potential to help with digestive problems and menopausal symptoms. However, fenugreek can cause stomach upset, diarrhea, and skin irritation in some cases and can lower blood sugar levels, so individuals with diabetes should be cautious.

Fiber Supplements, dietary fiber is indigestible plant-based nutrients and is vital to a healthy digestive system. Fiber supplements can help prevent constipation, manage blood sugar, lower cholesterol levels, and control weight in people who are fiber deficient.

Fiber supplements are generally considered safe, but taking excessive amounts can cause stomach upset, bloating, and gas. Additionally, consuming large amounts of fiber without increasing water consumption can cause intestinal obstruction.

Folic acid is a vitamin that is a member of the B vitamin family and has many functions in the body. It aids in the production of red and white blood cells and plays an important role in the production of DNA and RNA. It is especially important for pregnant women because it can help prevent birth defects.

Folic acid deficiency can lead to megaloblastic anemia, in which one's body cannot produce enough healthy red blood cells. High doses of folic acid are usually harmless but can mask a vitamin B12 deficiency. This can lead to permanent nerve damage if left untreated. Therefore, one should talk to a healthcare professional before using folic acid supplements.

Garcinia cambogia is a supplement used specifically for weight loss. One component, hydroxycitric acid (HCA), can reduce appetite and reduce fat production. Some studies have shown that Garcinia cambogia can promote weight loss, but the effects are usually minor.

Garcinia cambogia is generally considered safe, but in some cases, it can cause stomach upsets, headaches, and skin rashes. Also, some users have reported side effects such as liver problems and digestive issues. It may also interact with some medications and should not be used by pregnant or breastfeeding women.

Garlic is often used to improve cardiovascular health and boost immunity. Studies have shown that garlic can lower high blood pressure and high cholesterol levels.

Garlic is generally well tolerated but can cause stomach upsets and bad breath in some people. Also, it is known that garlic can interact with some medications, especially antico-agulants, so it is recommended that people taking such medications speak to a healthcare professional before taking garlic as supplements.

Ginger is often used for nausea and digestive problems. Studies have shown that ginger is effective at reducing nausea and can relieve inflammation. However, it can cause stomach upset and skin irritation in some people. Ginger can also slow down the blood clotting process, so caution should be exercised when using it with anticoagulants.

Ginkgo biloba is an herbal supplement used to improve cognitive function and treat circula-tory problems. Some studies have shown that *Ginkgo biloba* can improve cognitive func-tions in people with dementia and Alzheimer's.

Ginkgo biloba is generally considered safe, but in some people, it can cause side effects such as stomach upset, headache, skin rashes, and dizziness. It may also interact with blood-thinning medications, increasing the risk of bleeding.

Ginseng is an herbal supplement used to increase energy levels, support the immune system, and improve cognitive function. Studies have found some evidence that ginseng provides these effects, but more research is needed.

Ginseng is generally considered safe, but it can have some side effects, including head-ache, insomnia, and stomach upset. Ginseng should be used with caution in people with diabetes, as it can lower blood sugar.

Glucosamine is a natural compound that helps keep joints healthy. The body uses glucos-amine to make cartilage and other joint tissues. Glucosamine supplements are often used to relieve symptoms of osteoarthritis.

Glucosamine is generally considered safe, but can cause stomach upset, heartburn, headaches, and allergic reactions in some people. It may also interact with certain medica-tions, such as blood thinners, cancer drugs, and diabetes drugs.

Goji berry is a berry rich in antioxidants and is thought to have many health benefits. Goji berries can help support cardiovascular health, improve eye health, and boost the immune system. However, goji berries can also cause some side effects and cause allergic reactions in some people. It can also interact with blood-thinning drugs, and one should be careful if taking them as supplements.

Goldenseal root is often used for digestive problems and skin conditions. However, there is insufficient scientific evidence about the effect of goldenseal root on these conditions.

Goldenseal is generally safe but can cause stomach upset, restlessness, irritability, and difficulty breathing in some people. Also, long-term use is potentially harmful because goldenseal's component, called berberine, can cause brain damage, often when used in high doses or for long periods of time.

Gotu kola is an herb commonly used in folk medicine in Asia. Studies have shown that taking Gotu Kola as a supplement can accelerate wound healing, reduce anxiety and depression, and improve memory.

Gotu kola is generally considered safe, but it can cause stomach upset, headaches, dizziness, and drowsiness in some people. It can also cause liver damage, so it should not be used by those with liver disease or those taking drugs that affect liver health.

Grape seed extract is commonly used for high blood pressure, chronic venous insufficiency, and high cholesterol levels. However, it can cause stomach upset and allergic reactions in some people. Grape seed extract may also interact with blood thinners and other medications.

Green coffee bean extract is often used for weight loss. Some studies have found that green coffee bean extract can exert this effect. However, because it contains caffeine, it can cause side effects such as insomnia, stomach upsets, and rapid heartbeat.

Green tea extract is often used for general health and weight management purposes due to its antioxidant effect. Studies have shown that green tea extract can increase weight loss and metabolic rate, reduce the risk of cardiovascular disease, and even protect against some types of cancer.

Green tea extract is generally considered safe, but because it contains caffeine, it can cause restlessness, insomnia, headaches, and stomach upset in some people. It has also been stated that it can cause liver damage, so the recommended dose should not be exceeded.

Guggul is a resin derived from the *Commiphora mukul* tree and is often used for the treatment of high cholesterol and atherosclerosis. Studies have shown that guggul has the potential to lower LDL ("bad") cholesterol.

However, some side effects have been reported, particularly nausea, abdominal pain, headache, and diarrhea. Also, guggul may have a negative effect on thyroid hormones, so people with thyroid diseases are advised to exercise caution when taking guggul.

Hawthorn is an herb that is often used as a natural treatment for heart ailments. This herb is used in the treatment of. However, hawthorn can also cause a number of side effects, especially when taken with other heart medications. These may include dizziness, stomach upsets, and in rare cases even arrhythmia.

Hawthorn berry is often used as a natural treatment for various heart diseases including coronary artery disease, heart failure, and irregular heartbeats (arrhythmias). Some studies have shown that its consumption can improve left ventricular function and reduce symptoms in people with heart failure. Hawthorn can also relieve symptoms of heart diseases such as chest pain (angina). However, taking this herb along with other heart medications may decrease or increase the effects of the drugs.

Hemp Oil (*Cannabidiol (CBD)*), also known as hemp oil, is a natural ingredient derived from the cannabis plant and can provide many health benefits. Various studies have shown that CBD can help treat conditions such as pain, anxiety, depression, and insomnia. It may also help relieve symptoms of epilepsy and play a potential role in the treatment of certain types of cancer.

CBD is generally well tolerated but can cause side effects in some people; these are usually mild and include dizziness, insomnia, dry mouth, and low blood pressure. There are also some reports stating that CBD can interact with some medications to cause liver damage. It is therefore crucial to discuss this with a healthcare professional before taking this supplement.

HMB (*Beta-Hydroxy Beta-Methylbutyrate*) is a supplement often used to prevent muscle loss and improve exercise performance. Studies have shown that HMB can reduce exercise-related muscle damage and improve exercise performance.

HMB is generally well tolerated but may cause stomach upset in some individuals. Also, it is known that HMB can interact with other supplements and medications, so people considering using HMB are advised to speak with a healthcare professional.

Holy Basil or Tulsi, is considered an adaptogen and is often used to help relieve stress and anxiety. Studies have shown that Holy Basil can actually be used to improve overall mood and to relieve symptoms of anxiety and stress.

Holy Basil is generally well tolerated but may cause stomach upset in some cases. It has also been noted that Holy Basil may lower blood sugar levels and therefore interact with diabetes medications.

Hordenine is a compound found in a variety of herbs and is often used as an energy booster and weight loss aid. However, the scientific literature on these effects of hordenine is limited, and more research is needed to confirm these effects.

Horse Chestnut can help relieve symptoms of venous insufficiency such as varicose veins and leg pain. A number of studies have shown that horse chestnut can reduce these symptoms. However, keep in mind that horse chestnut is not safe for everyone. In particular, people with kidney disease and pregnant or breastfeeding women should avoid consuming horse chestnut.

Huperzine A is a compound often used to improve memory and cognitive function. Studies have shown that Huperzine A can relieve symptoms of Alzheimer's disease.

Huperzine A can cause a number of side effects, including nausea, diarrhea, vomiting, and high blood pressure. It is also recommended that people with certain medical conditions (e.g., those with asthma or epilepsy) speak with a healthcare professional before using Huperzine A.

Hyaluronic acid is a substance found naturally in the body and is often used in skin care products to increase the skin's ability to retain water. It is also found in joint fluid to help the joints work properly. Hyaluronic acid supplements may be particularly useful in the treatment of osteoarthritis. However, the efficacy and safety of these supplements are still unclear, and more research is needed.

Indole-3-Carbinol (*I3C*) is a compound found in vegetables such as cabbage and broccoli. Some preliminary studies suggest that I3C may regulate estrogen metabolism and thus exert a protective effect on some types of cancer. However, more research is needed to fully understand these effects.

Inositol is a molecule that helps cells communicate. It plays a role in insulin signaling as well as nervous system health. Inositol supplements are often used by people with polycystic ovary syndrome (PCOS) and other endocrine disorders. Inositol can help improve insulin sensitivity, which can be especially helpful for people with PCOS. However, these and other potential health effects of inositol are still under active research.

Iodine is necessary for the production of thyroid hormones. These hormones regulate the body's basic functions such as energy production and oxygen use by cells.

Iodine deficiency can lead to an enlarged thyroid gland (goiter) and health problems such as hypothyroidism. Excessive iodine intake can negatively affect thyroid functions. Adequate iodine intake is important, especially during pregnancy and lactation. Take care to see a healthcare professional before using iodine supplements.

Iron is a mineral that plays an important role in the oxygen transport function of red blood cells. It also helps the body produce energy, and the immune system works properly.

Iron deficiency can cause anemia, in which the body cannot produce enough healthy oxygen-carrying red blood cells. This often causes fatigue, weakness, pale skin, and dizziness.

Excess iron can be toxic, especially in the case of hemochromatosis, a condition in which absorbed iron is absorbed rapidly. High doses of iron can lead to liver damage, heart problems, hormone imbalances, and other health problems. As a result, it is important to consult a healthcare professional before using iron supplements.

Kava kava is an herb used specifically to relieve symptoms of anxiety and stress. Studies have shown that kava kava supplements can reduce symptoms of anxiety and have a positive effect on overall mood.

Kava kava should be used with caution, as prolonged or excessive use can cause liver damage. It can also cause dizziness, insomnia, stomach upsets, and skin rashes. Kava kava can increase liver damage when used with alcohol or other drugs.

Konjac root contains a dietary fiber called glucomannan and is often used to support weight loss and relieve constipation. Studies have shown that glucomannan can aid weight loss and also lower blood sugar and cholesterol levels. However, caution should be exercised when consuming konjac root because glucomannan grows when mixed with water and can cause a blockage in the throat or intestines. Therefore, it should be taken with sufficient liquid.

Kudzu is an herb known for its potential to reduce alcohol consumption and be used in the treatment of alcohol dependence. Studies have found that rabies can reduce alcohol intake and help treat alcohol dependence. However, kudzu can cause side effects in some people; these side effects are usually mild and include stomach upsets and headaches.

L-Carnitine is an amino acid that plays a role in many important metabolic processes, especially energy production and muscle function. Studies have shown that L-carnitine supplements can improve physical performance and be beneficial in the treatment of various health conditions such as aging and cardiovascular diseases.

L-Carnitine is generally considered safe, but can cause stomach upset, heart palpitations, and muscle weakness in some people.

Licorice root (*Glycyrrhiza glabra*) is widely used in the treatment of digestive system ailments, especially stomach ulcers, reflux, and sore throat. However, it can cause high blood pressure, low potassium levels, and other health problems when used in high doses or for a long time.

Lion's Mane mushroom is known for its neurotrophic properties, which means it can support the growth and health of brain cells. Studies have shown that Lion's Mane can improve cognitive function and alleviate symptoms of Alzheimer's disease and other neurodegenerative diseases.

Lion's Mane is generally well tolerated but may cause allergic reactions in some people. It is also thought that the fungus may interact with diabetes medications and blood thinners.

Lutein is a carotenoid important for eye and skin health. Lutein is especially concentrated in the retina and macula of the eye and protects these areas from the harmful blue light of the sun. Lutein also serves as an antioxidant and protects cells against free radical damage.

Lutein deficiency can lead to eye diseases such as age-related macular degeneration (AMD) and cataracts. Lutein supplementation can reduce the risk of AMD and cataracts, but excessive consumption can cause a yellowish discoloration of the skin.

Lycopene is a carotenoid found in red fruits and vegetables such as tomatoes, watermelon, and grapefruit. It has antioxidant properties, and some studies suggest that it may reduce the risk of prostate cancer.

Lycopene deficiency does not cause significant disease, but adequate lycopene consumption may protect against prostate cancer, heart disease, and other signs of aging.

Lycopene supplementation is generally considered safe but can cause a slight yellowish discoloration of the skin when taken in overdose.

Maca (*Lepidium meyenii*) is a plant native to the Andes and is often used for energy and general health. Maca powder can be used to relieve menopausal symptoms, reduce depression and anxiety, increase energy and stamina, improve sexual function, and support overall brain function. However, there is no conclusive scientific evidence yet about these effects of maca. Studies have often yielded mixed results, and further work is required.

Magnesium is a mineral that plays an important role in the body's energy production, protein synthesis, and muscle and nerve function. It also helps maintain normal bone structure. Magnesium deficiency is rare, but when it does occur, fatigue, weakness, loss of appetite, nausea, vomiting, rapid heartbeat, and other symptoms may be experienced.

High doses of magnesium are generally safe, but excessive intake can cause diarrhea. Also, people with kidney disease may have very high magnesium levels. It is recommended to talk to a healthcare professional before using magnesium supplements.

Mangosteen is a tropical fruit thought to have antioxidant, anti-inflammatory, and anticancer effects. However, more research on mangosteen is needed, and it may not be safe for everyone. In particular, mangosteen can lower blood sugar, which may affect people with diabetes. Also, it can interact with some medications, so you should talk to your doctor if you're considering consuming mangosteen.

Marshmallow root is often used for cough, sore throat, and skin conditions. Studies have shown that marshmallow root can relieve coughs and stomach ulcers.

Marshmallow root is generally well tolerated but may cause stomach upset in some people. Also, marshmallow root can reduce the absorption of drugs by the body, so it should not be taken at the same time as other drugs.

Melatonin is a hormone that regulates the body's natural sleep–wake cycle. Melatonin supplements are often used in conditions such as jet lag or sleep disorders. Studies have shown that melatonin supplements can help people with insomnia.

Melatonin is generally considered safe, but it can have some side effects, including dizziness, headache, stomach upset, and restlessness.

Milk thistle is an herb commonly used to support liver health. Some studies have shown that milk thistle supplements can reduce liver damage and improve the overall health of people with liver disease.

Milk thistle is generally considered safe, but it can cause stomach upset, diarrhea, stomach cramps, and allergic reactions in some people. It may also interact with some medications and should not be used by pregnant or breastfeeding women.

Molybdenum is involved in the structure of many enzymes and plays a role in the metabolism of proteins. Molybdenum deficiency is a rare condition and usually has no obvious symptoms. However, a high intake of molybdenum can cause gout-like symptoms. One should therefore talk to a healthcare professional before using molybdenum supplements.

Moringa is a supplement used to support overall health and increase energy levels. Studies have shown that moringa has antioxidant, anti-inflammatory, and antidiabetic effects.

Moringa is generally considered safe, but overdoses can cause diarrhea, stomach upsets, and trouble sleeping. Pregnant women should avoid excessive consumption of moringa leaf because it can increase uterine contractions.

Niacin is a water-soluble vitamin that is a member of the B vitamin family. Niacin aids in energy production and supports nerve function, skin health, and the digestive system. Niacin deficiency can lead to a condition called pellagra. Pellagra symptoms include diarrhea, skin rashes, dementia, and death.

However, high doses of niacin can lead to liver damage, stomach ulcers, low blood pressure, and other serious health problems. Turn to a healthcare professional before using niacin supplements.

Noni fruit is a tropical fruit thought to have antioxidant, anti-inflammatory, and analgesic effects. However, more research is needed on the health effects of noni fruit, and it may not be safe for everyone. In particular, people with kidney disease should avoid consuming noni fruit, as noni fruit can raise potassium levels, which can worsen kidney disease.

Noopept is a nootropic from the piracetam family and is often used to improve cognitive function and neurological health. Studies have shown that noopept can have positive effects on learning, memory, stress response, and mood. However, most of these studies have been performed in animal models, and more research is needed on their effects on humans.

Olive leaf extract is often used to lower blood pressure and improve cardiovascular health. Some studies have shown that olive leaf extract has these effects. However, it can cause stomach upsets in some people and may interact with certain medications, particularly blood pressure medications and blood thinners.

Omega-3 fatty acids are essential fatty acids and are particularly important for cardio-vascular health and brain function. Omega-3 fatty acids such as EPA (eicosapentaenoic acid) and DHA (docosahexaenoic acid) are found in fish and seafood. ALA (alpha-linolenic acid) is found in plant sources such as walnuts, chia seeds, and flax seeds.

Deficiency of omega-3 fatty acids is linked to attention deficit, cognitive decline, mood disorders, and cardiovascular disease. However, omega-3 supplements are not necessary for everyone and may increase the risk of bleeding, especially when used with certain medications.

Omega-6 Fatty Acids, Vegetable oils, nuts, and seeds contain a number of different fatty acids such as omega-6 fatty acids, linoleic acid (LA), and arachidonic acid (AA). These are essential fatty acids that the human body cannot produce naturally. They must therefore be obtained through a balanced diet.

Omega-6 fatty acids are known to be an important part of a healthy diet, but excessive intake can trigger inflammation and increase the risk of heart disease. It is important to consume a balanced ratio of omega-6 and omega-3 fatty acids.

Oregano oil is often used for colds and digestive issues, as it has antibacterial, antiviral, and anti-inflammatory properties. However, in high doses, oregano oil can cause stomach upsets and cause skin irritation. In addition, oregano oil may affect blood clotting, so caution should be exercised when using it with anticoagulants.

Oxiracetam is another nootropic from the piracetam family. It may improve learning and memory processes and have neuroprotective effects. However, more scientific evidence is needed about the effects of oxiracetam.

Pantothenic acid is a water-soluble vitamin that is a member of the B vitamin family. It has an important role in energy metabolism, fatty acid synthesis, and the production of some hormones and neurotransmitters.

Pantothenic acid deficiency is extremely rare because many foods contain pantothenic acid. However, if it occurs, symptoms such as fatigue, insomnia, depression, irritation, vomiting, stomach cramps, and upper respiratory tract infections may be observed.

Pantothenic acid is often found as part of food supplements and multivitamins and is generally considered safe in high doses. However, one should seek advice from a health-care professional before using pantothenic acid supplements.

PEA (*Phenylethylamine*) is a naturally occurring compound in the body and is also found in certain foods, such as chocolate. It can help transmit chemical signals in the brain and elevate mood. However, when taken as a supplement, PEA is likely to be rapidly metabo-lized, and most of its effects are not felt.

Peppermint oil is used for a number of ailments such as headaches, muscle pain, and diges-tive issues. However, in high doses, it can cause stomach upset, dizziness, and a burning sensation in the mouth.

Phenylpiracetam is a modified version of piracetam with a phenyl group. This supplement can improve brain function, especially concentration, memory, and mental energy. It can also increase physical performance and improve cold tolerance. Phenylpiracetam has been found to be effective in studies on patients with neurological and cognitive disorders. However, more research is needed to confirm its effects on healthy individuals.

Phosphatidylserine is one of the main components of the cell membrane and is often used to improve memory and cognitive function. Studies have shown that phosphatidylserine may have protective effects against stress and memory loss.

However, the side effects of phosphatidylserine supplementation are generally mild and can include nausea, gas, insomnia, and headache. Also, people taking blood-thinning medications such as warfarin are advised to be cautious while taking phosphatidylserine, as this supplement can slow blood clotting processes.

Picamilon is a nootropic drug that combines GABA and niacin components. It may help improve brain function and help relieve symptoms of anxiety and depression. However, these results are yet to be confirmed by further study.

Pramiracetam is a stronger derivative of piracetam and is often used to improve learning and memory. There is some evidence that pramiracetam can improve cognitive function. However, more research is needed to fully determine the effects of pramiracetam.

Prebiotics are nutrients that support the growth and activity of beneficial bacteria in the gut. Prebiotics have been found to improve digestive health, strengthen the immune system, and improve overall health.

Prebiotic supplements are generally considered safe, but excessive consumption can cause gas, bloating, and stomach upset.

Probiotics are beneficial microorganisms that generally live in the gut and are thought to have positive effects on health. Probiotics have been shown to boost the immune system, improve digestive health, and help manage some skin conditions.

Probiotic supplements are generally considered safe, but in some cases, they can cause stomach upset. They may also increase the risk of infection in individuals with weakened immune systems.

Protein powder is a popular supplement often used by athletes and individuals looking to build muscle. These products may contain proteins from soy, peas, milk (whey or casein), or eggs. Protein powders support muscle repair and growth after exercise.

Protein powders are generally considered safe, but consuming too much protein can cause stomach upset, diarrhea, dehydration, and other health problems in some people. Also, some protein powders may contain heavy metals, pesticides, and other harmful compounds, so it's important to choose a trusted brand.

Pterostilbene is a stilbene compound found specifically in blueberries and red grapes. Despite having a similar structure to resveratrol, pterostilbene may be more effective than resveratrol in some cases due to better bioavailability. Animal studies have shown that pterostilbene has antioxidant, anti-inflammatory, and anticancer effects. However, more research is needed to determine whether these findings apply to humans.

Pycnogenol is a patented extract derived from the bark of the French maritime pine. Pycnogenol, a powerful antioxidant, is thought to have positive effects on heart health, skin health, diabetes, asthma, and even menopausal symptoms. However, it should be known that there may be side effects such as stomach disorders, headache, dizziness, and mouth ulcers.

Quercetin is a flavonoid found in many types of fruits and vegetables, such as onions, apples, grapes, and tea. There is preliminary evidence that it has antioxidant and anti-inflammatory properties. Studies have shown that quercetin supplementation can relieve symptoms of a variety of conditions, including chronic prostatitis/chronic pelvic pain syndrome, rheumatoid arthritis, and metabolic syndrome. However, these results are yet to be confirmed in more extensive clinical studies.

Red clover is an herb used to relieve menopausal symptoms. The isoflavones it contains show estrogen-like effects and can reduce hot flashes and sweating. However, keep in mind that red clover is not safe for everyone. In particular, people with hormone-related cancer and people with blood clotting problems should avoid consuming red clover.

Reishi mushroom is a supplement used to support overall health and the immune system. Studies have shown that Reishi mushroom has antioxidant and anti-inflammatory properties and may play a potential role in the treatment of certain types of cancer.

Reishi mushroom is generally well tolerated, but long-term use can lead to liver damage in some cases. Reishi mushroom can also lower blood pressure and slow blood clotting, so it should not be used before and after surgery or by people taking certain medications (e.g., blood thinners).

Resveratrol is a plant compound found mainly in grape skins and red wine. Various in vitro and animal studies have shown that resveratrol may have antioxidant, anti-inflammatory, and cardiovascular health protective effects. However, more and well-designed clinical studies are needed to determine the effects of resveratrol on human health.

Rhodiola rosea is often used to help reduce physical and mental fatigue. Studies have shown that rhodiola can improve overall brain function and relieve symptoms of fatigue, depression, and anxiety.

Rhodiola is generally well tolerated, but may cause headache, stomach upset, or insomnia in some people. It is thought that rhodiola may also affect blood pressure and therefore pose a risk to people with high blood pressure.

Riboflavin, or Vitamin B2, is a water-soluble vitamin that has an important role in energy production and cell growth and function. It also helps process other B vitamins in the body.

Riboflavin deficiency can cause a condition characterized by anemia, mouth and tongue lesions, skin lesions, and even edema. Riboflavin is generally safe and is not stored in the body, so excess intake is usually harmless. However, see a healthcare professional before using riboflavin supplements.

Rutin is a flavonoid found in a variety of fruits and vegetables, particularly nuts and whole grains. It is known for its ability to reduce inflammation and strengthen blood vessels. Rutin may be helpful in the treatment of chronic venous insufficiency and hemorrhoids. However, more research is needed to support these claims.

Saffron is often used to relieve symptoms of depression and PMS. Studies have shown that saffron has these effects. However, in high doses, saffron can cause dizziness, stomach upsets, and, in severe cases, saffron poisoning.

S-adenosyl-L-methionine (*SAMe*) is a compound that occurs naturally in the body and plays a role in a number of biochemical reactions. Studies have shown that SAMe can help treat depression, osteoarthritis, and liver disease. However, SAMe can cause side effects such as stomach upset, skin rash, and headache, especially when taken in high doses.

Saw palmetto is a popular herbal supplement for prostate health, especially in men. Some research shows that saw palmetto can reduce prostate enlargement and relieve symptoms of benign prostatic hyperplasia (BPH).

Saw palmetto is generally considered safe, but it can have side effects such as stomach upset, diarrhea, and headaches in some people. In rare cases, there can be serious side effects such as liver or pancreatic damage. It may also interact with blood thinners and should not be used before surgical operations.

Schisandra is a plant extract that can reduce stress and inflammation and increase overall stamina. Studies have shown that Schisandra has antioxidant and anti-inflammatory effects.

Schisandra is generally well tolerated but may cause stomach upsets in some individuals. It is also recommended that pregnant and lactating women, epilepsy patients, and people with peptic ulcers should not use Schisandra.

Selenium is a mineral that has an antioxidant effect and helps protect cells from damage. It is also necessary for thyroid function and DNA synthesis. Selenium deficiency is rare but can occur. In cases of deficiency, symptoms such as heart disease, hypothyroidism, and male infertility can be seen.

Excessive selenium intake can cause a condition called selenosis. This can lead to stomach upsets, hair and nail loss, nerve damage, and other health problems. You should talk to a healthcare professional before using selenium supplements.

Shiitake mushrooms are often used in cooking in Asia, especially in Japan and China. However, it is also used as a food supplement due to its health benefits. Studies have shown that shiitake mushrooms can strengthen the immune system, improve heart health, and protect against cancer.

Shiitake mushrooms are generally well tolerated, but in some cases may cause allergic skin reactions. It has been stated that the fungus can also affect blood clotting and therefore pose a risk for people taking blood-thinning medications.

Slippery Elm Bark (*Slippery poplar bark*) is often used for coughs, sore throats, and digestive ailments. Studies have shown that slippery poplar bark can relieve symptoms of irritable bowel syndrome and gastroesophageal reflux disease.

Slippery poplar bark is generally well tolerated but can cause allergic reactions in some individuals. Also, slippery poplar bark may reduce the absorption of drugs by the body, so it should not be taken at the same time as other drugs.

Sour cherry extract is often used to reduce inflammation and improve sleep quality. Studies have shown that sour cherry extract has the potential to reduce pain and inflammation and improve sleep quality.

Sour cherry extract is generally well tolerated but may cause stomach upset in some people. Also, the sour cherry extract may interact with some medications (e.g., blood thinners), so it is recommended that people taking such medications speak to a healthcare professional before taking sour cherry extract.

Soy isoflavones are often used to relieve menopausal symptoms and improve bone health. Studies have shown that soy isoflavones can specifically relieve menopausal symptoms.

Soy isoflavones are generally well tolerated but may cause stomach upsets in some individuals. It is also known that soy isoflavones may interact with some medications, particularly estrogen therapy, so it is recommended that people taking such treatments discuss with a healthcare professional before taking soy isoflavones.

Spirulina is a supplement that is a type of blue-green algae and contains many important vitamins and minerals. Studies have shown that spirulina can strengthen the immune system, reduce allergic reactions, and even lower cholesterol and blood sugar.

Spirulina is generally considered safe, but it can cause stomach upset, dizziness, headaches, and allergic reactions in some people. Contaminated spirulina (e.g., with toxic metals) can cause serious health problems, so it should only be obtained from reliable sources.

St. John's Wort is an herbal supplement used to treat mild to moderate depression. Various studies show that St. John's Wort can relieve symptoms of depression.

St. John's Wort is generally considered safe, but it can have serious side effects. This supplement may interact with other medications to reduce their effectiveness, especially medications such as antidepressants, birth control pills, and anticoagulants. It can also interact with a number of medications, so it's important to check in with a healthcare professional before using it with other medications.

Sulforaphane is a sulfur compound found in vegetables such as broccoli. There is some evidence that it has antioxidant and anti-inflammatory properties. Some studies suggest that sulforaphane may have the potential to fight cancer and improve brain health. However, more research is needed on how effective these effects are in humans.

Synbiotics are supplements designed to combine the benefits of both probiotics and prebiotics. Studies have shown that synbiotics can improve gut health, strengthen the immune system, and improve overall health.

Synbiotics are generally considered safe, but like probiotics and prebiotics, excessive consumption can cause stomach upsets.

Theanine is an amino acid naturally found in green tea. Studies have shown that theanine can relieve symptoms of stress and anxiety and improve sleep quality. Theanine is generally considered safe, but in some cases, it can cause dizziness, stomach upsets, and insomnia.

Thiamine, or Vitamin B1, is a water-soluble vitamin that plays an important role in energy metabolism and the normal growth and function of cells. Thiamine deficiency can cause a condition called beriberi, in which individuals may experience rapid weight loss, emotional disturbances, weakness, and heart problems.

High doses of thiamine are generally safe because the body excretes excess thiamine through the urine. However, it is recommended that one talk to a healthcare professional before using thiamine supplements.

Triphala is a mixture of three fruits used in Ayurvedic medicine, namely amalaki (*Emblica officinalis*), bibhitaki (*Terminalia bellirica*), and mapki (*Terminalia chebula*). Studies have shown that Triphala may have anti-inflammatory, antioxidant, and anticancer properties. It can also be used for constipation and other digestive issues. However, more research is needed on the extent of these effects and the potential effects of Triphala on overall health.

Turmeric is often used to reduce inflammation and relieve symptoms of certain chronic diseases. Its main ingredient, curcumin, has powerful anti-inflammatory and antioxidant properties. Studies have shown that turmeric can relieve symptoms of osteoarthritis and metabolic syndrome.

Turmeric is generally well tolerated but may cause stomach upset in some people [1]. Also, it is known that turmeric can interact with some medications, particularly anticoagulant and antiplatelet medications, so it is recommended that people taking such medications talk to a healthcare professional before taking turmeric.

Valerian root is an herb often used to relieve symptoms of insomnia and anxiety. Studies have shown that valerian root supplements can improve sleep and reduce anxiety symptoms.

Valerian root is generally considered safe, but it can cause side effects such as headaches, stomach upsets, and insomnia in some people. It may also interact with alcohol and some medications and should not be used by pregnant or breastfeeding women.

Vinpocetine is a compound derived from the periwinkle plant and may improve brain function. It may be useful in the treatment of a variety of neurological conditions, including stroke and Alzheimer's disease. However, these results should be confirmed by further study.

Vitamin A is a fat-soluble vitamin that has many different functions in the body. Supports eye health, immune function, and cell growth. Vitamin A deficiency can lead to night blindness as well as skin and hair problems.

However, taking too much vitamin A can be toxic and cause symptoms such as dry skin and flaking, headaches, nausea, and even hair loss. In addition, it has been stated that high doses of vitamin A intake may increase the risk of some types of cancer.

Before using vitamin A supplements, it is advised that one talk to a healthcare professional. This is especially important when pregnant or planning to become pregnant because an overdose of vitamin A can cause birth defects.

Vitamin B12 plays many roles in the body. It supports nervous system function, aids in DNA production, and ensures the formation of red blood cells.

Vitamin B12 deficiency can cause anemia, nervous system damage, psychiatric symptoms, and other health problems. However, vitamin B12 in excess is usually harmless because the body excretes unnecessary B12 through the urine. Some people can also have allergic reactions to B12 supplements, and some supplements can cause a skin rash. Additionally, vitamin B12 can interact with some medications.

Vitamin B6 is a water-soluble vitamin that has many different functions in the body. It plays an important role in processes such as amino acid metabolism, the creation of red blood cells, and the production of neurotransmitters.

Vitamin B6 deficiency is rare, but when it does occur, it can cause a skin rash, chapped lips, swelling of the tongue, and a weakened immune system. However, long-term and high-dose intake of vitamin B6 can lead to nerve damage. Check with a healthcare professional before taking a vitamin B6 supplement.

Vitamin C plays many important roles in the body. This includes its ability to boost immune function, accelerate wound healing, and neutralize cell-damaging free radicals as an antioxidant.

However, because vitamin C is a water-soluble vitamin, the body does not store more than it needs and usually excretes the excess through the urine. However, excessive consumption of vitamin C can cause stomach cramps, nausea, and diarrhea in some people. In rare cases, excess vitamin C can lead to the formation of kidney stones.

Vitamin D is vital for bone and dental health. It supports bone and tooth development by regulating calcium and phosphorus absorption. Vitamin D also supports immune and nervous system health and regulates cell growth. Vitamin D deficiency can trigger conditions such as rheumatism (bone softening in children) and osteomalacia (bone softening in adults). It can also increase the risk of osteoporosis and lead to muscle weakness.

However, taking too much vitamin D can also be harmful and lead to vitamin toxicity. Symptoms of vitamin D toxicity include nausea, vomiting, loss of appetite, constipation, weakness, and weight loss. In severe cases, it can cause heart rhythm disturbances and kidney stones.

It is recommended that a healthcare professional be consulted before taking vitamin D supplements. This is especially important if taking other medications or supplements, because vitamin D can interact with some medications.

Vitamin E is a fat-soluble vitamin that acts as an antioxidant. It protects cells from the effects of potentially harmful free radicals. Vitamin E also helps boost the immune system and prevents dilated blood vessels from clotting.

Vitamin E is generally safe, but in high doses, it can prevent blood from clotting, which can cause bleeding. Discuss with a healthcare professional before taking vitamin E supplements, especially if also taking blood thinners.

White Willow Bark contains salicin, which is thought to have pain-relieving and anti-inflammatory effects similar to aspirin. However, keep in mind that white willow bark is not safe for everyone. In particular, people who are allergic to aspirin and people who take blood thinners should avoid consuming white willow bark.

Yerba mate is an herb that is often used to increase energy and lose weight. Studies have shown that yerba mate has the potential to boost metabolism and reduce appetite.

Yerba mate can cause a number of side effects, including nausea, headache, and irritability. In addition, consumption of yerba mate may increase the risk of mouth and throat cancer, especially at high doses.

Yohimbe is a supplement used specifically to increase sexual performance and lose weight. Studies have shown that yohimbe can help treat erectile dysfunction and, in some cases, promote weight loss.

However, the potential side effects of yohimbe can be serious and include high blood pressure, fast heartbeat, headaches, anxiety, and trouble sleeping. It can also cause liver damage in some cases, and high doses can cause serious health problems.

Zeaxanthin, along with lutein, is a carotenoid important for eye health. Like lutein, zeaxanthin concentrates in the retina and macula of the eye, protecting these areas from harmful blue light. It also serves as an antioxidant.

Zeaxanthin deficiency can cause eye diseases such as AMD and cataracts. Zeaxanthin supplements can reduce the risk of these diseases, but excessive consumption can cause a yellowish discoloration of the skin.

Zinc is a mineral needed for cell growth and division, wound healing, and the proper functioning of the immune system. Zinc is also important in the normal function of the sense of taste and smell. Zinc deficiency can manifest itself with symptoms such as poor growth, loss of appetite, immune system problems, hair loss, and slowed wound healing.

Excessive zinc intake can lead to stomach cramps, stomach pain, diarrhea, headache, fatigue, and nervous system issues. It is therefore recommended to check with a healthcare professional before using zinc supplements.

ZMA (*Zinc Monomethionine Aspartate*) is a supplement used to improve sports performance and recovery. Studies have shown that ZMA can increase exercise performance and muscle strength, as well as improve sleep quality.

ZMA is generally well tolerated but may cause stomach upset in some individuals. Also, ZMA can impair copper absorption, so long-term use may cause copper deficiency. It is recommended that people considering using ZMA speak with a healthcare professional.

REFERENCES

1. European Food Information Council EUFIC, "Dietary Supplements: Do We Need Them?," 2020.
2. National Institutes of Health NIH, "Dietary Supplements: What You Need to Know," 2021.
3. M. Holick, " Vitamin D Deficiency," *New England Journal of Medicine*, vol. 357, no. 3, pp. 266–281, 2007.
4. K. D. Tipton and R. R. Wolfe, "Protein and Amino Acids for Athletes," *Journal of Sports Sciences*, vol. 22, no. 1, pp. 65–79, 2004.
5. National Institutes of Health NIH, "Botanical Dietary Supplements," 2018.
6. Institute of Medicine, Dietary Reference Intakes for Calcium and Vitamin D, The National Academies Press, 2011.
7. A. Abdelhamid, T. Brown, J. Brainard, P. Biswas, G. Thorpe, H. Moore, K. Deane, C. Summerbell, H. Worthington, F. Song and L. Hooper, "Omega-3 Intake for Cardiovascular Disease," *Cochrane Systematic Review*, vol. 3, p. CD003177, 2020.
8. National Health Service NHS, "The Truth About Supplements: Do They Work and Are They Safe?," 2017.
9. Food and Drug Administration FDA, "Dietary Supplements," 2018.
10. National Institutes of Health NIH, " Talking with Your Healthcare Provider About Dietary Supplements," 2018.
11. Mayo Clinic, "Dietary Supplements: Do They Help or Hurt?," 2019.
12. National Institutes of Health NIH, "Quality of Dietary Supplements," 2017.
13. D. T. Thomas, K. A. Erdman and L. M. Burke, "Position of the Academy of Nutrition and Dietetics, Dietitians of Canada, and the American College of Sports Medicine: Nutrition and Athletic Performance," *Journal of the Academy of Nutrition and Dietetics*, vol. 116, no. 3, pp. 501–528, 2016.
14. Mayo Clinic, "Supplements: Nutrition in a Pill?," 2020.
15. Food and Drug Administration FDA, " Tips for Dietary Supplement Users," 2021.
16. Harvard Medical School, "Should You Take Dietary Supplements?," 2019.

12 Popular Natural Cures
Scientific Evidence and Myths

In recent years, there has been a notable increase in the popularity of natural cures, with a growing number of individuals seeking alternative remedies to address a range of health concerns. While some natural cures have been supported by scientific evidence, others remain based on myth. It is crucial to distinguish between these two concepts in order to make well-informed decisions regarding one's health. The objective of this chapter is to collate a list of these cures with brief explanations of the advantages and disadvantages of each.

12.1 POPULAR NATURAL TREATMENTS WITH SCIENTIFIC EVIDENCE

There are several natural treatments that have gained popularity due to their proven scientific evidence. These treatments have been extensively studied and shown to provide beneficial effects. Some of the popular natural treatments with scientific evidence include:

Acacia fiber is a soluble dietary fiber obtained from the resin of the acacia tree. Soluble fiber is fermented by beneficial bacteria in the intestines, which promotes gut health and regulates the digestive system.

   Acacia fiber has particularly prebiotic properties. Prebiotics feed the beneficial bacteria in the gut and help them multiply. This improves gut health, supports the immune system, and may reduce inflammation.

   Additionally, acacia fiber can help treat a variety of digestive issues, including constipation and diarrhea. It also regulates blood sugar levels and can help with weight control.

Almonds contain a number of nutrients that support heart health. These include healthy fats, fiber, protein, magnesium, and vitamin E. Vitamin E acts as an antioxidant, protecting against free radical damage [1]. Regular consumption of almonds can be particularly helpful in lowering LDL cholesterol levels and reducing the risk of heart disease [2].

Aloe vera is an herb with a variety of health benefits and is most commonly used for the treatment of skin conditions and burns. The active ingredients in aloe vera gels have anti-inflammatory and antimicrobial properties that help treat skin conditions and burns.

   Several scientific studies have shown that aloe vera can help treat skin burns. It has also been found that aloe vera can improve skin conditions, even slowing the signs of skin aging.

Arnica is noted for its topical pain and inflammation-relieving properties. Arnica is often used in the form of ointments and creams and applied on the skin. However, more research is needed on these effects of Arnica [3].

Artichoke (*Cynara scolymus*) is a plant species of Mediterranean origin and is popular worldwide as a vegetable and natural remedy. Artichokes have many health benefits, the most widely known of which are supporting digestive health and lowering cholesterol levels.

   To understand how artichoke supports digestive health, it is important to first understand the effect of fiber on the digestive system. Artichokes contain a type of fiber called

DOI: 10.1201/9781003520252-14

inulin. Inulin is a prebiotic, that is, a food source for beneficial microorganisms in the intestines.

These beneficial microorganisms form a community often referred to as the gut microbiome. This microbiome plays an important role in digestive processes, immune function, and overall health. Therefore, the presence of inulin contributes to the digestive health-promoting effect of artichoke.

Artichokes can also increase bile production by stimulating the stomach and intestines. Bile plays an important role in digesting fats, which supports overall digestive health. A good digestive system can increase energy levels and lead to improved overall health.

As for the benefits of artichoke for lowering cholesterol levels, it has been noted that artichoke extract can help lower LDL ("bad") cholesterol levels and increase HDL ("good") cholesterol levels. This may be due to the effects of artichoke on the liver because the liver is at the center of cholesterol metabolism. Artichokes can reduce the liver's own production of cholesterol while increasing bile flow. This effect may help lower overall cholesterol levels.

As a result, artichokes have the potential to manage digestive health and cholesterol levels. However, these effects are usually seen when artichokes are consumed regularly over a period of time. It's important to remember that each individual may have a different response to artichoke, and consuming artichokes is not a guarantee of solving any health problems.

Ashwagandha (*Withania somnifera*) is a type of herb that is considered an adaptogen. Adaptogens are herbs that can improve the body's ability to cope with stress. It has been used in Ayurvedic medicine for centuries and is used to relieve anxiety and stress, increase energy levels, and improve overall health.

The effects of Ashwagandha on anxiety have been investigated in a number of clinical studies. Studies show that Ashwagandha can relieve symptoms of anxiety and reduce the stress response. Ashwagandha can also improve sleep quality, raise energy levels, and improve cognitive functions.

B vitamins are a group of water-soluble vitamins and are important for energy production, cell metabolism, and nervous system function [3]. Vitamin B deficiency can cause symptoms such as fatigue, irritability, depression, and anemia.

B group of vitamins, including B1 (thiamine), B2 (riboflavin), B3 (niacin), B5 (pantothenic acid), B6 (pyridoxine), B7 (biotin), B9 (folate or folate acid), and B12 (cobalamin), contains eight different vitamins. These vitamins work together to keep all cells functioning properly [4].

Bee pollen is the microscopic dust of plant seeds that bees collect and carry to their hives. It contains pollen grains from a wide variety of plants, allowing bee pollen to offer a wide range of nutrients [4].

Bee pollen contains a wide variety of components such as proteins, amino acids, vitamins, minerals, enzymes, fatty acids, and flavonoids. It's also a powerful source of antioxidants, which means it can help prevent cell damage and reduce inflammation in the body.

Bee pollen can increase energy, improve digestion, reduce allergic reactions, and support overall health. However, bee pollen can cause allergic reactions in people who are allergic to pollen, so it is recommended that such individuals avoid bee pollen.

Berberine is an alkaloid obtained from plants of the *Berberis* genus and some other plants. Berberine is often used to support metabolic health. Various studies have shown that berberine is potentially useful in a variety of applications, such as the treatment of type 2 diabetes, cardiovascular disease, and hyperlipidemia.

Berberine helps reduce insulin resistance and improve insulin sensitivity. It may also exert insulin-like effects to lower blood sugar levels.

Many studies have shown that berberine can both lower HbA1c (average blood sugar) levels as well as lower blood glucose and insulin levels in patients with type 2 diabetes [5]. Berberine can also lower cholesterol and triglyceride levels and thus support overall cardiovascular health.

Beta-glucans are a type of polysaccharide found in the cell walls of various plants, particularly grains and fungi. It supports the immune system and can also help lower cholesterol levels.

Beta-glucans stimulate the activity of immune cells, especially macrophages, neutrophils, and natural killer cells. This in turn helps the body respond more effectively to pathogens and other harmful substances.

Beta-glucans may also help lower blood cholesterol levels. A number of clinical studies have found that foods containing beta-glucan (especially oats and barley) can lower cholesterol levels. This effect is particularly pronounced on LDL (bad) cholesterol levels, and therefore beta-glucans may play a potential role in reducing the risk of heart disease.

Birch leaves are a popular natural treatment for several different health problems. They are known for their diuretic properties, which can help regulate fluid balance in the body and prevent kidney stones. It is also thought to have antiseptic properties, which can speed up the healing of wounds and prevent skin infections.

Bitter melon (*Momordica charantia*) is a type of fruit that grows in tropical and subtropical regions. Used in Ayurveda and Traditional Chinese Medicine for centuries, bitter melon is particularly known for its ability to lower blood sugar levels.

Bitter melon may help lower blood sugar levels in people with type 2 diabetes. Animal studies containing bitter melon extract have shown that this extract lowers blood sugar levels and improves insulin sensitivity. Similar results have been found in some small-scale studies in humans.

However, these results are mostly from small-scale, short-term studies, so larger, longer-term studies are needed to confirm the full effects of bitter melon on blood sugar.

Black Cohosh (*Actaea racemosa or Cimicifuga racemosa*) is an herb often used for relief of menopausal symptoms. Native to North America, this herb has been used by native American peoples for a number of ailments for many centuries.

In various clinical studies, it has been found that Black Cohosh can alleviate symptoms associated with menopause, such as hot flashes, night sweats, and sleep disturbances in particular. However, these studies are generally small in scale, and their results are mixed. In addition, a larger meta-analysis of these effects of Black Cohosh found no evidence that Black Cohosh was more effective than placebo in relieving menopausal symptoms.

Black Cohosh can cause liver problems in some people, so it's important to talk to a healthcare professional before using it.

Black grape seed extract has powerful antioxidant properties. This extract specifically contains powerful antioxidant compounds called *proanthocyanidins*. Antioxidants help reduce oxidative stress in the body, which can help prevent aging and many chronic diseases.

Multiple scientific studies have confirmed the antioxidant effects of black grape seed extract. Additionally, this extract has been noted to benefit heart health and may protect against some types of cancer.

Black seed oil is derived from a plant called *Nigella sativa* and is often used as a health supplement for its antioxidant and anti-inflammatory properties. This oil contains a powerful antioxidant called thymoquinone. Thymoquinone may help reduce inflammation and oxidative stress, which may be useful in the treatment of a variety of health problems [6].

Black seed oil can be particularly effective in treating conditions such as asthma, high blood pressure, diabetes, and obesity. It may also strengthen the immune system and improve digestive health [7].

Blueberry (*Vaccinium myrtillus*) is known as a plant that supports eye health. Studies have shown that blueberries can especially improve night vision and help prevent retinal damage.

Blueberries contain powerful antioxidant compounds called anthocyanins, which can help prevent cell damage while promoting eye health. Several studies have found that blueberry extract can relieve eyestrain and eye pain. However, this area needs more research.

Blueberries are also known for their antioxidant properties and ability to support brain health. Blueberries contain powerful antioxidant compounds, including flavonoids, which may help reduce oxidative stress and fight aging and disease.

Furthermore, blueberries are known for their ability to improve cognitive function and strengthen memory. Several studies have shown that blueberries can slow cognitive decline in older adults.

Cranberry (*Vaccinium macrocarpon*) is used specifically to help prevent urinary tract infections (UTIs). Cranberry has been found to contain unique components that may help prevent the growth of bacteria (especially *E. coli*) that cause UTIs by adhering to the urinary tract walls.

A number of clinical studies have shown that regular consumption of cranberry juice can reduce the risk of UTIs, especially among women with recurrent UTIs [2]. However, there are conflicting results as to whether cranberry is effective for the treatment of UTIs, and so it is often used for prevention.

Borage oil is derived from the seeds of the borage plant (*Borago officinalis*) and is often used to improve skin health. This oil is rich in an omega-6 fatty acid called gamma-linolenic acid (GLA). GLA creates a type of chemical messenger in the body called prostaglandins. Prostaglandins can alleviate inflammation and pain.

Borage oil can also relieve skin redness and inflammation. This can relieve symptoms of skin conditions such as eczema, psoriasis, and rosacea. It can also increase moisture levels in the skin and improve the overall health and appearance of the skin.

Boswellia has health benefits such as reducing inflammation and improving skin health [8]. This resin is obtained from Boswellia trees and has been used for medicinal and religious purposes since ancient times.

Boswellia's anti-inflammatory properties may help manage inflammation-related conditions such as arthritis and asthma. Boswellia acid's ability to reduce inflammation can relieve pain and improve mobility.

Boswellia also supports skin health. It can moisturize the skin and reduce the signs of aging. It can accelerate the healing of wounds and cuts and prevent the formation of acne.

Butterbur is noted for its ability to relieve migraine and allergy symptoms. However, more research is needed to validate these effects of butterbur [9].

Calendula can help relieve skin irritations and inflammation. Calendula creams are often used to treat skin irritations, burns, acne, and mild skin infections [10]. Also, some studies have shown that calendula extracts have an anti-inflammatory effect [11]. However, it is important to consult a healthcare professional before using calendula, as some people may have an allergic reaction to calendula.

Cardamom is used to relieve stomach pain, reduce gas, and control nausea. With these properties, it can regulate the digestive system. It is also considered an antihypertensive that can help lower blood pressure. These benefits of cardamom have enabled it to be used in many traditional medicine practices around the world.

Chamomile is an herb that has been used for medicinal and beauty purposes for centuries. Its tea is used to treat insomnia and anxiety due to its calming effects. Some of these effects are due to the fact that chamomile contains high levels of flavonoids and other chemicals [12].

Also, chamomile can improve digestive health. It can relieve conditions such as constipation, gas, stomach pain, and irritable bowel syndrome (IBS). Chamomile tea can also relieve inflammation and skin conditions and boost overall immunity [13].

Chaste Tree Berry (*Vitex agnus-castus*), also known as Agnus Castus or Monk's Pepper, is an herb that can help relieve symptoms of premenstrual syndrome (PMS) and menopause.

Many studies have shown that chaste tree berry is particularly effective in managing PMS symptoms. Specifically, this herb can relieve symptoms such as mood swings, breast tenderness, insomnia, and irritability.

These effects of the plant occur by regulating hormones such as estrogen and progesterone. This regulation can reduce the symptoms of PMS caused by hormonal fluctuations during the menstrual cycle. It has also been observed that chaste tree berry can help alleviate the symptoms of menopause. However, more research is needed on this issue.

The side effects of chaste tree berry are usually mild and may include symptoms such as headache, nausea, and rash. It is not recommended to be used during pregnancy or in combination with hormonal drugs.

Chia seeds are rich in omega-3 fatty acids, fiber, and protein. In particular, chia seeds are an excellent source of alpha-linolenic acid (ALA), a plant-based omega-3 fatty acid. ALA is a fatty acid that the body cannot produce on its own and must be obtained from outside. This supports heart health and may reduce inflammation.

In addition, chia seeds are rich in fiber, which provides a feeling of fullness and regulates blood sugar. It also promotes muscle preservation and growth thanks to its high protein content.

Chicory root (*Cichorium intybus*) contains high amounts of a type of prebiotic fiber called inulin. Prebiotics nourish and support the beneficial bacteria living in the gut. For this reason, chicory root is used to support gut health and overall digestive health.

Inulin is a kind of soluble fiber that attracts water and makes stool soft and easy to pass. Chicory root can also help regulate blood sugar and control appetite.

Cinnamon is a spice known for its many health benefits. It is known for its ability to lower blood sugar, making it particularly beneficial for individuals with diabetes. It is thought to have anti-inflammatory properties, so it can help relieve inflammation in the body. Cinnamon also works as an antioxidant and provides protection against free radicals.

Clove is a powerful spice used both in the kitchen and medicine and has a variety of health benefits. It is known to have antioxidant, analgesic (painkiller), and antibacterial properties.

Cloves are often used to relieve toothache because they contain a compound called eugenol. Eugenol is a compound used to maintain oral health and relieve toothache. Cloves may also help relieve digestive ailments and improve overall digestive health.

Cocoa contains antioxidants that support heart health. Cocoa contains powerful antioxidant compounds, including flavonoids, which may help reduce oxidative stress and lower the risk of heart disease.

Several scientific studies have shown that cocoa flavonoids can improve heart health, lower blood pressure, improve the function of blood vessels, and lower blood lipids. Plus, cocoa contains compounds that are said to improve mood and enhance brain function.

Common hop (*Humulus lupulus*) is an herb that is often used for brewing, but also has medicinal properties. Scientific studies have shown that hops have soothing properties and can help alleviate sleep problems.

Hops also contain phytoestrogens, which may help relieve menopausal symptoms. Studies on its effect against menopausal symptoms have shown that hops can reduce sweating and hot flashes.

Coenzyme Q10 (*CoQ10*) is a compound found naturally in the body and plays a key role in cellular energy production. CoQ10 is located in the energy production centers of cells called mitochondria and helps the production of ATP (adenosine triphosphate) to meet the energy needs of the cells.

CoQ10 has the potential to improve heart health. Studies have shown that CoQ10 supplementation can improve the symptoms of patients with heart failure and reduce complications after a heart attack. Additionally, it has been stated that CoQ10 may protect against some types of cancer, alleviate migraine symptoms, and reduce the side effects of some drugs such as statins.

Cordyceps is a species belonging to the family of medicinal mushrooms. It has been used in traditional Chinese and Tibetan medicine for centuries and offers a variety of health benefits.

One of the most well-known effects of cordyceps is its ability to increase energy levels and physical performance. This mushroom can increase the production of ATP (adenosine triphosphate), which helps muscles last longer during exercise. Cordyceps may also have anti-inflammatory and antioxidant properties, which help support overall health.

Cordyceps is generally considered safe, but some people may report side effects such as stomach upset, dry mouth, and diarrhea.

Coriander (*Coriandrum sativum*) is an herb used both as a spice and as an herbal supplement. The leaves of the plant are often called "cilantro," while the seeds are known as "coriander."

Coriander can help relieve stomach ailments. One study found that coriander seed extract helped relieve stomach ulcer symptoms. Other research has shown that coriander can be effective in combating digestive issues such as gas and bloating.

There is also some evidence that coriander can help lower blood sugar levels. One study found that coriander seed extract reduced blood sugar and insulin levels in individuals with type 2 diabetes.

However, these results are often seen when using specific extracts and specific doses, and more research is needed. You should always start a new herbal supplement regimen by talking to a healthcare professional.

Cumin (*Cuminum cyminum*) is the seeds of a spice commonly used in many cuisines. It is thought to help improve digestive health and support the immune system.

Cumin is rich in antioxidants and phytochemicals, which may support overall health and protection against disease. In particular, cumin is thought to have carminative properties that reduce gas and bloating, which can help people with gastrointestinal conditions.

Some studies have also suggested that cumin may support immune system function as a result of its anti-inflammatory properties.

Curcumin is a component derived from the root of the turmeric plant and is often used as a cooking spice. It also has powerful anti-inflammatory and antioxidant properties.

Curcumin is often used to treat inflammatory conditions such as osteoarthritis and rheumatoid arthritis due to its anti-inflammatory properties. Studies have shown that curcumin can alleviate the symptoms of these diseases [14].

Curcumin can also reduce oxidative stress, which often contributes to aging and the development of many chronic diseases. Studies have shown that curcumin can increase antioxidant capacity in the body, thereby reducing oxidative stress [15].

Dandelion (*Taraxacum officinale*) is an herb known for its digestive health-promoting properties. It is usually consumed in the form of tea or extract and is generally well tolerated.

Dandelion may help support liver health. Studies have shown that dandelion extract can help regulate liver function and prevent liver damage. These effects are attributed to the antioxidant and anti-inflammatory properties of kale.

Additionally, dandelion can help the digestive system work properly. In particular, it can stimulate the production and secretion of bile, which can facilitate the digestion of fats and the absorption of nutrients.

Some types of dandelions may contain compounds with antidiabetic effects that can help lower blood sugar levels. However, the clinical significance of these effects is still unclear, and further research is needed.

Devil's Claw (*Harpagophytum procumbens*) is an herb often used to treat joint pain and inflammatory conditions. Its name comes from the distinctive spiny appearance of its fruits.

First used in local medicine in South Africa, Devil's Claw contains an ingredient called *harpagoside*, which has anti-inflammatory and analgesic (painkilling) properties. It is often used to treat inflammatory conditions such as arthritis, low back pain, and tendonitis.

The anti-inflammatory effect of Devil's Claw can help relieve symptoms of pain and inflammation. In some clinical studies, this herb has been found to have similar efficacy to standard treatments in reducing the symptoms of osteoarthritis.

The analgesic effect of Devil's Claw can be helpful in managing chronic pain. This herb has been proposed as a natural treatment option for low back pain and other non-inflammatory pain conditions.

However, Devil's Claw can have possible side effects and drug interactions. In particular, it may interact with blood thinners. Therefore, if considering using Devil's Claw, it's important to talk to a healthcare provider first.

Dong Quai is often used for its properties to relieve menopausal symptoms. However, further research is needed on these effects of Dong Quai [16].

Echinacea is an herb often used as a natural treatment for colds and other upper respiratory tract infections. There are several types of Echinacea, but *Echinacea purpurea*, *Echinacea angustifolia*, and *Echinacea pallida* are the most commonly used types.

Echinacea is thought to strengthen the immune system. Studies have shown that Echinacea can increase the immune response and, in this way, prevent various infections [17].

However, there is also some controversy over the effects of Echinacea.

Some other studies have found that Echinacea can relieve cold symptoms, but others have not found this effect [18]. It is generally accepted that more research is needed.

Elderberry (*Sambucus nigra*) is a kind of fruit used in herbal medicine. It is thought to be particularly helpful against cold and flu symptoms.

Many studies have found that elderberry fruit extract can reduce the duration and severity of flu and cold symptoms. These effects may be due to the fact that elderberry has high antioxidant and antiviral properties.

Eucalyptus is an herb used to relieve cough and respiratory ailments. This plant, whose homeland is Australia, grows worldwide, and the oil obtained from its leaves is used for medicinal purposes.

Eucalyptus oil can be particularly effective against cold and flu symptoms. When vaporized or inhaled, eucalyptus oil can open up the airways and facilitate the expulsion of mucus. Additionally, due to the antibacterial properties of eucalyptus oil, it can also be used in the treatment of respiratory infections.

Evening primrose oil is derived from the nightshade plant (*Oenothera biennis*) and contains high amounts of gamma-linolenic acid (GLA), making it a valuable natural supplement, especially for skin and joint health. GLA helps the body produce bioactive lipids called prostaglandins that regulate inflammation. It can help with ailments such as joint pain and inflammation.

In addition, evening primrose oil can help alleviate skin ailments. It has shown positive effects, especially on skin conditions such as atopic dermatitis and eczema. It can reduce inflammation in the skin and help strengthen the skin barrier. However, each person may respond differently to this herb, and thus it may not be effective for every skin condition.

Eyebright is used in traditional medicine for its properties to relieve eye irritation. More research is needed on these effects of Eyebright [19].

Motherwort is an herb often used in traditional herbal medicine to support the heart and nervous system. Thanks to its ability to relieve menopausal symptoms and lower the heart rate, it can have a soothing effect on a variety of emotional states (including anxiety and panic attacks) [20]. However, more scientific research on the effects of Motherwort should be done.

Fennel (*Foeniculum vulgare*) is an herb that helps improve digestive health and relieve menopausal symptoms. Fennel seeds have carminative properties, meaning they can reduce gas and bloating. For this reason, it is often used to relieve digestive ailments.

Also, several studies have found that fennel extract can relieve menopausal symptoms. In particular, fennel may be effective in reducing symptoms such as hot flashes, sleep problems, and anxiety.

Fenugreek is a spice obtained from the seeds of the *Trigonella foenum-graecum* plant and is used in traditional medicine for a number of health problems. Fenugreek is an herb especially known for its potential to help with digestive problems and menopausal symptoms. However, fenugreek can cause stomach upsets, diarrhea, skin irritation, and lower blood sugar levels in some cases, so individuals with diabetes need to be cautious.

The positive effects of fenugreek, especially on blood sugar control, have been supported by scientific research. Several studies have noted that fenugreek can lower blood sugar levels in people with type 2 diabetes. This effect occurs because fenugreek contains a high amount of fiber and thus slows glucose absorption.

Fenugreek can also lower cholesterol levels. Several studies have shown that fenugreek supplements lower both total cholesterol and "bad" LDL cholesterol levels.

It has also been found that Fenugreek can increase milk production in nursing mothers. This feature can help new mothers' needs to increase milk production. However, fenugreek can cause stomach upset and skin irritation in some people.

Furthermore, fenugreek may affect the blood clotting process, so caution should be exercised when using it with anticoagulants. Fenugreek is an herb especially known for its potential to help with digestive problems and menopausal symptoms.

Fenugreek is generally safe, but some people have reported side effects such as stomach upset, gas, and diarrhea.

Feverfew (*Tanacetum parthenium*) is an herb commonly used to relieve headaches and inflammation. It is especially used in the treatment of migraine headaches. Feverfew also contains a compound called Parthenolide, which has anti-inflammatory properties.

Many studies have found that feverfew can relieve migraine symptoms. Specifically, this herb can reduce the frequency and severity of headaches and alleviate migraine-related nausea and vomiting.

Flaxseeds are a rich source of nutrients that have a variety of health benefits. These include fiber, lignans, and omega-3 fatty acids. Fiber can help improve digestive health and also aid weight control because it keeps you feeling full for longer.

Flax seeds contain a type of phytoestrogen called lignans. Lignans have antioxidant and anti-inflammatory properties, which can help prevent a variety of diseases. Flaxseeds are also rich in a type of omega-3 fatty acid called alpha-linolenic acid (ALA). ALA may help improve heart health and reduce inflammation.

Garlic is an herb that has anti-inflammatory and antioxidant properties and supports heart health. Garlic may help lower blood pressure, balance cholesterol levels, and reduce the risk of heart disease.

In addition, the sulfur compounds found in garlic may also be important in the fight against cancer, due to its ability to reduce oxidative stress and alleviate inflammation. These effects are usually most pronounced when raw or fresh garlic is consumed, as heat treatment can destroy some of the sulfur compounds.

Garlic can cause stomach upset, bad breath, or skin odor in some people. It can also interact with blood-thinning medications, so care should be taken if taking this type of medication.

Ginger (*Zingiber officinale*) is an herb that specifically helps relieve nausea and inflammation. The antiemetic (anti-nausea) effect of ginger has been shown to be particularly effective on pregnancy-related nausea, chemotherapy, and postoperative nausea.

The anti-inflammatory properties of ginger may be especially beneficial for people with chronic inflammatory conditions such as osteoarthritis. Studies have shown that ginger extract can reduce pain and stiffness in people with osteoarthritis.

Ginger may also help with blood sugar control. One study found that when people with type 2 diabetes consumed ginger powder, their blood sugar dropped significantly [21].

Probiotics are live microorganisms known to benefit human health, usually bacteria and some types of yeast. These are often taken as supplements to support digestive health, but they can also help boost the immune system and improve overall health.

Scientific studies have shown that probiotics can help treat a variety of digestive disorders, including irritable bowel syndrome (IBS), inflammatory bowel disease (IBD), and certain infections. They may also be effective in preventing antibiotic-associated diarrhea.

Probiotics also have the ability to strengthen the immune system. Studies have shown that they can help prevent infections by modulating the immune response.

Ginkgo biloba is an herb often used to support memory and brain function. Studies have shown that *Ginkgo biloba* can have a positive effect on cognitive function and help prevent age-related memory loss in particular [22]. These effects of *Ginkgo biloba* are linked to its ability to increase blood circulation and reduce oxidative stress.

However, there is conflicting evidence about the effect of *Ginkgo biloba* on Alzheimer's disease or other types of dementia. Some studies have shown that this herb may be beneficial in alleviating such conditions, while others have found no benefit [23]. Therefore, if considering the use of *Ginkgo biloba* for these types of conditions, it is important to speak to a healthcare professional first.

Possible side effects of *Ginkgo biloba* may include headache, nausea, and diarrhea. Also, *Ginkgo biloba* may interact with blood-thinning medications, so caution should be exercised if you are taking this type of medication.

Ginseng is often used to increase physical and mental energy. There are several types, the two main types being *Panax ginseng* (Asian or Korean ginseng) and *Panax quinquefolius* (American ginseng).

Ginseng has the potential to boost overall energy levels and help cope with fatigue. This can improve sports performance and improve overall endurance. Additionally, ginseng may have a positive effect on cognitive function. Various studies have shown that ginseng can help improve memory, attention, and brain function.

Glucosamine is a popular dietary supplement, especially for joint health. It is a substance naturally found in the body and plays an important role in building healthy cartilage.

People with conditions affecting the joint, such as osteoarthritis, often use glucosamine supplements. Various studies have shown that glucosamine can relieve symptoms of osteoarthritis. However, these effects are usually mild and occur after prolonged use.

Glucosamine can also slow and in some cases even reverse the wear of articular cartilage. However, not all studies have demonstrated these effects of glucosamine, and further research is warranted.

Goji Berry (*Lycium barbarum or Lycium chinense*) is a fruit that is usually consumed dry and called a superfood because of its antioxidant properties. They are particularly rich in powerful antioxidants called carotenoids. These antioxidants can fight free radicals and reduce your body's oxidative stress, which can reduce the risk of chronic diseases.

Goji is also rich in vitamin A, vitamin C, and iron. These nutrients support overall health and improve immune system function.

Golden Seal (*Hydrastis canadensis*) is an herb known especially for its antibacterial properties. It is often used to relieve symptoms of colds, flu, and other respiratory infections. It can also be used to treat skin wounds and skin conditions such as eczema.

Golden Seal contains a compound called berberine, which may be effective against bacterial and fungal infections. However, more research is needed to confirm the health effects of goldenseal.

Gotu Kola (*Centella asiatica*) is a plant species that grows in Asia, Africa, and Australia. Used in Ayurveda and Traditional Chinese Medicine for centuries, Gotu Kola is known for a variety of health benefits, particularly its ability to support the nervous system and brain function.

Gotu Kola has the potential to improve brain health and cognitive function. In a number of animal and in vitro studies, Gotu Kola has been shown to improve memory function and have neuroprotective effects. In particular, it is seen as a potential candidate for the treatment of Alzheimer's disease and similar neurodegenerative diseases.

However, these results have been obtained at the animal and cell level, so more research is needed to confirm the full effects of Gotu Kola in humans.

Green coffee extract is a product obtained from unroasted coffee beans. Unroasted coffee beans contain a number of bioactive compounds, including caffeine and chlorogenic acid [24]. Both of these compounds can stimulate metabolism and accelerate fat burning, which means that green coffee extract can help with weight loss.

Also, green coffee extract has the ability to lower blood pressure. Some studies have shown that chlorogenic acid lowers blood pressure and improves heart health.

Green tea is derived from the leaves of the *Camellia sinensis* plant and is a widely consumed beverage around the world. Polyphenols are bioactive components with high amounts of antioxidant properties and are found in green tea to add to its positive effect on health.

The potential health benefits of green tea include reducing the risk of cardiovascular disease, preventing some types of cancer, and aiding weight loss. Some studies have shown that green tea can lower LDL ("bad") cholesterol and have a positive effect on the overall cholesterol profile.

The effect of green tea on type 2 diabetes has also been studied. Some studies have indicated that green tea consumption can lower blood sugar and reduce insulin resistance. However, this issue is still controversial, and more research is needed.

Hemp seeds are rich in vegetable protein, fiber, and omega-3 fatty acids. Omega-3 fatty acids may help improve heart health and reduce inflammation. Protein promotes muscle building and repair, while fiber improves digestive health [25].

Hemp seeds are also a rich source of magnesium, phosphorus, and potassium. These minerals support bone health, energy production, and overall cell function [26].

Hibiscus is often used to lower blood pressure. Hibiscus tea has been found to be effective in managing hypertension. Some studies have shown that regular consumption of hibiscus tea can significantly lower blood pressure [27].

The effects of hibiscus are comparable to medications often used to lower blood pressure. However, more research needs to be done on the effectiveness of hibiscus in lowering blood pressure, and it's important to speak with a healthcare professional before starting any treatment.

Honey, scientific evidence on the potential health benefits and harms of honey varieties is still limited today. Similarly, studies on specific species are also limited. Listed below are some examples of current research on specific types of honey:

1. *Flower Honey*: Flower honey is usually made from nectar collected from a number of flower species and is generally not specific to a particular flower type. In an in vitro study, it was shown that flower honey has antibacterial and antioxidant effects [28]. However, it is unclear whether these effects are consistent across all varieties of flower honey and whether they will show the same effects in humans.

2. *Manuka Honey*: Manuka honey is collected from the native Manuka tree of New Zealand and has attracted intense scientific research attention. It has been determined that Manuka honey accelerates wound healing and has antibacterial properties [29]. However, these benefits are often due to the "Unique Manuka Factor" (UMF) measurement, and not all Manuka honey types may have these effects.

3. *Acacia Honey*: Acacia honey is generally recommended for diabetics due to its low glycemic index [30]. However, it is still unclear what other health benefits this type of honey might have, and more research is needed.

4. *Chestnut Honey*: Chestnut honey is rich in antioxidants, and some in vitro studies suggest that antioxidants may reduce the risk of heart disease [31]. However, more research is needed to confirm these potential health benefits of chestnut honey.

5. *Alfalfa Honey*: Alfalfa honey is usually made from the nectar of clover flowers. Some studies have shown that alfalfa honey has anti-inflammatory and antioxidant effects [32]. However, more research is needed on the health effects of alfalfa honey.

6. *Carob Honey*: Carob honey is collected from carob trees and is usually found in the Mediterranean region. Carob honey has been found to have high antioxidant activity, but the specific health effects of this honey in humans still have limited research [33].

7. *Citrus Honey*: Citrus honey is collected from citrus trees (lemon, orange, tangerine, etc.). One study found that citrus honey showed antimicrobial and anti-inflammatory activity [34]. However, the results of this study may not be applicable to all varieties of citrus honey.

8. *Plum Honey*: Plum honey is collected from plum blossoms and is quite rare. Little scientific studies have been done on the health effects of this honey, and more research is needed.

9. *Pine Honey*: Pine honey is collected from pine trees and is common in the Mediterranean region. It has been found that pine honey has high antioxidant activity that can be used in the treatment of various diseases [35].

10. *Filtered Honey*: Filtered honey is generally obtained from various nectar sources and is not specific to a specific nectar source. The health effects of filtered honey depend on the various types of nectar it contains and are often less specific than a particular type of honey.

11. *Anzer Honey*: Anzer honey from Turkey is made from the nectar of the endemic flower species. This honey is known for having high antioxidant activity and antimicrobial, anti-inflammatory, and anticancer properties [36]. More research is needed on other possible health effects of Anzer honey.

12. *Mad Honey*: Mad honey is not actually a honey, but a nectar collected by bees from the nectar of the Rhododendron plant. It is obtained from the *Rhododendron ponticum* and *Rhododendron luteum* species found in Turkey, especially in the Black Sea region.

The nectar of this mad honey contains a toxin called grayanotoxin. Grayanotoxin can affect the central nervous system, causing dizziness, nausea, vomiting, excessive sweating, and low blood pressure. However, heating mad honey or storing it for a long time will cause the grayanotoxin to be largely destroyed.

It is known that mad honey is used against various health problems such as hypertension and some stomach disorders in Turkey, but these claims have not yet been scientifically proven [37].

Horny goat weed can help improve erectile function in men. The active ingredient of this plant, icariin, can improve blood circulation and relieve erectile dysfunction symptoms [38]. However, more research is needed on the safety and effectiveness of this herb.

Horse chestnut (*Aesculus hippocastanum*) is often used to relieve the symptoms of varicose veins and hemorrhoids. Horse chestnut contains a compound called *aescin*, which can strengthen vessel walls and have anti-inflammatory effects.

A number of clinical studies have found that horse chestnut extract can help relieve symptoms of chronic venous insufficiency (a condition underlying varicose veins). These symptoms may include pain, edema (swelling), itching, and heavy legs.

Horse chestnut can also help relieve the symptoms of hemorrhoids. Hemorrhoids are swelling of the veins in the lower part of the anus or rectum and can cause pain, itching, and bleeding. Some studies have found that horse chestnut may help relieve symptoms of hemorrhoids.

Horsetail is an herb that has historically been used to treat a number of different health problems. It is known to have diuretic properties, which can help regulate fluid balance in the body and reduce edema (excessive fluid buildup in the body).

Horsetail may also help improve skin health. Being rich in silica acid and silicon, these minerals can tighten skin, reduce wrinkles, and improve overall skin tone. It also promotes the production of collagen, which helps to increase the elasticity and suppleness of the skin.

Jasmine flower can help improve mood and sleep quality. Studies have shown that jasmine has relaxing and calming properties, which can reduce stress and anxiety and provide a better night's sleep [39]. Jasmine is also a popular option in aromatherapy.

Lemongrass is an herb that can improve digestive health and reduce stress. Its ingredients can relieve stomach pain and diarrhea, as well as reduce gas formation and bloating [40]. Lemongrass can also have a soothing effect on stress and anxiety and improve overall mood.

Kava Kava is a common herb, especially among island communities in the South Pacific, and is often consumed as a beverage or supplement. Kava Kava's most well-known benefits include relieving anxiety and insomnia [41].

These effects of Kava are due to the effects of the kavalactone active ingredient on the nervous system. Kavalactones create a sense of relaxation by binding to certain receptors in the nervous system, which can relieve symptoms of anxiety and insomnia.

There are many studies that show that Kava is effective in improving sleep quality. This effect is due to the relaxing effect of kava on the nervous system. However, Kava Kava should be used with caution as excessive and/or long-term use can cause liver damage. It is recommended that people considering using Kava Kava consult a healthcare professional first.

Kelp is a seaweed that is a large, multicellular species of algae. It contains large amounts of iodine, which is a vital mineral for thyroid function. One of the main minerals that the thyroid gland needs in order to produce thyroid hormones is iodine.

Thyroid hormones are important in many biological functions of the body, especially in energy production and metabolic rate control. Iodine deficiency can lead to health problems such as hypothyroidism (underactivity of the thyroid gland) and goiter (abnormal growth of the thyroid gland).

In addition to being a rich source of iodine, kelp also provides a number of vitamins and minerals. These include vitamin K, B vitamins, zinc, and iron. Kelp also contains antioxidant compounds such as polyphenols and flavonoids that support digestion and reduce inflammation.

However, when kelp is consumed in excess, it can lead to thyroid dysfunctions because too much iodine can overstimulate the thyroid gland. Therefore, it is important to talk to a healthcare professional before starting kelp consumption.

Kudzu is a plant species originating from Asia and has roots and flowers used for medicinal applications. Kudzu is particularly noted for its potential effects on alcohol addiction.

Some studies have suggested that kudzu root extract may reduce alcohol cravings and therefore reduce alcohol consumption. However, most of these findings come from animal studies, and results from studies in humans are mixed.

Several clinical studies have shown that kudzu extract can reduce alcohol intake, but other studies have found no effect. Therefore, more research is needed to fully understand kudzu's effects on alcohol dependence.

Lactobacillus acidophilus, also referred to as *L. acidophilus*, is a type of probiotic found naturally in the digestive tract. Probiotics are live microorganisms that help improve the gut microbiota (the community of microorganisms found in the gut).

L. acidophilus helps the gut microbiota maintain a healthy balance. This can help alleviate a number of digestive issues, particularly in conditions like diarrhea and irritable bowel syndrome (IBS).

In addition, *L. acidophilus* can help strengthen the immune system. The gut microbiota is an important part of the immune system, and probiotics such as L. acidophilus may have a positive effect on this system.

Lavender is an oil extracted from the flowers of *Lavandula angustifolia*, a popular herb for aromatherapy, bath products, and a variety of health applications. Lavender is thought to have many health benefits; two of the most widely known are its positive effects on anxiety and insomnia.

Scientific research has shown that lavender oil can relieve symptoms of anxiety and improve overall mood and quality of life [42]. There is also evidence that lavender inhalation can help treat insomnia and other sleep disorders [43].

Lemon balm (*Melissa officinalis*) is an herb often used for anxiety and insomnia. Studies have shown that balm can help reduce symptoms of anxiety. This effect may be linked to its ability to increase the activity of a brain chemical called GABA (gamma-aminobutyric acid). GABA is an inhibitory neurotransmitter that often aids relaxation and sleep [44].

Lemon balm may also help relieve symptoms of insomnia, especially when taken at bedtime. Lemon balm is usually consumed in tea form but is also available in extract or capsule form.

Lemon verbena (*Aloysia citriodora*) is often used to relieve digestive ailments and reduce anxiety symptoms. The leaves of lemon verbena are used to make teas, tinctures, and essential oils. This herb can relieve digestive problems such as stomach pain, gas, and diarrhea. Also, the relaxing effect of lemon verbena can help relieve symptoms of anxiety and insomnia.

Licorice root (*Glycyrrhiza glabra*) has been used throughout history to relieve symptoms of stomach ulcers and reflux. Licorice root promotes high production of mucus, which protects the lining of the stomach and intestines and repairs its damage. Also, the glycyrrhizin component in licorice root has anti-inflammatory and immunomodulatory properties.

Licorice root extract is also used to treat respiratory ailments such as coughs, colds, and viral infections. However, long-term and/or high-dose use may cause some side effects, so it is important to consult a healthcare professional before use.

Maca (*Lepidium meyenii*) is an herb used specifically to improve sexual health and increase energy levels. Native to the Andes Mountains, this herb is often consumed in powder form and added to a variety of foods and beverages.

A number of studies have shown that maca has positive effects on sexual function and libido. Also, maca root can help relieve fatigue and chronic fatigue and increase overall energy levels.

Magnesium is an essential mineral that helps cells perform many basic biological processes, such as energy production, protein creation, repair of genetic material DNA, and new cell formation.

In terms of cardiovascular health, magnesium can help lower blood pressure and reduce the risk of heart attack and stroke. Magnesium is also important for the prevention and treatment of heart conditions such as arrhythmias and heart muscle function.

Magnesium also supports the health conditions of the nervous system. Magnesium can increase the activity of a neurotransmitter called *GABA*, which calms nerve activity in the brain and provides a sense of relaxation. For this reason, magnesium supplements are often used to treat insomnia and anxiety.

Maitake mushroom is a mushroom with properties that can strengthen the immune system. Maitake contains a type of polysaccharide called beta-glucans, which activates the immune system and thus helps the body better resist diseases.

Manuka honey is produced with nectar collected from New Zealand's native manuka tree (*Leptospermum scoparium*). Unlike other types of honey, manuka honey contains a particularly high level of a natural antibiotic called methylglyoxal (MGO) [45].

The high antibiotic activity of Manuka honey has made it a popular choice for treating a handful of health conditions. These conditions include wounds, burns, infections, stomach ulcers, and other digestive problems.

Despite these health benefits of Manuka honey, it may not be suitable for everyone. For example, people with diabetes should carefully consider their consumption, as it contains sugar.

Marshmallow root (*Althaea officinalis*) is an herb that has been used for medicinal purposes for hundreds of years. The most distinctive properties of marshmallow root are that it is used to provide relief in the throat and mouth and to relieve cough. This herb can coat mucous membranes and reduce irritation, thanks to the mucopolysaccharides in it.

Marshmallow root is also used to reduce inflammation in the digestive tract and relieve stomach ulcers. However, more scientific research is needed to confirm these effects of marshmallow roots.

Milk thistle (*Silybum marianum*) is an herb often used to support liver health. The seeds of Milk Thistle contain active ingredients called silymarin. Milk thistle has antioxidant and anti-inflammatory properties and can help regenerate liver cells.

A number of clinical studies have found that milk thistle can reduce inflammation and oxidative stress associated with liver diseases. Milk thistle could potentially help treat alcoholic and non-alcoholic liver disease, hepatitis, and even liver cancer. However, many of these studies have been done on animals, and more research is needed on the effects of milk thistle on humans.

Moringa (*Moringa oleifera*) is a type of tree that grows mainly in South Asia. The whole tree is used for medicinal purposes, including its leaves, bark, flowers, fruits, seeds, and roots.

Moringa contains a number of vitamins and minerals, including Vitamin A, Vitamin C, and Vitamin E. It is also rich in important nutrients such as calcium, potassium, and protein. It has been found that moringa has antioxidant and anti-inflammatory properties and can help lower blood sugar levels and cholesterol [46].

Mullein is an herb with properties that support respiratory health. In particular, it has an expectorant and cough-relieving effect. These effects are based on the plant's ability to soften the bronchi and facilitate the expulsion of phlegm. However, more scientific research is needed to confirm the accuracy of these claims [47].

Neem is an herb that can improve skin health and protect against parasites. Neem can help treat skin conditions such as acne, eczema, and psoriasis and can cleanse and moisturize the skin. Also, the neem plant has antifungal, antibacterial, and antiparasitic properties.

Noni juice is obtained from the fruits of the noni tree (*Morinda citrifolia*). This tree grows on the islands of the Pacific, the Caribbean, and parts of Asia. Noni fruit has been used in traditional medicine to treat many ailments.

Noni juice is rich in antioxidants and therefore helps the body fight oxidative stress and inflammation [48]. These antioxidants help prevent cell damage and improve overall health. Noni juice is also thought to be able to boost the immune system and increase energy levels.

Olive leaf, while the leaves of the olive tree are less well known than the fruit and oil of the olive, they offer many potential health benefits. Olive leaf has antioxidant properties and may help lower blood pressure [49].

The antioxidant effect of olive leaf is due to the phenolic components it contains, especially a component called oleuropein. Antioxidants are substances that help prevent cell damage and can help prevent many diseases associated with aging.

The blood pressure lowering effect is based on the olive leaf's ability to dilate blood vessels. This effect can be especially beneficial for people with high blood pressure. However, it is important to see a healthcare professional before using any herbal supplement.

Omega-3 fatty acids are polyunsaturated fatty acids that are vital for human health. The best known and most researched types are known as eicosapentaenoic acid (EPA), docosahexaenoic acid (DHA), and alpha-linolenic acid (ALA). Fish oil is one of the best sources, especially rich in EPA and DHA, while vegetable sources often contain ALA.

Scientific studies have shown that Omega-3 fatty acids can help support heart health. In particular, it has benefits such as protection from cardiovascular diseases, lowering triglyceride levels and lowering blood pressure.

Omega-3 fatty acids also have anti-inflammatory properties, which may be beneficial for people with inflammatory conditions such as rheumatoid arthritis. Some studies have shown that Omega-3 fatty acids can alleviate the symptoms of these conditions [50].

Oregano oil is an essential oil extracted specifically from the *Origanum vulgare* species and has antifungal, antibacterial, antiviral, and anti-inflammatory properties. The phenolic compounds in thyme oil, especially carvacrol and thymol, are responsible for these properties. Thanks to these properties, thyme oil can be used in the treatment of various bacterial and fungal infections.

However, there are some important notes regarding the use of oregano oil. First, oregano oil can often cause irritation to the skin or mucous membranes, so it should not be used undiluted with a carrier oil. Second, oregano oil can potentially cause allergic reactions, so it's important to perform a small skin test before using it.

Parsley is an herb that most people use extensively in the kitchen, but its health benefits are often overlooked. Parsley has diuretic properties and supports overall health.

The diuretic effect of parsley helps the body expel excess fluid. This feature can be useful in cases such as edema (water retention in the body). In addition, parsley's ability to remove toxins from the body also supports overall health.

Parsley also contains a number of important vitamins and minerals, including vitamin C, vitamin K, iron, and folate. These nutrients help strengthen the immune system, maintain bone health, and help cells function properly.

Passionflower (*Passiflora incarnata*) is often used to relieve symptoms of anxiety and insomnia. Various studies have found that passionflower has a calming effect on anxiety. Additionally, passionflower can help relieve insomnia. One study found that taking passionflower extract shortened the time it took to fall asleep and improved the overall quality of sleep.

Pau D'Arco is a South American herb with a variety of health benefits. The bark of the plant has antimicrobial and anti-inflammatory properties. However, these effects have generally been observed in laboratory conditions, and more studies are needed to determine their effects in humans [5].

Pecans are a rich source of antioxidants. Antioxidants help protect cells against free radical damage, which slows the aging process and may reduce the risk of chronic diseases [51]. Plus, pecans contain healthy fats that can help support heart health. Therefore, it makes sense to consider these delicious nuts as part of a balanced diet.

Pectin is a type of soluble dietary fiber found naturally in the cell walls of fruits and vegetables. This type of fiber forms a gel-like substance when mixed with water, which slows down digestion.

This property explains how pectin supports digestive health. Pectin regulates bowel movements and prevents constipation. It can also relieve reflux symptoms by neutralizing stomach acid.

Some studies have also shown that pectin can lower blood sugar levels in people with type 2 diabetes. Pectin achieves this effect by slowing the rapid rise in postprandial blood sugar levels.

Peppermint (*Mentha piperita*) is an herb that provides a number of health benefits. In particular, peppermint oil and peppermint tea are often used to treat digestive ailments. Many studies have shown that peppermint oil can especially relieve symptoms of irritable bowel syndrome (IBS).

Also, peppermint can be used as a refreshing mouthwash and improve oral health. The antimicrobial properties of peppermint can reduce bacterial growth in the mouth, which may help prevent tooth decay and periodontal disease.

Pine bark extract is a nutritional supplement obtained from the bark of various types of pine trees. It is often used for a variety of health benefits. The most overlooked health benefit of pine bark extract is its antioxidant capacity. Pine bark extract is rich in powerful antioxidants called *proanthocyanidins.*

Antioxidants help protect the body against free radical damage, which improves overall health, including heart disease and brain health. However, research on the specific health effects of pine bark extract has generally been conducted on animals or cell cultures, and more research in humans is needed.

Plantain leaf is known for its ability to relieve skin irritation and support digestive health. It can protect mucous membranes and relieve irritation. It can also be beneficial to digestive health because it relieves constipation and regulates bowel movements [52].

Propolis is a kind of resin mixture produced by bees and collected mainly from tree buds and other plant sap. Bees use propolis to narrow the entrance to the hive, to keep out strangers diseases, and to coat the inside of the hive.

Propolis is one of the oldest known natural antibiotics and is thought to have a number of health benefits. It contains a number of active ingredients such as flavonoids and phenolic acids. These ingredients have been shown to have antioxidant and antibacterial properties.

The health benefits of propolis include boosting the immune system, preventing colds and other infections, improving oral health, accelerating the healing of wounds, and treating skin problems.

Despite these benefits of propolis, it may cause allergic reactions in some people, so first-time users should be careful.

Psyllium is a source of fiber obtained from the bark of the Plantago ovata plant. It is widely used to improve digestive health and lower cholesterol levels. Its fibrous structure relieves constipation by softening and enlarging stool.

Also, psyllium might lower cholesterol levels. A number of studies have found that taking regular psyllium supplements can lower overall cholesterol levels, especially LDL ("bad") cholesterol.

Pumpkin seeds are rich in magnesium and antioxidants. Magnesium is a mineral that regulates more than 300 enzymatic reactions in the body [53]. This supports a number of vital functions such as energy production, protein synthesis, and nerve function. Pumpkin seeds also contain a number of antioxidants that help prevent free radical damage. These antioxidants may contribute to many health benefits, from heart health to cancer risk reduction [54].

Pycnogenol is a patented extract consisting of flavonoid compounds specifically derived from the bark of the French maritime pine (*Pinus pinaster*) tree. It is known for its wide-ranging antioxidant properties, and with this feature, it protects cells against oxidative damage. It is especially used to support heart and brain health.

Various studies have shown that pycnogenol lowers heart disease risk factors, particularly high blood pressure, and lowers levels of bad LDL cholesterol. In addition, there is some evidence that pycnogenol can improve brain function and cognitive abilities.

Quercetin is a flavonoid commonly found in many fruits and vegetables, such as onions, apples, grapes, red wine, broccoli, and tea. Due to its anti-inflammatory and antihistamine effects, it is thought to have the potential to combat allergies, asthma, and autoimmune diseases.

Quercetin plays an important role in many biochemical pathways that work to control inflammation. It also alleviates allergic responses by stabilizing mast cells and basophils and inhibiting histamine release. In addition, quercetin has antioxidant properties, the ability to fight free radicals, and reduce oxidative stress, which may be beneficial in preventing various chronic diseases.

Red clover is an herb that is especially used to relieve the symptoms of menopause. Studies show that this herb can relieve hot flashes in particular. However, more studies are needed on this subject [55].

Red yeast rice is produced from rice fermented with *Monascus purpureus*, a type of yeast. It is a product that has been used in Traditional Chinese Medicine (TCM) for thousands of years and is widely used to support cardiovascular health.

Red yeast rice contains monacolin K, an ingredient in a group of medicines known as statins and used to lower LDL ("bad") cholesterol levels [56]. Studies have shown that red yeast rice supplements can effectively lower LDL cholesterol levels [57]. However, the amount of monacolin K in red yeast rice can vary widely and may be absent in some products. Therefore, it is important to read product labels carefully.

Possible side effects of red yeast rice are similar to those associated with statins and can include abdominal pain, muscle pain, and, rarely, liver damage.

Reishi mushroom (*Ganoderma lucidum*) is a type of mushroom that is often used in Traditional Chinese Medicine (TCM) for health and longevity. Reishi mushrooms can strengthen the immune system and protect against certain types of cancer, high blood pressure, and blood sugar levels.

Reishi mushroom contains many active ingredients, but polysaccharides and triterpenoids are considered the most important bioactive components. These components are thought to have anti-inflammatory, antiallergic, antioxidant, and anti-tumor properties [6]. It has been said that Reishi mushroom may additionally possess antiviral and antibacterial properties that increase overall immune functions.

Resveratrol is a natural phenol compound found especially in red grapes, blueberries, peanuts, and cocoa. Various studies have shown that resveratrol has antiaging, anticancer, anti-inflammatory, and heart-healthy properties.

Resveratrol stands out with research that it can improve heart health. A number of studies have shown that resveratrol can lower blood pressure and reduce heart disease risk factors.

The antiaging effects of resveratrol relate specifically to the activation of sirtuin genes. These genes may help slow the aging of cells and prolong their lifespan.

Rhodiola rosea is an adaptogen herb that can increase the body's ability to cope with stress. Clinical studies have shown that *Rhodiola rosea* can be effective in reducing symptoms of fatigue, depression, and anxiety [58].

This herb works by regulating the body's response to stress hormones (cortisol), which can reduce overall stress levels and signs of fatigue. *Rhodiola rosea* is often used to increase energy levels and improve mental performance.

Possible side effects of *Rhodiola rosea* may include insomnia, dizziness, and dry mouth. Also, this herb may interact with certain medications, such as antidepressants, so it's important to check with your healthcare provider before starting any supplement.

Rooibos or red tea is obtained from the leaves of the *Aspalathus linearis* plant. Native to South Africa, this herb is widely used in tea making and is grown in warm climates.

Perhaps the most well-known benefit of rooibos is its high antioxidant content. These antioxidants can help the body cope with oxidative stress, which can slow the aging process and reduce the risk of developing chronic diseases. Antioxidants include flavonoids and phenolic compounds.

Additionally, rooibos may help support heart health. Studies have shown that regular consumption of rooibos can lower blood pressure and cholesterol levels. However, these effects are often seen in conjunction with regular consumption and other healthy lifestyle changes.

Rosehip is the fruit of various rose species and is often appreciated for its intense vitamin C content and antioxidant effects. Vitamin C supports the immune system, improves skin health, and protects against free radicals.

Rosehip may also have anti-inflammatory properties. Some studies have shown that taking rosehip supplements can alleviate inflammatory conditions such as arthritis.

Rosemary (*Rosmarinus officinalis*) is an herb with some evidence that it helps support brain function. Specifically, rosemary contains rosmarinic acid, an ingredient thought to improve memory and increase concentration.

Studies have shown that rosemary extract can improve memory performance and reduce symptoms of cognitive decline [59]. It has also been shown that rosemary extract can help support memory function, especially in older adults [60].

Royal jelly is a highly nutritious substance produced by worker bees and used for the feeding of queen bees and larvae. The queen bee grows by eating only royal jelly throughout her life. This results in them being larger and longer lasting than any other bee [61].

Royal jelly is rich in amino acids, vitamins, enzymes, and fatty acids and is also a source of B vitamins. It is especially rich in vitamins B5 and B6. It also supports collagen production and is beneficial for skin health.

Royal jelly's health benefits include boosting overall health and stamina, boosting energy levels, hydrating and protecting the skin, relieving menopausal symptoms, and lowering cholesterol levels. However, more research is needed on the effects of royal jelly, and it may cause allergic reactions for some people.

Saffron is a type of spice obtained from the *Crocus sativus L.* plant. This herb is particularly notable for its ability to relieve symptoms of depression. These effects of saffron have been supported in several clinical trials. For example, in a meta-analysis, saffron was found to significantly alleviate the symptoms of patients with major depressive disorder [62].

Sage (*Salvia officinalis*) is used to support memory and brain function and relieve menopausal symptoms. Sage contains several active ingredients with antioxidant and anti-inflammatory properties.

In particular, there is some evidence that sage has positive effects on memory. One study found that sage extract can improve the memory and cognitive abilities of Alzheimer's patients.

Sage is also used to relieve menopausal symptoms, especially to reduce hot flashes and sweating. One study found that sage extract can significantly reduce these symptoms.

Saw Palmetto is a small palm species that usually grows in the southeastern United States. For centuries, it has been used in traditional medicine to support prostate health in men.

It is often used to relieve symptoms of prostate conditions such as benign prostatic hyperplasia (BPH). Many clinical studies have focused on Saw Palmetto's ability to reduce BPH symptoms. A meta-analysis found that Saw Palmetto supplementation can improve urine flow rate and reduce nighttime urination frequency.

However, the American Urological Association (AUA) stated in a guideline published in 2011 that there is insufficient evidence that Saw Palmetto is effective in the treatment of BPH. Therefore, more research is needed to confirm the full effects of Saw Palmetto on prostate health.

Schisandra (*Schisandra chinensis*) is a plant that is the fruit of the Schisandra chinensis plant. Used in traditional Chinese medicine, this herb is often recognized for its ability to reduce stress and increase overall stamina. Schisandra is considered an adaptogen, meaning it can help regulate the body's stress response.

Various studies have shown that Schisandra can improve physical performance, endurance, and stress response. For example, one study found that Schisandra can reduce feelings of fatigue during exercise and improve exercise performance.

Senna is a plant extract derived from the *Senna alexandrina* plant. It is often used to relieve constipation. Senna contains sennosides, an ingredient that improves motility in the gastrointestinal tract. This helps stool pass through the intestines faster, which relieves the symptoms of constipation.

Senna is commonly used for constipation and is generally safe for short-term use. However, long-term use can cause intestinal irritation or a reduced ability to maintain regularity of bowel movements.

Sesame seeds are rich in a number of nutrients, particularly magnesium and copper.

Magnesium is an essential mineral for more than 300 enzymatic reactions and plays a role in many bodily functions such as energy production, protein synthesis, cell communication, and DNA synthesis [63].

Copper also performs a number of important functions in the body, particularly important in energy production and iron metabolism [64]. Also, sesame seeds contain B vitamins, which are important for energy metabolism, nerve function, and cell growth and division.

Shepherd's Purse is an herb known especially for its ability to alleviate menstrual bleeding. The herb has hemostatic (stopping bleeding) properties. This can help control heavy menstrual bleeding. However, more scientific evidence is needed in this regard [65].

Skullcap is an herb known for its ability to relieve anxiety and insomnia. In traditional Chinese medicine, the plant is believed to have calming effects on the nervous system. However, more scientific research is needed to confirm these claims [66].

Slippery Elm is known for its digestive health-promoting properties. The plant produces a mucus-like substance that coats and relaxes the stomach and intestines. Thanks to this feature, it can alleviate conditions such as irritable bowel syndrome (IBS) and reflux [67].

Spirulina is a seaweed that supports immune functions and has detoxification properties. Spirulina contains a number of nutritional components, including vitamins B and C, beta-carotene, iron, magnesium, and gamma-linolenic acid.

Some studies have shown that spirulina can strengthen the immune system and protect the body from toxins. Additionally, there is research showing that spirulina has the potential to reduce inflammation, improve lipid and blood sugar levels, and exhibit anticancer properties [68].

St. John's Wort (*Hypericum perforatum*) is an herb that can help relieve symptoms of depression. This effect may be due to the herb's ability to increase serotonin levels in the brain, serotonin, a *feel-good* neurotransmitter.

Various studies have shown that St. John's wort can help relieve mild to moderate symptoms of depression [69]. However, it is important to note that people with severe symptoms of depression may need medication or other professional healthcare.

Stinging nettle (*Urtica dioica*) is an herb that offers a number of health benefits, including its anti-inflammatory effects and ability to reduce pain. These properties suggest that stinging nettle may help relieve symptoms of arthritis and similar conditions.

Several scientific studies have shown that stinging nettle can relieve arthritis symptoms. For example, one study found that nettle extract can improve pain and mobility symptoms in people with osteoarthritis [70]. However, more research is needed on these effects of stinging nettle.

Nettle (*Urtica dioica*) is also an herb used to support prostate health and relieve allergy symptoms. It can be found in various forms and has been used by many cultures throughout history to treat a variety of ailments.

When it comes to prostate health, stinging nettle is often used to relieve symptoms of a condition called benign prostatic hyperplasia (BPH). BPH is an enlarged prostate condition that usually develops with age and can make urination difficult. Several clinical studies have shown that stinging nettle can help relieve BPH symptoms [71].

Stinging nettle may also help relieve allergy symptoms. Some studies have shown that stinging nettle has antihistamine properties and can therefore help relieve allergy symptoms [72].

Sunflower seeds are particularly rich in vitamin E and selenium. Vitamin E is an antioxidant that helps the body fight free radicals [73]. This can help prevent cell damage and slow aging. Selenium also acts as an antioxidant and supports thyroid function, DNA production, and the body's defense against infections [74].

Brazil nuts are an extraordinarily rich source of selenium. Selenium is a mineral that performs a number of important functions in the body. In particular, it plays a role in the production of several important proteins with antioxidant properties, helps the normal functioning of the thyroid gland, and supports the immune system. Selenium deficiency can lead to a number of health problems, so it's important to consume a sufficient amount [74].

Thyme has powerful antioxidant and antimicrobial properties. Studies have shown that thyme can protect against bacteria, fungi, and even some viruses. In addition, thyme contains important antioxidants that are effective in reducing oxidative stress that causes various diseases [75].

Tribulus (*Tribulus terrestris*) is an herb that grows in tropical and temperate regions. The fruit and root of Tribulus are used for a variety of health benefits and are often used to boost libido and sports performance [76].

Tribulus is used specifically to increase sexual function in men, and some studies have shown that Tribulus can increase libido and erectile function. There is also some evidence that Tribulus can improve muscle growth and sports performance.

However, more information is needed about the side effects and safety of Tribulus. Side effects such as stomach upset, sleep problems, and menstrual irregularities have been reported.

Valerian root is an herb often used to relieve symptoms of insomnia and anxiety. Valerian works by calming the nervous system and supporting the body's relaxation response.

Various scientific studies have shown that valerian root can relieve insomnia symptoms and improve sleep quality. In addition, some studies have also indicated that valerian root can relieve anxiety symptoms.

Chicory (*Cichorium intybus*) is an herb that helps improve digestive health. In particular, a prebiotic called inulin, found in the root of chicory, supports the digestive system by promoting the growth of healthy bacteria in the intestines. Some studies have shown that chicory can improve digestive health and especially relieve symptoms of irritable bowel syndrome (IBS) and constipation.

Velvet Bean (*Mucuna pruriens*) is an herb with a high content of L-dopa. L-dopa is a compound that converts in the brain to a neurotransmitter called dopamine [77]. Dopamine regulates the reward and pleasure centers in the brain and provides motor control, so dopamine deficiency is linked to Parkinson's disease.

There are several benefits to using *Mucuna pruriens*. By increasing dopamine production, it can reduce symptoms of depression and anxiety, regulate sleep, and improve overall mood and energy. It also has the potential to alleviate Parkinson's disease symptoms. However, the consumption of *Mucuna pruriens* has side effects and potential side effects such as drowsiness, headache, and tension, and caution should be exercised in its consumption.

Walnuts are nutritious nuts and contain valuable nutrients such as omega-3 fatty acids, antioxidants, fiber, protein, and various vitamins and minerals. Omega-3 fatty acids may help heart health, brain function, and reduce inflammation.

Antioxidants help prevent cellular damage caused by free radicals and may reduce the risk of chronic diseases. Walnuts contain both of these components, which are important for healthy heart and brain function.

Waterhyssop, scientifically known as *Bacopa monnieri* and popularly known as Brahmi, is a plant that usually grows in aquatic environments. It has been used in Ayurveda and traditional Indian medicine for centuries to support nervous system and brain function.

One of the most researched potential benefits of bacopa is memory enhancement. Clinical studies have found that waterhyssop is effective in improving memory and cognitive abilities. A number of studies, especially in elderly individuals, have shown that waterhyssop can improve memory performance and alleviate the symptoms of neurodegenerative diseases such as dementia and Alzheimer's.

However, not all effects of waterhyssop are seen immediately. Many studies have found that the memory-enhancing effects of waterhyssop usually appear within a few weeks or months of regular use.

Wheat germ is the embryo of a wheat grain, which enables the seed to develop into a new plant. Wheat contains most of the vitamin and mineral content, although the germ makes up only a small part of the seed.

Wheat germ is packed with important nutrients such as B vitamins (B1, B2, B3, and B6), vitamin E, folic acid, magnesium, phosphorus, zinc, manganese, selenium, and iron. These vitamins and minerals support energy production, strengthen the immune system, and may reduce the risk of heart disease.

In addition, wheat germ contains the mineral chromium, which helps reduce the body's insulin resistance and reduces the risk of type 2 diabetes. Due to its high fiber content, wheat germ improves digestive health, provides a feeling of satiety, and can help with weight control.

Wheatgrass is a plant rich in vitamins and minerals. When consumed as grass juice, wheatgrass provides several health benefits, but more research is needed on these effects.

White willow bark is an extract from the plant called *Salix alba* and is used as a natural pain reliever and anti-inflammatory. White willow bark contains a compound called salicin. In the body, salicin is converted to salicylate, a substance that relieves pain and inflammation.

White willow bark has been used to treat conditions such as headaches, arthritis, and osteoarthritis. However, the effects of this herb are usually mild and short-lived, and prescription drugs are often more effective in cases of severe pain or chronic inflammation.

Wild yam is often used for its properties to relieve menopausal symptoms. However, these effects are still controversial, and further research is needed on these effects of wild yam [78].

Witch hazel is an herb often used to improve skin health. It can help relieve various skin conditions, especially skin conditions such as acne, eczema, and psoriasis.

Witch hazel also has powerful anti-inflammatory properties and can help reduce skin irritation and inflammation. Because of these properties, it is often used in the treatment of sunburn, insect bites, and various skin conditions.

Wood Betony is known for his ability to relieve neurological pain. The herb has the potential to relieve headaches, nerve pain, and migraines. However, these effects are generally supported by anecdotal evidence, and further scientific research is needed [79].

Yarrow (*Achillea millefolium*) is used as a medicinal herb and is believed to provide many different health benefits. Yarrow has anti-inflammatory properties and may also be helpful in stopping bleeding.

Yarrow can be used topically to help heal skin wounds. Additionally, yarrow tea is used by some people to relieve digestive issues, pain, and fever.

Yerba mate is a beverage derived from *Ilex paraguariensis*, a plant native to South America. Yerba mate contains caffeine and can therefore increase physical and mental energy. It also contains many important vitamins and minerals, which contribute to overall health and energy levels.

Although yerba mate contains caffeine, it has generally been reported to cause fewer jitters and other side effects compared to coffee. It also contains, besides caffeine, other natural stimulants such as theobromine and theophylline, which can lead to a more balanced and long-lasting energy boost.

Yogurt is a dairy product formed as a result of bacterial fermentation of milk. The two main bacterial species, *Lactobacillus delbrueckii* subsp. *bulgaricus* and *Streptococcus thermophilus*, are used to make yogurt, and these bacteria provide the acidic taste, consistency, and probiotic properties of yogurt.

Yogurt is a source of important nutrients such as protein, calcium, B vitamins, and probiotics. Probiotics are beneficial bacteria that are important for digestive health. Various studies have shown that yogurt consumption can reduce the risk of digestive disorders, obesity, heart disease, and type 2 diabetes [80].

Yogurt is also generally more tolerable for people who are lactose intolerant because during fermentation bacteria break down milk's lactose. However, it's important to note that not all yogurts offer the same health benefits. Some yogurts may contain unhealthy additional ingredients such as sugar or artificial sweeteners.

Zinc is a mineral that has many different functions in the human body. Zinc supports the growth and division of cells, the formation of proteins and DNA, the proper functioning of the immune system, and the healing of wounds.

Zinc deficiency can lead to an inadequate immune response, slow wound healing, and, in some cases, hair loss. Zinc can be found in a variety of foods, including seafood, meat, grains, dairy products, and legumes.

The above information is for general information purposes only and should not replace professional medical advice. A healthcare professional should always be consulted before deciding on a particular treatment or medication.

12.2 POPULAR NATURAL TREATMENTS WITH CONFLICTING SCIENTIFIC EVIDENCE

Research for each of most of these examples is often ambiguous and sometimes shows conflicting results. Therefore, consultation with a healthcare professional is recommended before recommending the use of a particular treatment. Some examples of such natural treatments are listed below:

1. St John's Wort: This herb is often used to treat mild to moderate depression. However, there is mixed evidence about its efficacy and side effects.
2. Kava: Evidence on the efficacy and safety of this widely used herb for anxiety shows mixed results.
3. Gingko Biloba: This herb is often used for memory disorders, but the evidence on its effectiveness shows mixed results.
4. Black Cohosh: This herb is frequently used for menopausal symptoms, but the evidence shows mixed results.
5. Saw Palmetto: This herb is used for prostate enlargement, but evidence on its effectiveness shows mixed results.
6. Echinacea: This herb is used against colds and flu, but the evidence on its effectiveness shows mixed results.
7. Glucosamine: This natural ingredient is commonly used for osteoarthritis, but the evidence on its effectiveness shows mixed results.

8. Chondroitin: This natural ingredient is often used for osteoarthritis, but the evidence on its effectiveness shows mixed results.
9. Melatonin: This natural hormone is often used for insomnia, but the evidence on its effectiveness shows mixed results.
10. Pedigree 10: This herb is commonly used for menopausal symptoms and heart health, although evidence on its effectiveness shows mixed results.
11. Cat's Claw: Used for arthritis and other inflammatory diseases, but the evidence is mixed.
12. SAM-e (S-adenosylmethionine): Used for the treatment of depression, but research on its effectiveness has yielded conflicting results stating that it can interact negatively with antidepressant medications.
13. Tea Tree Oil: A popular remedy for acne treatment, but evidence shows mixed results.
14. Sugar Grass: Claimed to help lower blood sugar levels, but the evidence is not yet clear.
15. Acupuncture: Used for a variety of conditions including pain, migraine, and blood pressure reduction, but evidence shows mixed results.
16. Homeopathy: Used for a variety of health conditions, but evidence is conflicting about its effectiveness.
17. Magnesium Supplements: Recommended for a variety of conditions such as heart health and sleep patterns, but the evidence for its effectiveness is mixed.
18. Chromium Picolinate: Claimed to help support metabolism, but the evidence is mixed.
19. Garlic Supplements: Used to support heart health, but research on its effectiveness has yielded mixed results.

The examples above are general guidelines and should not be used without considering individual health conditions, possible side effects, and drug interactions. The evidence on natural health treatments is constantly updated. Therefore, it is very important to stay up-to-date with information related to this and to consult a health professional.

12.3   POPULAR NATURAL TREATMENTS LACKING SCIENTIFIC EVIDENCE

There are several popular natural treatments that lack scientific evidence to support their effectiveness. These include:

1. Black seed: It is used for various health conditions, but there is insufficient evidence.
2. Detox teas: Claimed to help flush out harmful toxins from the body, solid scientific evidence is lacking.
3. Facial acupuncture: Claimed to improve skin health, but there is insufficient evidence.
4. Colostrum supplements: It is claimed to strengthen the immune system and improve digestive health, but there is insufficient evidence.
5. Reiki: Claimed to reduce stress and improve overall health, but there is insufficient evidence.
6. Ayurveda: The traditional medicine system of India. However, there is insufficient scientific evidence for many applications and treatments.
7. Crystal therapy: It is used for the treatment of physical and emotional ailments, but scientific evidence is lacking in this regard.
8. Healing stones: Claimed to have a positive effect on mood and overall health, but there is no solid scientific evidence.
9. Kinesiology tapes: Claimed to relieve pain and inflammation, but insufficient evidence is available.
10. Chakra balance: Claimed to improve mood and overall health, but there is no solid scientific evidence.
11. Bioenergy therapy: It is used for a variety of health conditions, but there is insufficient scientific evidence.

These are examples based on current research in the natural health sciences and popular treatments. When seeking information on natural treatments and alternative medicine, it is always important to carefully check your sources and seek professional medical advice.

The above information is for general information purposes only and should not replace professional medical advice. It is always recommended to consult a healthcare professional before making a decision on a particular treatment or medication.

12.4 ANIMAL-DERIVED NATURAL TREATMENTS

The use of animal-derived products in natural health products is quite common. However, research on their efficacy and safety often yields mixed results. Some examples are given below.

These examples should be used as a general guide and should not be used without considering the health status of each individual, possible side effects, and drug interactions. The evidence on natural health treatments is constantly being updated, and it is essential to get the most up-to-date information and consult a healthcare professional.

12.4.1 Scientifically Proven

1. Honey: It has been scientifically proven that honey has wound-healing properties.
2. Omega-3 Fatty Acids: It has been scientifically proven that Omega-3 fatty acids, especially from fish, improve heart health and reduce the risk of depression.
3. Glucosamine and Chondroitin: These compounds, usually derived from shellfish, have been shown to support joint health.
4. Bee Pollen: Bee pollen has been shown to boost immunity and alleviate some allergic reactions.

12.4.2 Scientifically Unproven

1. Horned Deer Extract: Claimed by some to improve performance, this product receives little scientific support.
2. Hai Shark Cartilage: Despite its claim to prevent cancer, the effectiveness of this product is still unclear.
3. Snake Oil: This product, used to treat skin problems, is not scientifically supported.
4. Emu Oil: Although claimed to have anti-inflammatory properties, the effectiveness of this oil is still unclear.

REFERENCES

1. M. Traber, "Vitamin E Inadequacy in Humans: Causes and Consequences," *Advances in Nutrition*, vol. 5, no. 5, pp. 503–514, 2014.
2. D. Jenkins, C. Kendall and A. Marchie, "Dose Response of Almonds on Coronary Heart Disease Risk Factors: Blood Lipids, Oxidized Low-Density Lipoproteins, Lipoprotein(a), Homocysteine, and Pulmonary Nitric Oxide: A Randomized, Controlled, Crossover Trial," *Circulation*, vol. 106, no. 11, pp. 1327–1332, 2002.
3. P. Kriplani, K. Guarve and U. Baghael, "*Arnica montana* L. – A Plant of Healing: Review," *Journal of Pharmacy and Pharmacology*, vol. 69, no. 8, pp. 925–945, 2017.
4. K. Komosinska-Vassev, P. Olczyk, J. Kaźmierczak, L. Mencner and K. Olczyk, "Bee Pollen: Chemical Composition and Therapeutic Application," *Evidence-Based Complementary and Alternative Medicine*, vol. 2015, p. 297425, 2015. doi: 10.1155/2015/297425.
5. B. Park, H. Lee, S. Lee, X. Piao, G. Takeoka, R. Wong, Y. Ahn and J. Kim, "Antibacterial Activity of *Tabebuia impetiginosa* Martius Ex DC (Taheebo) Against *Helicobacter pylori*," *Journal of Ethnopharmacology*, vol. 105, no. 1-2, pp. 255–262, 2006.

6. A. Ahmad, A. Husain and M. Mujeeb, "A Review on Therapeutic Potential of *Nigella sativa*: A Miracle Herb," *Asian Pacific Journal of Tropical Biomedicine*, vol. 3, no. 5, pp. 337–352, 2013.

7. A. F. Majdalawieh and M. W. Fayyad, "Immunomodulatory and Anti-Inflammatory Action of *Nigella sativa* and Thymoquinone: A Comprehensive Review," *International Immunopharmacology*, vol. 28, no. 1, pp. 295–304, 2015.

8. H. P. Ammon, "Modulation of the Immune System by *Boswellia serrata* Extracts and Boswellic Acids," *Phytomedicine*, vol. 17, no. 11, pp. 862–867, 2010.

9. R. Oelkers-Ax, A. Leins, P. Parzer, T. Hillecke, H. V. Bolay, J. Fischer, S. Bender, U. Hermanns and F. Resch, "Butterbur Root Extract and Music Therapy in the Prevention of Childhood Migraine: An Explorative Study," *European Journal of Pain (London, England)*, vol. 12, no. 3, pp. 301–313, 2008.

10. V. Duran, M. Matic, M. Jovanović, N. Mimica, Z. Gajinov, M. Poljacki and P. Boza, "Results of the Clinical Examination of an Ointment with Marigold (*Calendula officinalis*) Extract in the Treatment of Venous Leg Ulcers," *International Journal of Tissue Reactions*, vol. 27, no. 3, pp. 101–106, 2005.

11. P. Chandran and R. Kuttan, "Effect of Calendula officinalis Flower Extract on Acute Phase Proteins, Antioxidant Defense Mechanism and Granuloma Formation During Thermal Burns," *Journal of Clinical Biochemistry and Nutrition*, vol. 43, no. 2, pp. 58–64, 2008.

12. J. D. Amsterdam, Y. Li, I. Soeller, K. Rockwell, J. J. Mao and J. Shults, "A Randomized, Double-Blind, Placebo-Controlled Trial of Oral *Matricaria recutita* (chamomile) Extract Therapy for Generalized Anxiety Disorder," *Journal of Clinical Psychopharmacology*, vol. 29, no. 4, pp. 378–382, 2009.

13. J. K. Srivastava, E. Shankar and S. Gupta, "Chamomile: A Herbal Medicine of the Past With a Bright Future (Review)," *Molecular Medicine Reports*, vol. 3, no. 6, pp. 895–901, 2010.

14. J. W. Daily, M. Yang and S. Park, "Efficacy of Turmeric Extracts and Curcumin for Alleviating the Symptoms of Joint Arthritis: A Systematic Review and Meta-Analysis of Randomized Clinical Trials," *Journal of Medicinal Food*, vol. 19, no. 8, pp. 717–729, 2016.

15. V. P. Menon and A. R. Sudheer, "Antioxidant and Anti-Inflammatory Properties of Curcumin," *The Molecular Targets and Therapeutic Uses of Curcumin in Health and Disease*, vol. 595, pp. 105–125, 2007.

16. J. Liu, J. E. Burdette, H. Xu, C. Gu, R. B. van Breemen, K. P. Bhat, N. Booth, A. I. Constantinou, J. M. Pezzuto, H. H. Fong, N. R. Farnsworth and J. L. Bolton, "Evaluation of Estrogenic Activity of Plant Extracts for the Potential Treatment of Menopausal Symptoms," *Journal of Agricultural and Food Chemistry*, vol. 49, no. 5, pp. 2472–2479, 2001.

17. S. A. Shah, S. Sander, C. M. White, M. Rinaldi and C. I. Coleman, "Evaluation of Echinacea for the Prevention and Treatment of the Common Cold: A Meta-Analysis," *The Lancet. Infectious Diseases*, vol. 7, no. 7, pp. 473–480, 2007.

18. M. Karsch-Völk, B. Barrett and K. Linde, "Echinacea for Preventing and Treating the Common Cold," *The Cochrane Database of Systematic Reviews*, 2014.

19. R. Paduch, A. Woźniak, P. Niedziela and R. Rejdak, "Assessment of Eyebright (*Euphrasia officinalis* L.) Extract Activity in Relation to Human Corneal Cells Using in Vitro Tests," *Balkan Medical Journal*, vol. 31, no. 1, pp. 29–36, 2014.

20. S. Zevin and S. Benavides, "Herbs and Alternative Therapies in the Hypertension Clinic," *American Journal of Hypertension*, vol. 17, no. 9, pp. 818–820, 2004.

21. P. Azimi, R. Ghiasvand, A. Feizi, M. Hariri and B. Abbasi, "Effect of Cinnamon, Cardamom, Saffron and Ginger Consumption on Blood Pressure and a Marker of Endothelial Function in Patients with Type 2 Diabetes Mellitus: A Randomized Controlled Clinical Trial," *Blood Pressure*, vol. 25, no. 3, pp. 133–140, 2016.

22. R. F. Santos, J. C. Galduroz, A. Barbieri, M. L. Castiglioni, L. Y. Ytaya and O. F. Bueno, "Cognitive Performance, SPECT, and Blood Viscosity in Elderly Non-Demented People Using Ginkgo biloba," *Pharmacopsychiatry*, vol. 36, no. 4, pp. 127–133, 2003.

23. S. Weinmann, S. Roll, C. Schwarzbach, C. Vauth and S. N. Willich, "Effects of Ginkgo biloba in Dementia: Systematic Review and Meta-Analysis," *BMC Geriatrics*, vol. 10, p. 14, 2010.

24. E. Thom, "The Effect of Chlorogenic Acid Enriched Coffee on Glucose Absorption in Healthy Volunteers and Its Effect on Body Mass When Used Long-Term in Overweight and Obese People," *Journal of International Medical Research*, vol. 35, no. 6, pp. 900–908, 2007.

25. J. C. Callaway, "Hempseed as a Nutritional Resource: An Overview," *Euphytica*, vol. 140, pp. 65–72, 2004.

26. C. Leizer, D. Ribnicky, A. Poulev, S. Dushenkov and I. Raskin, "The Composition of Hemp Seed Oil and Its Potential as an Important Source of Nutrition," *Journal of Nutraceuticals, Functional & Medical Foods*, vol. 2, no. 4, pp. 35–53, 2000.

27. D. McKay, C. Chen, E. Saltzman and J. Blumberg, "Hibiscus Sabdariffa L. Tea (tisane) Lowers Blood Pressure in Prehypertensive and Mildly Hypertensive Adults," *Journal of Nutrition*, vol. 140, no. 2, pp. 298–303, 2010.

28. M. D. Mandal and S. Mandal, "Honey: Its Medicinal Property and Antibacterial Activity," *Asian Pacific Journal of Tropical Biomedicine*, vol. 1, no. 2, pp. 154–160, 2011.

29. J. M. Alvarez-Suarez, M. Gasparrini, T. Y. Forbes-Hernández, L. Mazzoni and F. Giampieri, "The Composition and Biological Activity of Honey: A Focus on Manuka Honey," *Foods*, vol. 3, no. 3, pp. 420–432, 2014.

30. S. Bogdanov, T. Jurendic, R. Sieber and P. Gallmann, "Honey for Nutrition and Health: A Review," *Journal of the American College of Nutrition*, vol. 27, no. 6, pp. 677–689, 2008.

31. A. Pascoal, S. Rodrigues, A. Teixeira, X. Feás and L. M. Estevinho, "Biological Activities of Commercial Bee Pollens: Antimicrobial, Antimutagenic, Antioxidant and Anti-Inflammatory," *Food and Chemical Toxicology*, vol. 63, pp. 233–239, 2014.

32. T. Eteraf-Oskouei and M. Najafi, "Traditional and Modern Uses of Natural Honey in Human Diseases: A Review," *Iranian Journal of Basic Medical Sciences*, vol. 16, no. 6,pp. 731–742, 2013.

33. Z. Can, "An Investigation of Turkish Honeys: Their Physico-Chemical Properties, Antioxidant Capacities and Phenolic Profiles," *Food Chemistry*, vol. 141, pp. 338–345, 2013.

34. E. Mavric, S. Wittmann, G. Barth and T. Henle, "Identification and Quantification of Methylglyoxal as the Dominant Antibacterial Constituent of Manuka (*Leptospermum scoparium*) Honeys from New Zealand," *Molecular Nutrition & Food Research*, vol. 52, no. 4, pp. 483–489, 2008.

35. N. Al-Waili, "Topical Application of Natural Honey, Beeswax and Olive Oil Mixture for Atopic Dermatitis or Psoriasis: Partially Controlled, Single-Blinded Study," *Complementary Therapies in Medicine*, vol. 20, no. 6, pp. 305–313, 2012.

36. M. Malkoç, H. Çakır, Y. Kara, Z. Can and S. Kolayli, "Phenolic Composition and Antioxidant Properties of Anzer Honey from Black Sea Region of Turkey," *Uludağ Arıcılık Dergisi*, vol. 19, pp. 143–151, 2019.

37. G. Tel-Çayan, B. H. Çiftçi, M. Taş-Küçükaydın, Y. Temel, F. Çayan, S. Küçükaydın and M. E. Duru, "Citrus Honeys from Three Different Regions of Turkey: HPLC-DAD Profiling and In Vitro Enzyme Inhibition, Antioxidant, Anti-Inflammatory and Antimicrobial Properties with Chemometric Study," *Chemistry & Biodiversity*, vol. 20, no. 9, p. e202300990, 2023. doi:10.1002/cbdv.202300990.

38. A. W. Shindel, Z. C. Xin, G. Lin, T. M. Fandel, Y. C. Huang, L. Banie, B. N. Breyer, M. M. Garcia, C. S. Lin and T. F. Lue, "Erectogenic and Neurotrophic Effects of Icariin, a Purified Extract of Horny Goat Weed (Epimedium Spp.) In Vitro and In Vivo," *The Journal of Sexual Medicine*, vol. 7, pp. 1518–1528, 2010.

39. K. Kuroda, N. Inoue, Y. Ito, K. Kubota, A. Sugimoto, T. Kakuda and T. Fushiki, "Sedative Effects of the Jasmine Tea Odor and (R)-(-)-Linalool, One of Its Major Odor Components, on Autonomic Nerve Activity and Mood States," *European Journal of Applied Physiology*, vol. 95, pp. 107–114, 2005.

40. G. Shah, R. Shri, V. Panchal, N. Sharma, B. Singh and A. S. Mann, "Scientific Basis for the Therapeutic Use of *Cymbopogon citratus*, Stapf (Lemon Grass)," *Journal of Advanced Pharmaceutical Technology and Research*, vol. 2, no. 1, pp. 3–8, 2011.

41. J. Sarris, C. Stough, C. Bousman, Z. Wahid, G. Murray, R. Teschke, K. Savage, A. Dowell, C. Ng and I. Schweitzer, "Kava in the Treatment of Generalized Anxiety Disorder: A Double-Blind, Randomized, Placebo-Controlled Study," *Journal of Clinical Psychopharmacology*, vol. 33, no. 5, pp. 643–648, 2013.

42. S. Kasper, M. Gastpar, W. E. Müller, H. P. Volz, H. J. Möller, S. Schläfke and A. Dienel, "Lavender Oil Preparation Silexan Is Effective in Generalized Anxiety Disorder—A Randomized, Double-Blind Comparison to Placebo and Paroxetine," *The International Journal of Neuropsychopharmacology*, vol. 17, no. 6, pp. 859–869, 2014.

43. A. S. Lillehei and L. L. Halcon, "A Systematic Review of the Effect of Inhaled Essential Oils on Sleep," *The Journal of Alternative and Complementary Medicine*, vol. 20, no. 6, pp. 441–451, 2014.

44. D. O. Kennedy, W. Little and A. B. Scholey, "Attenuation of Laboratory-Induced Stress in Humans After Acute Administration of *Melissa officinalis* (Lemon Balm)," *Psychosomatic Medicine*, vol. 66, no. 4, pp. 607–613, 2004.

45. D. A. Carter, S. E. Blair, N. N. Cokcetin, D. Bouzo, P. Brooks, R. Schothauer, and E. J. Harry, "Therapeutic Manuka Honey: No Longer So Alternative," *Frontiers in Microbiology*, vol. 7, no. 569, p. 194754, 2016.

46. S. Stohs and M. Hartman, "Review of the Safety and Efficacy of Moringa oleifera," *Phytotherapy Research*, vol. 29, no. 6, pp. 796–804, 2015.

47. A. Turker and N. Camper, "Biological Activity of Common Mullein, a Medicinal Plant," *Journal of Ethnopharmacology*, vol. 82, no. 2-3, pp. 117–125, 2002.

48. B. West, S. Deng, F. Isami, A. Uwaya and C. Jensen, "The Potential Health Benefits of Noni Juice: A Review of Human Intervention Studies," *Foods*, vol. 7, no. 4, 2018.

49. T. Perrinjaquet-Moccetti, A. Busjahn, C. Schmidlin, A. Schmidt, B. Bradl and C. Aydogan, "Food Supplementation with an Olive (*Olea europaea* L.) Leaf Extract Reduces Blood Pressure in Borderline Hypertensive Monozygotic Twins," *Phytotherapy Research*, vol. 22, no. 9, pp. 1239–1242, 2008.

50. R. J. Goldberg and J. Katz, "A Meta-Analysis of the Analgesic Effects of Omega-3 Polyunsaturated Fatty Acid Supplementation for Inflammatory Joint Pain," *Pain*, vol. 129, pp. 210–223, 2007.

51. S. Rajaram, K. Burke, B. Connell, T. Myint and J. Sabaté, "A Monounsaturated Fatty Acid-Rich Pecan-Enriched Diet Favorably Alters the Serum Lipid Profile of Healthy Men and Women," *Journal of Nutrition*, vol. 131, no. 9, pp. 2275–2279, 2001.

52. A. Samuelsen, "The Traditional Uses, Chemical Constituents and Biological Activities of Plantago Major L. A Review," *Journal of Ethnopharmacology*, vol. 71, no. 1–2, pp. 1–21, 2000.

53. J. de Baaij, J. Hoenderop and R. Bindels, "Magnesium in Man: Implications for Health and Disease," *Physiological Reviews*, vol. 95, no. 1, pp. 1–46, 2015.

54. D. Stevenson, F. Eller, L. Wang, J. Jane, T. Wang and G. Inglett, "Oil and Tocopherol Content and Composition of Pumpkin Seed Oil in 12 Cultivars," *Journal of Agricultural and Food Chemistry*, vol. 55, no. 10, 2007.

55. M. Lipovac, P. Chedraui, C. Gruenhut, A. Gocan, M. Stammler and M. Imhof, "The Effect of Red Clover Isoflavone Supplementation Over Vasomotor and Menopausal Symptoms in Postmenopausal Women," *Gynecological Endocrinology*, vol. 28, no. 3, pp. 203–207, 2012.

56. Y. Li, L. Jiang, Z. Jia, W. Xin, S. Yang, Q. Yang and L. Wang, "A Meta-Analysis of Red Yeast Rice: An Effective and Relatively Safe Alternative Approach for Dyslipidemia," *PloS One*, vol. 9, no. 6, p. e98611, 2014.

57. M. C. Gerards, R. J. Terlou, H. Yu, C. H. Koks and V. E. Gerdes, "Traditional Chinese Lipid-Lowering Agent Red Yeast Rice Results in Significant LDL Reduction but Safety Is Uncertain – A Systematic Review and Meta-Analysis," *Atherosclerosis*, vol. 240, no. 2, pp. 415–423, 2015.

58. S. K. Hung, R. E. Perry, and E. Ernst, "The Effectiveness and Efficacy of *Rhodiola rosea* L.: A Systematic Review of Randomized Clinical Trials," *Phytomedicine*, vol. 18, no. 4, pp. 235–244, 2011.

59. A. Pengelly, J. Snow, S. Y. Mills, A. Scholey, K. Wesnes and L. R. Butler, "Short-Term Study on the Effects of Rosemary on Cognitive Function in an Elderly Population," *Journal of Medicinal Food*, vol. 15, no. 1, pp. 10–17, 2012.

60. M. Moss, J. Cook, K. Wesnes and P. Duckett, "Aromas of Rosemary and Lavender Essential Oils Differentially Affect Cognition and Mood in Healthy Adults," *International Journal of Neuroscience*, vol. 113, no. 1, pp. 15–38, 2003.

61. M. F. Ramadan, and A. Al-Ghamdi, "Bioactive Compounds and Health-Promoting Properties of Royal Jelly: A Review," *Journal of Functional Foods*, vol. 4, no. 1, pp. 39–52, 2012.

62. H. A. Hausenblas, D. Saha, P. J. Dubyak and S. D. Anton, "Saffron (*Crocus sativus* L.) and Major Depressive Disorder: A Meta-Analysis of Randomized Clinical Trials," *Journal of Integrative Medicine*, vol. 11, no. 6, pp. 377–383, 2013.

63. R. Swaminathan, "Magnesium Metabolism and Its Disorders," *The Clinical Biochemist Reviews*, vol. 24, no. 2, pp. 47–66, 2003.

64. L. Harvey, K. Ashton, L. Hooper, A. Casgrain and S. Fairweather-Tait, "Methods of Assessment of Copper Status in Humans: A Systematic Review," *The American Journal of Clinical Nutrition*, vol. 89, no. 6, pp. 2009S–2024S, 2009.

65. M. Zamani, N. Neghab and S. Torabian, "Therapeutic Effect of *Vitex agnus* and *Crataegus oxyacantha* on Cardiovascular Diseases: A Traditional Use and Modern Evidence," *Frontiers in Pharmacology*, vol. 11, no. 486, 2020.

66. C. Brock, J. Whitehouse, I. Tewfik and T. Towell, "American Skullcap (*Scutellaria lateriflora*): A Randomised, Double-Blind Placebo-Controlled Crossover Study of Its Effects on Mood in Healthy Volunteers," *Phytotherapy Research*, vol. 285, pp. 692–698, 2014.

67. L. Langmead, C. Dawson, C. Hawkins, N. Banna, S. Loo and D. Rampton, "Antioxidant Effects of Herbal Therapies Used by Patients With Inflammatory Bowel Disease: An in Vitro Study," *Alimentary Pharmacology & Therapeutics*, vol. 16, no. 2, pp. 197–205, 2002.

68. Q. Wu, L. Liu, A. Miron, B. Klímová, D. Wan and K. Kuča, "The Antioxidant, Immunomodulatory, and Anti-Inflammatory Activities of Spirulina: An Overview," *Archives of Toxicology*, vol. 90, no. 8, pp. 1817–1840, 2016.

69. K. Linde, M. Berner and L. Kriston, "St John's Wort for Major Depression," *Cochrane Database of Systematic Reviews*, 2008.

70. J. E. Chrubasik, B. D. Roufogalis, H. Wagner and S. A. Chrubasik, "A Comprehensive Review on the Stinging Nettle Effect and Efficacy Profiles. Part II: Urticae Radix," *Phytomedicine*, vol. 14, pp. 568–579, 2007.

71. T. Schneider and H. Rübben, "Stinging Nettle Root Extract (Bazoton-Uno) in Long Term Treatment of Benign Prostatic Syndrome (BPS). Results of a Randomized, Double-Blind, Placebo-Controlled Multicenter Study After 12 Months," *Der Urologe. Ausg. A*, vol. 43, no. 3, p. 302–306.

72. B. J. Roschek, R. Fink, M. McMichael and R. Alberte, "Nettle Extract (Urtica dioica) Affects Key Receptors and Enzymes Associated with Allergic Rhinitis," *Phytotherapy Research: PTR*, vol. 23, no. 7, pp. 920–926, 2009.

73. M. Traber and J. Stevens, "Vitamins C and E: Beneficial Effects from a Mechanistic Perspective," *Free Radical Biology and Medicine*, vol. 51, no. 5, pp. 1000–1013, 2011.

74. M. Rayman, "The Importance of Selenium to Human Health," *Lancet*, vol. 356, no. 9225, pp. 233–241, 2000.

75. H. O. Elansary, A. Szopa, P. Kubica, H. Ekiert, M. A. Mattar, F. A. Al-Mana and D. O. El-Ansary, "Bioactivities of Traditional Medicinal Plants in Alexandria," *Evidence-Based Complementary and Alternative Medicine*, vol. 2018, 2018.

76. T. M. Sellandi, A. B. Thakar, M. S. Baghel, "Clinical Study of *Tribulus terrestris* Linn. in Oligozoospermia: A Double Blind Study," *Ayu*, vol. 33, no. 3, pp. 356–364, 2012.

77. L. R. Lampariello, A. Cortelazzo, R. Guerranti, C. Sticozzi and G. Valacchi, "The Magic Velvet Bean of *Mucuna pruriens*," *Journal of Traditional and Complementary Medicine*, vol. 2, no. 4, pp. 331–339, 2012.

78. W. H. Wu, L. Y. Liu, C. J. Chung, H. J. Jou and T. A. Wang, "Estrogenic Effect of Yam Ingestion in Healthy Postmenopausal Women," *Journal of the American College of Nutrition*, vol. 24, no. 4, pp. 235–243, 2005.

79. M. Wichtl, Herbal Drugs and Phytopharmaceuticals: A Handbook for Practice on a Scientific Basis, CRC Press, 2004.

80. G. Y. Tang, X. Meng, R. Y. Gan, C. N. Zhao, Q. Liu, Y. B. Feng, S. Li, X. L. Wei, A. G. Atanasov, H. Corke and H. B. Li, "Health Functions and Related Molecular Mechanisms of Tea Components: An Update Review," *International Journal of Molecular Sciences*, vol. 20, no. 24, p. 6196, 2019. https://doi.org/10.3390/ijms20246196.

13 Aromatherapy

Aromatherapy is a holistic healing practice that utilizes the therapeutic properties of essential oils to promote physical and emotional well-being. These essential oils are derived from various parts of plants, such as flowers, leaves, stems, and roots, and are known for their distinct fragrances. Listed below are the various aromatherapy sources discussed in the current scientific literature.

13.1 ESSENTIAL OILS

This section examines a number of essential oils and their various applications, with a particular focus on their potential therapeutic effects. While the scientific evidence supporting the efficacy of these oils is inconclusive, their historical and contemporary uses in perfumery, skincare, and aromatherapy reflect their enduring appeal and versatility. The objective of this guide is to examine the source, benefits, and practical applications of each oil in order to elucidate the multifaceted roles these fragrant extracts play in enhancing health and well-being.

Amber essential oil is derived from fossilized resins and is often used in perfumery and aromatherapy applications. This oil is thought to have anti-inflammatory and analgesic (pain-relieving) properties [1]. However, there is not much scientific research on amber essential oil.

Anise essential oil is derived from the plant *Pimpinella anisum* and usually has a sweet, fruity scent. Anise oil is known to have antispasmodic, antiseptic, and digestive health-promoting properties [2]. Additionally, some studies have shown that anise oil can help ease breathing and relieve asthma symptoms [3].

Avocado essential oil is derived from the pulp of the avocado fruit (*Persea americana*) and is widely used in skincare products. It mainly contains monounsaturated fatty acids that preserve the skin's natural moisture and strengthen the skin barrier.
In addition, it can increase the elasticity of the skin and alleviate the signs of aging. However, avocado oil is not an "essential oil" because it is not obtained by steam distillation and does not exhibit the characteristics of a typical essential oil [4].

Bay leaf essential oil is obtained by steam distillation from the Laurus nobilis plant. This oil is used in the treatment of various skin conditions due to its anti-inflammatory, antiseptic, antibacterial, and antifungal properties [5]. Bay leaf oil is also used to relieve muscle pain and increase blood circulation. Moreover, the pleasant scent of this oil helps in reducing anxiety and stress.

Bergamot essential oil is obtained from the fruit of the *Citrus bergamia* tree. It is often used in aromatherapy because of its antiseptic, antidepressant, and anti-inflammatory properties. Studies have shown that bergamot essential oil can help relieve stress, anxiety, and even certain pain conditions [6].

Black pepper essential oil is obtained by steam distillation from the *Piper nigrum* plant and is thought to have anti-inflammatory, antiviral, antimicrobial, and antioxidant properties. It also has benefits such as relieving pain and supporting digestion [7].

DOI: 10.1201/9781003520252-15

Blueberry essential oil is often used in skin care products and aromatherapy applications. This oil is known to have antioxidant, anti-inflammatory, and antiaging properties [8]. However, there isn't much scientific research on blueberry essential oil.

Cardamom essential oil is obtained by steam distillation from the plant *Elettaria cardamomum*. It supports the digestive system and has antispasmodic and anti-inflammatory properties [9]. It also facilitates breathing and relieves respiratory ailments such as coughing.

Cinnamon essential oil is usually derived from cinnamon bark or leaves and has a spicy, warm scent. Cinnamon is known to have antimicrobial, anti-inflammatory, and antioxidant properties [10]. Additionally, cinnamon oil may help regulate blood sugar, a potential benefit for patients with type 2 diabetes [11].

Citron essential oil is usually derived from the peel of the Citrus lemon plant and is known for its invigorating and energizing effects. Some studies have shown that citron oil can relieve symptoms of stress and anxiety and even improve focus [12].

Clary sage essential oil, also known as yellow sage, is obtained by steam distillation from the *Salvia sclarea plant*. It is known to have antidepressant, antispasmodic, and aphrodisiac properties [13]. It can also help relieve menopausal symptoms and promote skin health.

Cocoa essential oil is obtained by steam distillation from *Theobroma cacao* seeds. This oil is often used in the manufacture of perfumes and chocolate-flavored food products. However, there isn't much scientific research on cocoa essential oil [14].

Coconut oil, technically, is not an essential oil, but it's widely used in aromatherapy because it's an excellent carrier oil. Coconut oil is extracted from the meat of mature coconuts. It's high in medium-chain fatty acids, which can have numerous health benefits. These include improving brain function, boosting heart health, and increasing fat loss. Coconut oil is also renowned for its moisturizing benefits, making it a popular choice for skin and hair care [15].

Eucalyptus essential oil is derived from the *Eucalyptus globulus* tree and is often used to relieve respiratory ailments due to its antiseptic, decongestant, and anti-inflammatory properties. Eucalyptus oil has been found to have antimicrobial, antiviral, and antifungal properties in many studies. Studies have also found that eucalyptus oil can help reduce pain and inflammation [16, 17].

Ginger essential oil is derived from the Zingiber officinale plant and usually has a warm, spicy scent. Ginger oil is known to have anti-inflammatory and antioxidant properties. It may also help relieve nausea and digestive upsets [18].

Grapefruit essential oil is derived from the Citrus paradisi plant and has an invigorating, fresh scent. This oil is known to have antiseptic, anti-inflammatory, and antidepressant properties. Studies show that grapefruit oil can increase energy levels and have a positive effect on mood [19, 20].

Jasmine essential oil is obtained by steam distillation of jasmine flowers. This oil is used to relieve anxiety and depression because of its relaxing and sedative properties. Jasmine oil also improves skin health and evens out skin tone. Also, this oil is believed to have aphrodisiac effects [21].

Jojoba essential oil is a liquid wax derived from the seeds of the *Simmondsia chinensis* plant. Jojoba oil helps maintain the skin's moisture balance and is used against a variety of skin problems. It has anti-inflammatory properties and can be used to treat skin conditions such as acne, psoriasis, and sunburn but does not fall into the "essential oil" category [22].

Lavender aromatherapy Soaps containing lavender oil offer calming and relaxing effects while cleansing the skin. Lavender oil is known to have antiseptic and anti-inflammatory properties, so it can relieve skin irritations and inflammation. Additionally, this type of soap is often used at bedtime because lavender oil promotes a better quality of sleep [23].

Lavender essential oil, Lavender, Latin name *Lavandula angustifolia*, usually grows in certain parts of Europe and Asia and is often used in aromatherapy. Lavender essential oil is obtained from the flowers of the plant, usually by steam distillation. Lavender is often considered the "universal oil" in the aromatherapy world as it has a stimulating effect.

Lavender oil has relaxing and calming properties that can help relieve symptoms of anxiety and stress in particular [24]. For example, one study showed that lavender essential oil significantly reduced symptoms of stress and anxiety [25]. Lavender may also help relieve insomnia symptoms. One study in particular found that participants exposed to lavender essential oil fell asleep faster into a deep sleep and woke up more energetic [26].

Lavender essential oil can also be used to treat skin ailments as it has antiseptic and anti-inflammatory properties. Studies have shown that lavender oil also assists in speeding up wound healing [27].

Lemongrass essential oil, also known as balm oil, is obtained by steam distillation from the Melissa officinalis plant. Due to its sedative and relaxing properties, this oil is known to be used to reduce anxiety and insomnia [28]. It can also help heal skin infections and wounds due to its antiviral and antimicrobial properties. Lemongrass essential oil is also used to support digestion and reduce gas formation.

Linden essential oil is an essential oil often used in aromatherapy and skin care products. It can reduce inflammation and calm the skin. However, good scientific studies are lacking on the well-documented effects of linden essential oil.

Myrrh (*Commiphora myrrha*) is a plant extract that has been used throughout history in cosmetic, perfumery, and medicinal applications. It is thought to have anti-inflammatory, antibacterial, and antifungal properties. It is also stated to have positive effects on wound healing and oral health [29].

Olive essential oil is obtained from the fleshy part of the olive fruit (*Olea europaea*) and has been used for health and beauty for centuries [30, 31]. However, olive oil is not considered an "essential oil" because essential oils contain volatile aroma compounds from plant material, often by distillation. Olive oil does not fall into this category, but it has many benefits.

Olive oil contains high levels of oleic acid, which helps moisturize the skin. It also contains antioxidants and vitamin E, which help protect the skin against the aging process. In addition to skin health, olive oil provides many health benefits. For example, it is commonly used in diets to support heart health, and some studies have shown that olive oil may protect against certain types of cancer.

However, olive oil is often used in pure form or in skin care products. When used in pure form, it is often applied directly to the skin or added to skin care products. When used in skin care products, olive oil is often added to moisturizers, lotions, face masks, and soaps.

Olive oil might not be considered an essential oil but is widely used in both health and beauty fields due to its many benefits.

Orange essential oil is derived from the peel of the orange tree and usually has a pleasant, uplifting scent. Studies have shown that orange essential oil can have anti-inflammatory and antimicrobial as well as antidepressant effects that can reduce anxiety levels [32, 33].

Patchouli essential oil is derived from the *Pogostemon cablin* plant and usually has a rich, earthy scent. Patchouli oil is known to have anti-inflammatory, antimicrobial, and anti-fungal properties. In addition, patchouli essential oil has shown the potential to relieve symptoms of anxiety and depression [34, 35].

Peach essential oil is obtained from peach kernels by cold pressing method. This oil moisturizes and softens the skin. However, peach oil is not an essential oil and is often mixed with other essential oils and used in skin care products. There is not much research on peach essential oil in the scientific literature [36].

Peppermint essential oil is extracted from the leaves of Mentha piperita. Peppermint oil is known for its refreshing and invigorating effect, making it a popular choice in aromatherapy. Peppermint essential oil can be used to relieve headaches, increase energy levels, and alleviate digestive issues [37].

Studies find that peppermint oil inhalation may help relieve migraine symptoms [38]. Peppermint essential oil also has antibacterial, antiviral, and anti-inflammatory properties, making it a popular ingredient in skin care products and oral care products.

Peppermint essential oil is suitable for topical use as well as aromatherapy applications but should always be diluted with a carrier oil because it can cause a burning sensation on the skin. Keep in mind that peppermint oil can also cause allergic reactions, so it is important to do a skin patch test before trying a new product [39].

Red cedar essential oil is obtained by steam distillation from the wood of the *Juniperus virginiana* tree. This oil is used in the treatment of various skin diseases as it has antiseptic, antifungal, and anti-inflammatory properties [40]. It can also reduce stress and anxiety and improve sleep. Red cedar oil is also used as an insect repellent.

Rose essential oil is an oil obtained by steam distillation from Rosa damascena flowers, which is generally used in the making of rose water and perfumes. It is thought to have anti-inflammatory, antiseptic, antispasmodic, and calming properties. It may also help in relieving menopausal symptoms [41].

Rosemary essential oil is a powerful oil, derived from the plant Rosmarinus officinalis. It is known to have antioxidant and anti-inflammatory properties and is often used for memory enhancement, relieving muscle soreness, and promoting hair growth. Also, several studies have shown that rosemary essential oil can help improve memory and concentration [42].

Sage essential oil is derived from the Salvia officinalis plant and generally has a fresh, herbal scent. Sage oil is known to have antimicrobial, anti-inflammatory, and antifungal properties. Furthermore, sage oil has shown a potential to relieve symptoms of anxiety and depression in one study [43].

Sandalwood oil is an essential oil obtained from the *Santalum album* tree. This oil can help calm the mind, reduce stress, and improve sleep quality. There is also evidence that sandalwood oil has antimicrobial properties [44].

Tea tree essential oil is derived from the *Melaleuca alternifolia* plant and is often used in skincare products. The antiseptic, antimicrobial, and anti-inflammatory properties of tea tree oil can help manage a range of skin conditions and issues, from acne treatment to wound healing and dandruff control. One study found that when tea tree oil is applied to skin lesions, it provides rapid healing and reduced symptoms [45].

Thyme essential oil is derived from the *Thymus vulgaris* plant and often has a pungent, spicy scent. Thyme oil is known to have antimicrobial, antioxidant, and anti-inflammatory properties [46]. Thyme oil may also help relieve symptoms of respiratory ailments [47].

Ylang ylang essential oil is derived from the flowers of the *Cananga odorata* tree and is often used in aromatherapy for its calming and relaxing effects. It can also help moisturize the skin and improve skin health. There is evidence that ylang ylang oil has hypotensive and anxiolytic effects [48].

13.2 PRACTICAL USES OF AROMATHERAPY PRODUCTS

Aromatherapy products are not merely scented; they are designed to enhance well-being and relaxation. This section examines the various applications of these products, including bath bubbles, salts, and candles, and elucidates the specific therapeutic benefits associated with each.

Aromatherapy bath bubbles containing essential oils turn bathing into a pleasant and relaxing experience. Various essential oils provide different benefits. For example, lavender is relaxing, mint is energizing, and Eucalyptus opens the airways. Such products are part of aromatherapy practice that promotes general health and well-being [39].

Aromatherapy bath salts consist of a number of salt types (usually Epsom salts, Himalayan salts, or Sea salts) mixed with essential oils. These salt combinations are then added to bath water to provide aromatherapeutic benefits.

Bath salts can help reduce muscle aches and stiffness, reduce stress, and provide an overall sense of relaxation [49]. Additionally, the choice of essential oils can be geared toward different kinds of health benefits. For example, bath salts infused with lavender oil can reduce anxiety and improve sleep quality [50].

Aromatherapy candles are candles that are usually combined with one or more essential oils. When these candles are lit, the essential oils evaporate due to the heat and fill the air. This allows users to enjoy both the light of the candle and the aromatic benefits of the essential oil.

Essential oils, depending on their properties and choice, can provide a variety of therapeutic benefits. For example, lavender essential oil can reduce stress and promote sleep, while rosemary essential oil can improve focus and memory [51].

Aromatherapy diffusers are devices in which essential oils are vaporized when mixed with air. This steam aromatizes the air in the room and offers the benefits of aromatherapy.

Diffusers can offer the health benefits of essential oils as well as emitting a pleasant scent into rooms [39].

Aromatherapy dim lamps usually include a heat source (usually a candle or electric heater) and a ceramic or metal dish that heats and vaporizes essential oils. This vapor disperses into the surrounding air and provides therapeutic effects. The use of dim lamps often balances the energy of a room and can aid relaxation, concentration, or sleep [52].

Aromatherapy facial steam is a treatment that usually combines some type of essential oil with water vapor. Applying this steam to the face provides skin cleansing and a relaxing experience. Essential oils offer a variety of benefits, depending on their properties and choice. For example, eucalyptus oil may help open up the sinuses, while lavender oil may reduce anxiety and provide relief [53].

Aromatherapy hair masks containing essential oils can improve the overall health and shine of the hair. For example, lavender oil may promote hair growth, while tea tree oil may help prevent dandruff [54].

Aromatherapy incense sticks infused with essential oils are used to fill a room or space with a specific aroma. These are widely used in aromatherapy practice and offer the potential therapeutic benefits of various oils. However, there is some concern that the continued and heavy use of incense sticks may adversely affect air quality, especially indoors [55].

Aromatherapy massage oils are usually a blend of one or more essential oils and a carrier oil (such as jojoba, avocado, or sweet almond oil). These oils are absorbed by the body by being rubbed into the skin during the massage. Research has shown that aromatherapy massage can be effective in reducing stress and anxiety and improving overall quality of life [56].

Aromatherapy pillow sprays usually contain essential oils with a relaxing effect such as lavender, bergamot, and ylang ylang. It is used to facilitate the transition to sleep and to improve the quality of sleep. Some essential oils, such as lavender oil, have been shown in scientific studies to reduce anxiety and improve sleep [39].

Aromatherapy serums containing essential oils are often used in skin care routines. Different oils provide various benefits according to skin types and needs. For example, tea tree oil can help treat acne, while rose oil can help maintain skin moisture balance and alleviate signs of aging [39].

Aromatherapy shampoos often contain a variety of essential oils. These shampoos offer the aromatic benefits of these oils while washing and also provide therapeutic benefits for various skin and hair types. For example, tea tree essential oil may help reduce dandruff and improve hair health [45].

Aromatherapy Skin lotions containing essential oils can be used to support skin health and alleviate various skin problems. For example, lotions containing lavender oil can calm the skin, while products containing tea tree oil can help treat acne [39].

The entirety of the above information should be used as a general guide and should not be used without considering the health status of each individual, possible side effects, and drug interactions. It is extremely important to consult a healthcare professional about aromatherapy practices.

REFERENCES

1. F. M. Dugan, S. L. Lupien and B. D. Gossen, "Selected Essential Oil Compounds and a New Potential Bioherbicide Inhibitor Polar Growth in Sclerotinia Sclerotiorum," *Biological Control*, vol. 24, no. 2, pp. 149–155, 2002.
2. K. Koriem, "Approach to Pharmacological and Clinical Applications of Anisi Aetheroleum," *Asian Pacific Journal of Tropical Biomedicine*, vol. 5, no. 1, pp. 60–67, 2015.
3. H. M. M. Ahmed, "The Potential Effect of Anise Oil on the Bronchial Smooth Muscle of Asthmatic Mice," *Alexandria Journal of Medicine*, vol. 53, no. 4, pp. 351–359, 2017.
4. M. L. Dreher and A. J. Davenport, "Has Avocado Composition and Potential Health Effects," *Critical Reviews in Food Science and Nutrition*, vol. 53, no. 7, pp. 738–750, 2013.
5. X. Han and T. L. Parker, "Anti-Inflammatory, Tissue Remodeling, Immunomodulatory, and Anticancer Activities of Oregano (*Origanum vulgare*) Essential Oil in a Human Skin Disease Model," *Biochimie Open*, vol. 4, pp. 73–77, 2017.
6. X. Han, J. Gibson, D. L. Eggett and T. L. Parker, "Bergamot (*Citrus bergamia*) Essential Oil Inhalation Improves Positive Feelings in the Waiting Room of a Mental Health Treatment Center: A Pilot Study," *Phytotherapy Research*, vol. 31, no. 5, pp. 812–816, 2017.
7. G. S. Bae, M. S. Kim, W. S. Jung, S. W. Seo, S. W. Yun, S. G. Kim and H. J. Song, "Inhibition of Lipopolysaccharide-Induced Inflammatory Responses by Piperine," *European Journal of Pharmacology*, vol. 642, no. 1–3, pp. 154–162, 2012.
8. V. G. Rodrigues, P. T. V. Rosa, M. O. M. Marques, A. J. Petenate and M. A. A. Meireles, "Supercritical Extraction of Essential Oil from Aniseed (*Pimpinella anisum* L) Using CO_2: Solubility, Kinetics, and Composition Data," *Journal of Agricultural and Food Chemistry*, vol. 51, no. 6, pp. 1518–1523, 2003.
9. H. Al-Zuhair, A. A. Abd el-Fattah and H. A. Abd el Latif, "Efficacy of a Herbal Mixture (Cardamom and Saffron) in the Treatment of Obesity: A Randomized, Triple-Blind, Placebo-Controlled Trial," *Global Journal of Health Science*, vol. 8, no. 8, pp. 175–181, 1996.
10. J. C. Liao, J. S. Deng, C. S. Chiu, W. C. Hou, S. S. Huang, P. H. Shie and G. J. Huang, "Anti-Inflammatory Activities of Cinnamomum Cassia Constituents In Vitro and In Vivo," *Evidence-Based Complementary and Alternative Medicine*, vol. 2012, p. 429320, 2012.
11. R. W. Allen, E. Schwartzman, W. L. Baker, C. I. Coleman and O. J. Phung, "Cinnamon Use in Type 2 Diabetes: An Updated Systematic Review and Meta-Analysis," *Annals of Family Medicine*, vol. 11, no. 5, pp. 452–459, 2013.
12. J. K. Kiecolt-Glaser, J. E. M. W. B. Graham, K. Porter, S. Lemeshow and R. Glaser, "Olfactory Influences on Mood and Autonomic, Endocrine, and Immune Function," *Psychoneuroendocrinology*, vol. 33, no. 3, pp. 328–339, 2008.
13. N. Perry and E. Perry, "Aromatherapy in the Management of Psychiatric Disorders: Clinical and Neuropharmacological Perspectives," *CNS Drugs*, vol. 20, no. 4, pp. 257–280, 2006.
14. S. Y. K. Chee, S. N. A. Malek and N. Ramli, "Essential Oils in the Leaves of Cocoa (*Theobroma cacao* L.) Clone UITI and NA33," *Journal of Essential Oil Research*, vol. 17, no. 3, pp. 312–313, 2005.
15. K. G. Nevin and T. Rajamohan, "Effect of Topical Application of Virgin Coconut Oil on Skin Components and Antioxidant Status During Dermal Wound Healing in Young Rats," *Skin Pharmacology and Physiology*, vol. 23, no. 6, pp. 290–297, 2010.
16. D. Mieres-Castro, S. Ahmar, R. Shabbir and F. Mora-Poblete, "Antiviral Activities of Eucalyptus Essential Oils: Their Effectiveness as Therapeutic Targets Against Human Viruses," *Pharmaceuticals (Basel, Switzerland)*, vol. 14, no. 12, p. 1210, 2021.
17. Y. S. Jun, P. Kang, S. S. Min, J. M. Lee, H. K. Kim and G. H. Seol, "Effect of Eucalyptus Oil Inhalation on Pain and Inflammatory Responses After Total Knee Replacement: A Randomized Clinical Trial," *Evidence-Based Complementary and Alternative Medicine*, vol. 2013, p. 502727, 2013.
18. M. Ozgoli, "Effects of Ginger Capsules on Pregnancy, Nausea, and Vomiting," *Journal of Alternative and Complementary Medicine*, vol. 15, no. 3, pp. 243–246, 2009.
19. M. C. Ou, Y. H. Liu, Y. W. Sun and C. F. Chan, "The Composition, Antioxidant and Antibacterial Activities of Cold-Pressed and Distilled Essential Oils of *Citrus paradisi* and *Citrus grandis* (L.) Osbeck," *Evidence-Based Complementary and Alternative Medicine*, vol. 2015, pp. 1–9, 2015.
20. T. Matsumoto, H. Asakura and T. Hayashi, "Effects of Olfactory Stimulation from the Fragrance of the Japanese Citrus Fruit Yuzu (Citrus Junos Sieb. Ex Tanaka) on Mood States and Salivary Chromogranin A as an Endocrinologic Stress Marker," *Journal of Alternative and Complementary Medicine*, vol. 20, no. 6, pp. 500–506, 2014.

21. T. Hongratanaworakit, "Stimulating Effect of Aromatherapy Massage With Jasmine Oil," *Natural Product Communications*, vol. 5, no. 1, pp. 157–162, 2010.

22. N. Pazyar, R. Yaghoobi, M. R. Ghassemi, A. Kazerouni, E. Rafeie and N. Jamshydian, "Jojoba in Dermatology: A Succinct Review," Italian Journal of Dermatology and Venereology: Official Organ, *Italian Society of Dermatology and Syphilography*, vol. 148, no. 6, pp. 687–691, 2013.

23. P. H. Koulivand, M. Khaleghi Ghadiri and A. Gorji, "Lavender and the Nervous System," *Evidence-Based Complementary and Alternative Medicine*, vol. 2013, p. 681304, 2013.

24. S. Kasper, M. Gastpar, W. E. Müller, H. P. Volz, H. J. Möller, S. Schläfke and A. Dienel, "Lavender Oil Preparation Silexan Is Effective in Generalized Anxiety Disorder—A Randomized, Double-Blind Comparison to Placebo and Paroxetine," *The International Journal of Neuropsychopharmacology*, vol. 17, no. 6, pp. 859–869, 2014.

25. Y. L. Lee, Y. Wu, H. W. Tsang, A. Y. Leung and W. M. Cheung, "A Systematic Review on the Anxiolytic Effects of Aromatherapy in People with Anxiety Symptoms," *The Journal of Alternative and Complementary Medicine*, vol. 17, no. 2, pp. 101–108, 2011.

26. A. S. Lillehei and L. L. Halcon, "A Systematic Review of the Effect of Inhaled Essential Oils on Sleep," *The Journal of Alternative and Complementary Medicine*, vol. 20, no. 6, pp. 441–451, 2014.

27. R. Samuelson, M. Lobl, S. Higgins, D. Clarey and A. Wysong, "The Effects of Lavender Essential Oil on Wound Healing: A Review of the Current Evidence," *Journal of Alternative and Complementary Medicine (New York, N.Y.)*, vol. 26, no. 8, pp. 680–690, 2020.

28. D. O. Kennedy, W. Little and A. B. Scholey, "Attenuation of Laboratory-Induced Stress in Humans After Acute Administration of *Melissa officinalis* (Lemon Balm)," *Psychosomatic Medicine*, vol. 66, no. 4, pp. 607–613, 2004.

29. S. Su, T. Wang, J. A. Duan, W. Zhou, Y. Q. Hua, Y. P. Tang and L. Yu, "Anti-Inflammatory and Analgesic Activity of Different Extracts of *Commiphora myrrha*," *Journal of Ethnopharmacology*, vol. 141, no. 2, pp. 667–672, 2012.

30. S. Cicerale, X. A. Conlan, A. J. Sinclair and R. S. Keast, "Chemistry and Health of Olive Oil Phenolics," *Critical Reviews in Food Science and Nutrition*, vol. 49, no. 3, pp. 218–236, 2009.

31. R. W. Owen, A. Giacosa, W. E. Hull, R. Haubner, G. Würtele, B. Spiegelhalder and H. Bartsch, "Olive-Oil Consumption and Health: The Possible Role of Antioxidants," *The Lancet Oncology*, vol. 1, pp. 107–112, 2000.

32. P. Sun, L. Zhao, N. Zhang, C. Wang, W. Wu, A. Mehmood, L. Zhang, B. Ji and F. Zhou, "Essential Oil and Juice from Bergamot and Sweet Orange Improve Acne Vulgaris Caused by Excessive Androgen Secretion," *Mediators of Inflammation*, vol. 2020, p. 8868107, 2020.

33. J. Choi, J. H. Kim, M. Park and H. J. Lee, "Effects of Flavonoid-Rich Orange Juice Intervention on Major Depressive Disorder in Young Adults: A Randomized Controlled Trial," *Nutrients*, vol. 15, no. 1, p. 145, 2022.

34. A. El-Massry, "Chemical Composition and Anti-Inflammatory Activity of *Pogostemon cablin* Essential Oil," *American Journal of Essential Oils and Natural Products*, vol. 5, no. 1, pp. 21–25, 2017.

35. M. H. Woo, "Antidepressant-Like Effect of Essential Oil Isolated from *Pogostemon cablin* in Mice," *Journal of Essential Oil Research*, vol. 31, no. 4, pp. 323–332, 2019.

36. Aromatics International, "Peach Kernel Carrier Oil," [Online]. Available: https://www.aromatics.com/products/peach-kernel-carrier-oil.

37. D. L. McKay and J. B. Blumberg, "A Review of the Bioactivity and Potential Health Benefits of Peppermint Tea (*Mentha piperita* L)," *Phytotherapy Research: An International Journal Devoted to Pharmacological and Toxicological Evaluation of Natural Product Derivatives*, vol. 20, no. 8, pp. 619–633, 2006.

38. H. Göbel, A. Heinze, K. Heinze-Kuhn, A. Göbel and C. Göbel, "Peppermint Oil in the Acute Treatment of Tension-Type Headache," vol. 30, no. 3, pp. 295–310, 2016.

39. A. Orchard and S. van Vuuren, "Commercial Essential Oils as Potential Antimicrobials to Treat Skin Diseases," *Evidence-Based Complementary and Alternative Medicine*, vol. 2017, p. 4517971, 2017.

40. D. Wilson, "What You Need to Know About Cedarwood Essential Oil," [Online]. Available: https://www.healthline.com/health/cedarwood-essential-oil.

41. M. H. Boskabady, M. N. Shafei, Z. Saberi and S. Amini, "Pharmacological Effects of *Rosa damascena*," *Iranian Journal of Basic Medical Sciences*, vol. 14, no. 4, p. 295, 2011.

42. M. Moss, J. Cook, K. Wesnes and P. Duckett, "Aromas of Rosemary and Lavender Essential Oils Differentially Affect Cognition and Mood in Healthy Adults," *International Journal of Neuroscience*, vol. 113, no. 1, pp. 15–38, 2003.

43. A. L. Lopresti, "Salvia (Sage): A Review of Its Potential Cognitive-Enhancing and Protective Effects," *Drugs in R&D*, vol. 17, no. 1, pp. 53–64, 2017.
44. B. B. Mishra and D. D. Singh, "Microbial and Phytochemical Screening of the Sandalwood Oil of *Santalum album* L," *Industrial Crops and Products*, vol. 108, pp. 48–57, 2017.
45. C. F. Carson, K. A. Hammer and T. V. Riley, "*Melaleuca alternifolia* (Tea Tree) Oil: A Review of Antimicrobial and Other Medicinal Properties," *Clinical Microbiology Reviews*, vol. 19, no. 1, pp. 50–62, 2006.
46. S. Aazza, S. El-Guendouz, M. G. Miguel, M. D. Antunes, M. L. Faleiro, A. I. Correia and A. C. Figueiredo, "Antioxidant, Anti-Inflammatory and Anti-Hyperglycaemic Activities of Essential Oils from *Thymbra capitata, Thymus albicans, Thymus caespititius, Thymus carnosus, Thymus lotocephalus* and *Thymus mastichina* from Portugal," *Natural Product Communications*, vol. 11, no. 7, pp. 1029–1038, 2016.
47. A. Saad, "Anti-Inflammatory and Antioxidant Effects of *Thymus capitata* Essential Oil," *Journal of Essential Oil Bearing Plants*, vol. 19, no. 5, pp. 1127–1139, 2016.
48. T. Hongratanaworakit and G. Buchbauer, "Relaxing Effect of Ylang Ylang Oil on Humans After Transdermal Absorption," *Phytotherapy Research*, vol. 20, no. 9, pp. 758–763, 2006.
49. S. G. Biradar, S. B. Sreenivas and A. S. Hiremathad, "Recent Advances in Bath Salts," *Drug Discovery Today*, vol. 25, no. 2, pp. 195–200, 2020.
50. C. Dunn, J. Sleep and D. Collett, "Sensing an Improvement: An Experimental Study to Evaluate the Use of Aromatherapy, Massage and Periods of Rest in an Intensive Care Unit," *Journal of Advanced Nursing*, vol. 21, no. 1, pp. 34–40, 1995.
51. K. Hirokawa, T. Nishimoto and T. Taniguchi, "Effects of Lavender Aroma on Sleep Quality in Healthy Japanese Students," *Perceptual and Motor Skills*, vol. 114, pp. 111–122, 2012.
52. E. S. Choi, "Effects of Inhalation Aromatherapy on Symptoms of Sleep Disturbance in the Elderly With Dementia," *Evidence-Based Complementary and Alternative Medicine*, vol. 2017, p. 902807, 2017.
53. B. Ali, "Essential Oils Used in Aromatherapy: A Systemic Review," *Asian Pacific Journal of Tropical Biomedicine*, vol. 5, no. 8, pp. 601–611, 2015.
54. Y. Panahi, M. Taghizadeh, E. T. Marzony and A. Sahebkar, "Rosemary Oil vs Minoxidil 2% for the Treatment of Androgenetic Alopecia: A Randomized Comparative Trial," *Skinmed*, vol. 13, no. 1, pp. 15–21, 2015.
55. L. P. Naeher, M. Brauer, M. Lipsett, J. T. Zelikoff, C. D. Simpson, J. Q. Koenig and K. R. Smith, "Woodsmoke Health Effects: A Review," *Inhalation Toxicology*, vol. 19, no. 1, pp. 67–106, 2007.
56. S. K. Tang and M. Y. Tse, "Aromatherapy: Does It Help to Relieve Pain, Depression, Anxiety, and Stress in Community-Dwelling Older Persons?," *BioMed Research International*, vol. 2014, p. 430195, 2014.

14 Integrative Approaches to Healing

In recent years, integrative approaches to health and wellness have garnered increasing attention, particularly those that blend traditional therapeutic modalities with spiritual and natural health practices. Music therapy and bioresonance therapy represent two such modalities that have shown promising results in enhancing overall well-being. Music therapy leverages the therapeutic properties of sound and rhythm to address emotional, cognitive, and physical challenges, while bioresonance therapy uses electromagnetic frequencies to promote healing and balance within the body. Both approaches are increasingly recognized for their potential to complement conventional medical treatments and support holistic health.

The intersection of these therapies with religious and spiritual frameworks offers an intriguing perspective on health. Many religious traditions emphasize the importance of spiritual balance and harmony, which can be harmoniously aligned with the principles underlying music therapy and bioresonance. By exploring how these therapeutic practices integrate with spiritual beliefs and natural health principles, we gain a deeper understanding of their potential to contribute to a more comprehensive approach to wellness. This chapter aims to elucidate the roles of music therapy and bioresonance therapy within this broader context, highlighting their benefits and exploring their intersection with religious and spiritual dimensions of health.

14.1 MUSIC THERAPY

Music therapy is a treatment approach that uses music to improve the physical and emotional health of patients. This approach includes both active (making or singing) and passive (listening to music) methods.

A number of scientific studies have shown that music therapy can be effective in relieving various conditions such as anxiety, depression, and pain. For example, a meta-analysis found that music therapy can significantly reduce anxiety and pain in cancer patients [1].

Additionally, music therapy can help improve memory abilities in Alzheimer's patients. A study has shown that music therapy is effective in rejuvenating memories and increasing communication skills in Alzheimer's patients [2].

However, the effectiveness of music therapy depends on the method applied and the health problem targeted. These subjects need more scientific research.

14.1.1 Music Therapy Approaches

There are various types and approaches to music therapy. Below are examples of various music therapy approaches:

1. Active Music Therapy: It is a form of therapy in which the individual actively participates by playing a musical instrument or singing.
2. Passive Music Therapy: It involves the therapist playing music and the individual listening to this music. Its purpose may be relaxation and stress reduction.
3. Resonance Music Therapy: While balancing the emotional state and energy level of the individual, it activates the inner subconscious processes.
4. Recreational Music Therapy: It is aimed at developing group work and social skills.

DOI: 10.1201/9781003520252-16

5. Psychodynamic Music Therapy: It is used to reveal the subconscious thoughts and feelings of the individual.

6. Neurological Music Therapy: It focuses on improving brain functions; it is usually applied to individuals with stroke, Parkinson's, or brain damage.

7. Cognitive-Behavioral Music Therapy: It is used to learn or change certain behaviors.

8. Psycho-Educational Music Therapy: It helps the individual learn certain skills; it is usually applied to people on the autism spectrum.

9. Bonny Method of Guided Imagery and Music (GIM): Promotes self-awareness and growth using music and guided imagination.

10. Improvisational Music Therapy: It is based on a musical dialogue between the therapist and the individual and often encourages emotional expression.

11. Vibrational Sound Therapy: The body's energy is balanced by using the vibrations of musical instruments.

12. Community Music Therapy: It involves the participation of all members of the community and aims to increase social cohesion within the community.

13. Nordoff-Robbins Music Therapy: It is aimed at increasing the creativity and self-expression of individuals with special needs.

14. The Kodály Method: It aims at musical education and the development of musical abilities.

15. The Orff Approach: It focuses on the development of musical skills using rhythm, movement, drama, and language.

16. Dalcroze Method: It helps to develop musical abilities by combining music and movement.

17. The Suzuki Method: It focuses on ear-based learning and is often used to improve children's musical skills.

18. Mantra Meditation: It is a type of therapy in which music and mantra repetition are combined for meditation.

19. Music Biofeedback: Music is used as a response mechanism; and music changes based on the person's physical or emotional state.

20. Notation Therapy: It is a type of music therapy in which musical notes are used therapeutically.

Each music therapy approach can be customized to the individual's needs and therapeutic goals. Also, many approaches combine different therapy techniques. Therefore, there are numerous ways in which music therapy can be applied. It is difficult to generalize about which of these methods will be most effective because each person's needs are different. Before starting any music therapy program, it is important to consult with a professional.

14.2   BIORESONANCE THERAPY

Bioresonance therapy is an alternative medicine treatment that aims to restore energy balance in the body. This form of therapy claims that the different cells and organs of the body have unique frequencies, and that good health depends on these frequencies being in the right range [3].

Bioresonance therapy is usually done using electrodes and a bioresonance device. The device aims to detect "wrong" frequencies caused by disease and restore the body's natural frequencies [4].

However, there is disagreement in the scientific community about bioresonance therapy. Many studies question the efficacy and safety of this treatment modality [5, 6]. Some studies have suggested that bioresonance may be helpful for certain conditions, while others have noted that treatment is ineffective [7].

Often, we see bioresonance therapy used primarily to treat certain allergic reactions. However, available evidence has not shown that treatment is effective for these conditions [8].

Therefore, caution is advised when considering bioresonance therapy or any alternative therapy before speaking to a healthcare professional.

Bioresonance therapy has been used for a number of different health problems. However, the scientific evidence is limited and in some cases contradictory.

Some examples of the situations where bioresonance therapy is used are listed below:

1. Allergies and Food Intolerances: Bioresonance has been used by some healthcare providers to diagnose and treat allergies and food intolerances. Some preliminary studies have suggested that bioresonance therapy may alleviate allergy symptoms. However, these studies often have minor and methodological problems, and more research is needed in this regard.
2. Smoking Cessation: Some people have used bioresonance therapy to help them quit smoking. However, scientific evidence supporting the effectiveness of bioresonance in smoking cessation is very limited, and more research is needed on this subject.
3. Chronic Pain: Bioresonance therapy has also been used for a variety of chronic pain conditions, including fibromyalgia and migraine. However, research in this area is often incomplete and contradictory, and definitive conclusions on this issue have not been reached.

The examples above illustrate several situations where bioresonance therapy is used. However, stronger scientific evidence is needed on these topics. It is important for individuals considering using bioresonance therapy to prioritize speaking to a healthcare professional and evaluate each treatment in its own context.

14.3   RELIGION AND NATURAL HEALTH

Religion is an organized system of beliefs, practices, symbols, customs, and ceremonies associated with facilitating a sense of proximity to the divine as well as cultivating an understanding of one's connection and obligations to others in communal living. Religion is a multidimensional concept that may be observed privately or publicly and often involves aspects of the mystical or supernatural [9].

Religion plays an important role in the lives of many people, and a number of scientific studies have been conducted on the impact of religion on health. Many studies show that religion and spirituality have positive effects on various aspects of health.

Religion functions as an important stress reduction and coping mechanism for many people. These potential advantages for one's psychological well-being and mental health have physiological ramifications that affect one's physical well-being, impact the susceptibility to illnesses, and shape the response to medical interventions.

For example, one study found that people who are more observant of religious practices tend to have better mental health and adapt more quickly to health problems compared to those who are less observant of religious practices [9].

It has also been observed that religiously observant individuals generally have healthier lifestyle habits and consume less alcohol and tobacco. This can further positively affect their general health status [10].

However, the effects of religious practices can vary from person to person and depending on personal interpretations of religion and spirituality. Thus, research on this topic is often complex and multifaceted.

REFERENCES

1. J. Bradt, C. Dileo, L. Magill and A. Teague, "Music Interventions for Improving Psychological and Physical Outcomes in Cancer Patients," *Cochrane Database of Systematic Reviews*, vol. 8, p. CD006911, 2016.
2. N. A. Foster and E. R. Valentine, "The Effect of Auditory Stimulation on Autobiographical Recall in Dementia," *Experimental Aging Research*, vol. 27, no. 3, pp. 215–228, 2001.

3. F. Wandtke, "Bioresonance Allergy Testing Versus Prick Testing and RAST," *Allergologie*, vol. 16, no. 144, 1993.

4. J. Hennecke, Bioresonance: A New View of Medicine: Scientific Principles and Practical Experience, Books On Demand, 2012.

5. E. Ernst, "Bioresonance, a Review of the Evidence," *International Journal of Clinical Practice*, vol. 58, no. 1, pp. 49–51, 2004.

6. M. S. Lee, B. C. Shin and E. Ernst, "Bioresonance for Allergic Diseases: A Systematic Review," *Journal of Allergy and Clinical Immunology*, vol. 124, no. 4, pp. 705–706, 2009.

7. P. Karakos, T. Grigorios, K. Theodoros and L. Theodoros, "The Effectiveness of Bioresonance Method on Human Health," *Open Journal of Epidemiology*, vol. 8, no. 1, pp. 1–8, 2019.

8. E. Ernst, "Bioresonance: A New Energy Medicine," *Journal of Bioelectromagnetics*, vol. 15, no. 3, pp. 295–301, 2014.

9. H. G. Koenig, "Religion, Spirituality, and Health: The Research and Clinical Implications," *ISRN Psychiatry*, vol. 2012, p. 278730, 2012.

10. H. Koenig, D. King and V. Carson, Handbook of Religion and Health, New York, NY: Oxford University Press, 2012.

Index

For Product Safety Concerns and Information please contact our EU
representative GPSR@taylorandfrancis.com
Taylor & Francis Verlag GmbH, Kaufingerstraße 24, 80331 München, Germany

www.ingramcontent.com/pod-product-compliance
Lightning Source LLC
Chambersburg PA
CBHW061418210326
41598CB00035B/6259